Epidemiology

Leon Gordis, M.D., M.P.H., Dr.P.H.
Professor of Epidemiology
Johns Hopkins School of Hygiene
    and Public Health
Professor of Pediatrics
Johns Hopkins School of Medicine
Baltimore, Maryland

W.B. SAUNDERS COMPANY
A Division of Harcourt Brace & Company
Philadelphia   London   Toronto
Montreal   Sydney   Tokyo

W.B. SAUNDERS COMPANY
A Division of Harcourt Brace & Company

The Curtis Center
Independence Square West
Philadelphia, Pennsylvania 19106

Library of Congress Cataloging-in-Publication Data
Gordis, Leon
Epidemiology / Leon Gordis.
p.   cm.
ISBN 0–7216–5137–2
1. Epidemiology.   I. Title.
RA651.G58 1996   614.4–dc20
DNLM/DLC   95–16680

EPIDEMIOLOGY   ISBN 0–7216–5137–2

Printed in the United States of America.

Last digit is the print number: 9   8   7   6   5   4   3   2

For Dassy

Preface

In recent years, epidemiology has become an increasingly essential approach in both public health and clinical practice. The discipline is the basic science of disease prevention, and it plays major roles in the development and evaluation of public policy as well as in the social and legal arenas. Epidemiology is now used together with laboratory research to identify risk factors for disease and to shed light on the mechanisms involved in pathogenesis. Epidemiologic studies are receiving increasing attention in the public media, and this heightened visibility carries major implications for health care providers and policy makers as well as for epidemiologists themselves. As a result, the approaches, methodology, and uses of epidemiology have become of increasing interest to an ever-broadening group of professionals as well as to the public at large.

This book is an introduction to epidemiology and to the epidemiologic approach to problems of health and disease. The basic principles and methods of epidemiology are presented together with many of the applications of epidemiology to public health and clinical practice. The book is organized in three sections: Section I focuses on the epidemiologic approach to understanding disease and to developing the basis for interventions designed to modify and improve its natural history. After an introductory chapter that provides a broad context and perspective for the discipline, Chapter 2 discusses how disease is transmitted and acquired. The measures we use to assess the frequency of disease are presented in Chapter 3. Chapter 4 addresses the critical issue of how to distinguish persons who have a disease from those who do not and how to assess the quality of the diagnostic and screening tests used. Once persons who have a certain disease have been identified, how do we characterize the natural history of their disease in quantitative terms? Such characterization is essential if we are to identify any changes over time that take place in survival and severity or changes that result from preventive or therapeutic interventions (Chapter 5). Because our ultimate objective is to improve human health by modifying the natural history of disease, the next step is to select an appropriate and effective intervention measure—a selection that is ideally made using the results of randomized trials of prevention and treatment (Chapters 6 and 7).

Section II deals with the use of epidemiology to identify the causes of disease. It discusses the design of cohort, case-control, and other types of studies (Chapters 8 and 9). Chapters 10 and 11 discuss how the results of these studies are used to estimate risk in order to determine whether there is an association of an exposure and a disease as reflected by an increase in risk in exposed persons. After a brief review (Chapter 12), Chapter 13 discusses how we move from such evidence of an association to answering the important question, Does the association reflect a causal relationship? (Chapter 13). In so doing, it is critical to take into account issues of bias, confounding, and interaction, which are discussed in Chapter 14. Chapter 15 describes the use of epidemiology, often in conjunction with molecular biology, to assess the relative contributions of genetic and environmental factors to disease causation.

Section III discusses several important applications of epidemiology to major health issues. Chapter 16 addresses how epidemiology is used to evaluate health services, Chapter 17 reviews the use of epidemiology in evaluating screening programs, and Chapter 18 the use of epidemiology in formulating and evaluating public policy. These diverse applications have enhanced the importance of epidemiology but at the same time given rise to an array of new problems, both ethical and professional, in the conduct of epidemiologic studies and in the use of the results of such studies. Some of these problems are discussed in the final chapter of the book (Chapter 19).

The sequence of the three sections of this book is designed to provide the reader with a basic understanding of epidemiologic methods and study design and of the place of epidemiology both in preventive and clinical medicine and in disease investigation. Extensive illustrations are used to clarify the concepts, methods, and examples described in the text, and review questions are included at the end of most chapters or topics. After finishing this book, the reader should be able to assess the adequacy of the design and conduct of reported studies and the validity of the conclusions reached in published articles. It is my hope that this book will convey to its readers the excitement of epidemiology, its basic conceptual and methodologic underpinnings, and an appreciation of its increasingly vital and expanding roles in enhancing the health of both individuals and communities through effective prevention and treatment.

Leon Gordis

Acknowledgments

This book is based on my experience in teaching two courses in introductory epdemiology at Johns Hopkins for over 20 years—Principles of Epidemiology to students in the School of Hygiene and Public Health and Clinical Epidemiology to students in the School of Medicine. To quote the Talmudic sage, Rabbi Hanina, ''I have learned much from my teachers, and even more from my colleagues, but most of all from my students.'' I am grateful to the more than 7,000 students whom I have been privileged to teach during this time. Through their questions and critical comments they have contributed significantly to the content, style, and configuration of this book.

I was first stimulated to pursue studies in epidemiology by my mentor and friend, Dr. Milton Markowitz. To this day he remains a guide and inspiration to me. Years ago, when we were initiating a study to evaluate the effectiveness of a comprehensive care clinic for children in Baltimore, he urged me to obtain the training needed to evaluate the program rigorously; even at that time he recognized that epidemiology was an essential approach for evaluating health services. He therefore suggested I speak with Dr. Abraham Lilienfeld, who was at the time Chairman of the Chronic Diseases Department at the Johns Hopkins School of Hygiene and Public Health. I then came as a student to Abe's department where he became my doctoral advisor and friend. Over many years, until his death in 1984, Abe had the wonderful talent of being able to communicate to his students and colleagues the excitement he found in epidemiology and he shared with them the thrill of discovering new knowledge using population-based methods. To both Milt Markowitz and Abe Lilienfeld I owe tremendous debts of gratitude.

In preparing this book I have been fortunate to have had assistance from many wonderful colleagues and friends. My deepest thanks are expressed to my colleague Allyn Arnold, Research Associate in the Department of Epidemiology at Johns Hopkins. We have worked closely over many years in the two introductory courses that formed the basis for this book. As I prepared this book, she was an excellent advisor, editor, and critic. She utilized her superb skills in computer graphics to refine and finalize many of the illustrations that I first developed for classroom teaching and then revised for this volume. All this she has done with great skill, dedication, and caring, and I am very grateful to her.

I wish to thank Drs. Lechaim Naggan and Jonathan Samet for their critical reviews of the manuscript and for their many valuable suggestions, and Dr. Gloria Petersen for critiquing the chapter on genetic factors in disease causation. I am also very grateful to Laurie Pratt, a doctoral student in our department, who carefully reviewed and proofread the manuscript and made many perceptive and valuable suggestions. Over the years my colleagues and friends Drs. Haroutune Armenian, Moyses Szklo, and Paul Whelton have spent many hours with me discussing a variety of conceptual issues and in doing so helped me find better ways of presenting them in an introduction to epidemiology. Many other colleagues, both in our department and elsewhere, have also been generous with their time and talents in discussing many of the issues that arose first in teaching and then in preparing and revising the manuscript. All of their efforts have contributed significantly to improving this volume.

Since joining the faculty at Johns Hopkins over 20 years ago, I have been privileged to work under outstanding leaders in the Johns Hopkins School of Public Health and

School of Medicine. Deans John C. Hume, D.A. Henderson, and Alfred Sommer in the School of Public Health, and Deans Richard Ross and Michael M.E. Johns in the School of Medicine have always enthusiastically supported the teaching of epidemiology in both schools.

I also deeply appreciate the outstanding contribution of Barbara Ewing in typing the manuscript of this book and its seemingly endless revisions. She also handled many of the crucial details involved in preparing the manuscript and did so with great dedication. I also wish to thank Dann Tjomsland, who typed early drafts of the manuscript.

I have had the good fortune to work with an outstanding group at W.B. Saunders. I have benefited from the strong and enthusiastic support of my editor, Larry McGrew. His gracious, sensitive, and appropriately firm guidance coupled with his thorough knowledge of the publishing process were critical to my completing the manuscript and to the subsequent steps leading to publication. Deborah Thorp has been a superb copy editor. She has a wonderful critical eye and pen and spared no efforts to identify errors and enhance the clarity and readability of this book. Other outstanding members of the W.B. Saunders staff with whom I have had the pleasure of working included Denise LeMelledo, Production Manager, Nicholas Rook, Designer, and Renée Gagliardi, Editorial Assistant. I am indebted to all of them for their fine efforts and for the warm and caring way in which they have contributed to the quality of this book.

Finally, my family has been a constant source of love, inspiration, and encouragement to me. My children urged me to write this book and lent enthusiastic support as I did so. Years ago, my wife Hadassah strongly supported my pursuing studies both in medicine and in epidemiology, and since that time she has constantly encouraged me in all my professional activities, even when this has involved personal sacrifices on her part. She was enthusiastic from the start about my preparing this book, and facilitated my writing it through her seemingly limitless patience and optimistic outlook. With her keen critical mind she has always left me thinking and reconsidering issues that I first thought simple and later came to recognize as being considerably more complex and challenging. Her love and support have made completion of this book possible. I have truly been very fortunate, and I thank her more than these words can express.

LEON GORDIS

Contents

ix

The Epidemiologic Approach to Disease and Intervention

This section begins with an overview of the objectives and approaches of epidemiology and presents some examples of the applications of epidemiology to human health problems (Chapter 1). It then discusses how diseases are transmitted (Chapter 2). Diseases do not arise in a vacuum; they result from an interaction of human beings with their environment. An understanding of the concepts and mechanisms underlying the transmission and acquisition of disease is critical to exploring the epidemiology of human disease.

To discuss the epidemiologic concepts presented in this book, we need to develop a common language, particularly for the descriptions and comparisons of morbidity and mortality that follow. Chapter 3 therefore discusses rates and related issues, as well as how measures of morbidity and mortality are used in both clinical medicine and public health.

Armed with knowledge of how to describe morbidity and mortality in quantitative terms, we then turn to the question of how to assess the quality of diagnostic and screening tests that are used to determine which persons in the population have a certain disease (Chapter 4). After this is determined, we need ways of describing in quantitative terms the natural history of disease; this is essential for assessing the severity of an illness and for evaluating the possible effects on survival of new therapeutic and preventive interventions (Chapter 5).

Having identified persons who have a disease, how do we decide what treatments or preventions to use to modify the natural history of the illness? Chapters 6 and 7 present the randomized trial, an invaluable and critical study design that is generally considered the ''gold standard'' for evaluating the effectiveness as well as the potential side effects of new therapeutic or preventive interventions.

CHAPTER 1

Introduction

THE OBJECTIVES OF EPIDEMIOLOGY

Epidemiology is the study of how disease is distributed in populations and of the factors that influence or determine this distribution. Why does a disease develop in some people and not in others? The premise underlying epidemiology is that disease, illness, and ill health are not randomly distributed in a population. Rather, each of us has certain characteristics that predispose us to, or protect us against, a variety of different diseases. These characteristics may be primarily genetic in origin or may be the result of exposures to certain environmental hazards.

A broader definition of epidemiology than that given in the preceding paragraph has been widely accepted. It defines epidemiology as

the study of the distribution and determinants of health-related states or events in specified populations and the application of this study to control of health problems.[1]

What is noteworthy about this definition is that it incorporates both a description of the content of the discipline and the purpose or application for which epidemiologic investigations are carried out.

What are the specific objectives of epidemiology?

First, to identify the etiology or the cause of a disease and the risk factors—that is, factors that increase a person's risk for a disease. We want to know how the disease is transmitted from one person to another or from a nonhuman reservoir to a human population. Our ultimate aim is to intervene to reduce morbidity and mortality from the disease. We want to develop a rational basis for prevention programs. If we can identify the etiologic or causal factors for disease and reduce or eliminate exposure to those factors, we can develop a basis for prevention programs.

Second, to determine the extent of disease found in the community. What is the burden of disease in the community? This question is critical for planning health services and facilities and for training future health care providers.

Third, to study the natural history and prognosis of disease. Clearly, certain diseases are more severe than others; some may be rapidly lethal, and others may have longer or shorter durations of survival. We want to define the baseline natural history of a disease in quantitative terms so that as we develop new modes of intervention, either through treatments or new ways of preventing complications, we can compare the results of using such new modalities to the baseline data to see whether our new approaches have truly been effective.

Fourth, to evaluate new preventive and therapeutic measures and new modes of health care delivery. For example, has the establishment of maximum lengths of stay in hospitals had any impact on health outcome in the patients discharged and on the quality of their lives after hospital discharge? Has the growth of managed care and other new approaches to health care delivery had an impact on health outcome?

Fifth, to provide the foundation for developing public policy and regulatory decisions relating to environmental problems. For example, is the electromagnetic radiation that is emitted by electric blankets, heating pads, and other household appliances a hazard to human health? Are high levels of atmospheric ozone or particulate matter a cause of adverse acute or chronic health effects in human populations? Is radon in homes a significant risk to humans beings? Which occupations are associated with increased risks of disease in workers and what types of regulation are required?

CHANGING PATTERNS OF COMMUNITY HEALTH PROBLEMS

A major role of epidemiology is to provide a clue to changes that take place over time in the

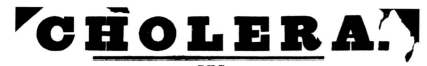

CHOLERA.

THE
DUDLEY BOARD OF HEALTH,

HEREBY GIVE NOTICE, THAT IN CONSEQUENCE OF THE

Church-yards at Dudley

Being so full, no one who has died of the CHOLERA will be permitted to be buried after *SUNDAY* next, (To-morrow) in either of the Burial Grounds of *St. Thomas's*, or *St. Edmund's*, in this Town.

All Persons who die from CHOLERA, must for the future be buried in the Church-yard at Netherton.

BOARD of HEALTH, DUDLEY.
September 1st, 1832.

W. MAURICE, PRINTER, HIGH STREET, DUDLEY.

Figure 1–1. Sign in cemetery in Dudley, England, in 1839. (From the Dudley Public Library, Dudley, England.)

health problems that present in the community. Figure 1–1 shows a sign in a cemetery in Dudley, England, in 1839. At that time, cholera was the major cause of death in England; the churchyard was so full that no burials of persons who died of cholera would henceforth be permitted. The sign conveys an idea of the importance of cholera in the public's consciousness and in the spectrum of public health problems in the early 19th century. Clearly, cholera is not a major problem in the United States today; but in many countries of the world it remains a serious threat, and many countries periodically report outbreaks of cholera that are characterized by high death rates.

Let us compare the major causes of death in the United States in 1900 and in 1990 (Fig. 1–2). In 1900, the leading cause of death was influenza and pneumonia, the next was tuberculosis, and the third was gastroenteritis. In 1990, the leading causes of death were heart disease, cancer, cerebrovascular disease or stroke, and unintentional injuries. What change has occurred? Over a period of 90 years there has been a dramatic shift in the causes of death in this country. At the turn of the century,

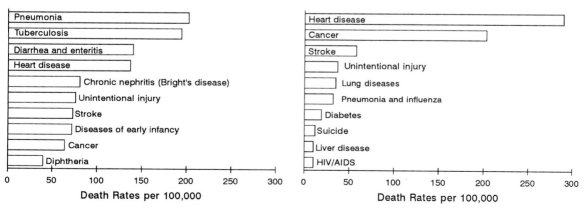

Figure 1–2. Ten leading causes of death in the United States, 1900 and 1990. (Adapted from Grove RD, Hetzel AM: Vital Statistics Rates of the United States, 1940–1960. Washington DC, US Government Printing Office, 1968; and National Center for Health Statistics: Advance Report of Final Mortality Statistics: 1990. Monthly Vital Stat Rep 41, no. 7 (suppl), 1993.)

the three leading causes of death were infectious diseases; now we are dealing with chronic diseases that in most situations do not appear to be communicable or infectious in origin. Consequently, the kinds of research, intervention, and services we need today differ from those that were required in the United States in 1900. The pattern seen in developing countries today is often similar to that seen in the United States in 1900: infectious diseases are the largest problems. But, as countries become industrialized they increasingly manifest the mortality patterns currently seen in developed countries, with chronic disease mortality becoming the major challenge. However, even in industrialized countries, as acquired immunodeficiency syndrome (AIDS) and human immunodeficiency virus (HIV) infections have emerged and tuberculosis has increased, infectious diseases are again becoming major public health problems.

Another demonstration of changes that have taken place over time is seen in Figure 1–3, which shows the remaining years of expected life in the United States at birth and at age 65 years for the years 1900, 1950, and 1985, for white females, nonwhite females, white males, and nonwhite males. The years of life remaining at birth have dramatically improved in all of these groups, with most of the improvement having occurred from 1900 to 1950, and much less having occurred since 1950. If we look at the remaining years of life at age 65 years, very little improvement is seen from 1900 to 1985. What primarily accounts for the increase in remaining years of life at birth are the

decreases in infant mortality and childhood diseases. In terms of diseases that afflict adults, we have been much less successful in extending the span of life, and this remains a major challenge.

EPIDEMIOLOGY AND PREVENTION

A major goal of epidemiology is to identify subgroups in the population who are at high risk for disease. Why should we identify such high-risk groups? First, if we are able to identify such groups, we may be able to identify the specific factors or characteristics that put them at high risk and try to modify those factors. Second, if we can identify high-risk groups we could direct preventive efforts, such as screening programs for early disease detection, to populations who are most likely to benefit from any interventions that are developed for the disease.

In discussing prevention it is helpful to distinguish between primary and secondary prevention. *Primary prevention* denotes an action taken to prevent the development of a disease in a person who is well and does not have the disease in question. For example, we can immunize a person against certain diseases so that the disease never develops. Or, if a disease is environmentally induced, we can prevent a person's exposure to the environmental factor involved and thereby prevent the development of the disease. Primary prevention is our ultimate goal. We know for example that most lung cancer is preventable. If we can get people to stop

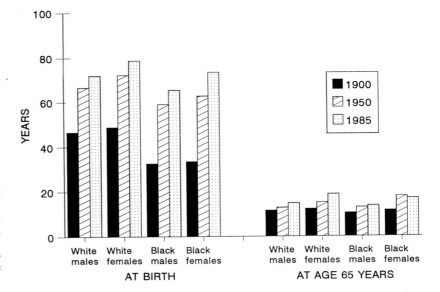

Figure 1–3. Life expectancy at birth and at 65 years of age, by race, and sex, United States, 1900, 1950, and 1985. (Redrawn from National Center for Health Statistics: Health, United States, 1987 DHHS publication no. 88–1232. Washington, DC, Public Health Service, March 1988.)

smoking we can eliminate about 70% to 80% of lung cancer in human beings. However, although we aim to prevent disease from occurring in human populations, we do not have the information needed for implementing effective primary prevention for many diseases. Often we do not have the biologic, clinical, and epidemiologic data on which to base a primary prevention program.

Secondary prevention denotes the identification of people who have already developed a disease, at an early stage in the disease's natural history, through screening and early intervention. For example, most cases of breast cancer in women can be detected through breast self-examination and mammography. Many believe that routine testing of the stool for occult blood can detect treatable colon cancer early in its natural history. The rationale for secondary prevention is that if we can identify disease earlier in its natural history, intervention measures will be more effective. Perhaps we can prevent mortality or complications of the disease and use less invasive or less costly treatment to do so.

Two possible approaches to prevention are a *population-based approach* and a *high-risk approach*.[2] In a population-based approach, a preventive measure is widely applied to an entire population. For example, prudent dietary advice for preventing coronary disease or advice against smoking may be provided to an entire population. An alternate approach is to target a high-risk group with the preventive measure. Thus, screening for cholesterol in children might be restricted to children who come from high-risk families. Clearly, a measure that will be applied to an entire population must be relatively inexpensive and non-invasive. A measure that is to be applied to a high-risk subgroup of the population may be more expensive and is often more invasive or inconvenient. Population-based approaches can be considered public health approaches, whereas high-risk approaches more often require a clinical action to identify the high-risk group to be targeted. In most situations, a combination of both approaches is ideal.

EPIDEMIOLOGY AND CLINICAL PRACTICE

Epidemiology is critical not only to public health but also to clinical practice. The practice of medicine is dependent on population data. For example, if a physician hears an apical systolic murmur, how does she know that it represents mitral regurgita-

tion? Where did this knowledge originate? The diagnosis is based on correlation of the auscultatory findings with the findings of surgical pathology or autopsy in a large group of patients. Thus the process of *diagnosis* is population-based. The same holds for *prognosis*. A patient asks his physician, "How long do I have to live, doctor?" and the doctor replies, "Six months to a year." On what basis does the physician prognosticate? He or she does so on the basis of experience with large groups of patients who had the same disease, were observed at the same stage of disease, and received the same treatment. Again, prognostication is based on population data. Finally, *selection of appropriate therapy* is also population based. Randomized clinical trials studying the effects of a treatment in large enough groups of patients are the ideal way to identify appropriate therapy. Thus, population-based concepts and data underlie the critical processes of clinical practice, including diagnosis, prognostication, and selection of therapy. In effect, the physician applies a population-based probability model to the patient who is lying on the examining table.

Figure 1–4 shows a physician demonstrating that the practice of clinical medicine relies heavily on population concepts. What is portrayed humorously is a true commentary on one aspect of pediatric practice: a pediatrician often makes a diagnosis based on what the parent tells him or her over the telephone and what illnesses, such as viral and bacterial diseases, the pediatrician knows to be "going around" the community. Thus, the data available about illness in the community can be very helpful in suggesting a diagnosis, even if they are not conclusive. Data regarding the etiology of sore throats according to a child's age are particularly

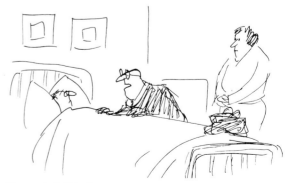

Figure 1–4. "You've got whatever it is that's going around." (Drawing by Ross; copyright 1975. The New Yorker Magazine, Inc.)

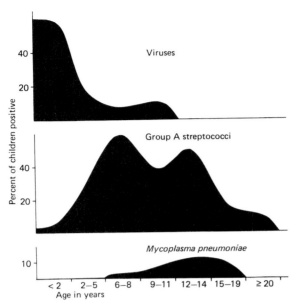

Figure 1–5. Frequency of agents by age of children with pharyngitis, 1964–1965. (From Denny FW: The replete pediatrician and the etiology of lower respiratory tract infections. Pediatr Res 3:464–470, 1969.)

relevant (Fig. 1–5). If the infection occurs early in life, it is likely to be viral in origin. If it occurs at ages 4 to 7 years, it is likely to be streptococcal in origin. In an older child it is more likely to be due to *Mycoplasma*. Although these data do not make the diagnosis, they do provide the physician or other health care provider with a good clue as to what agent or agents to suspect.

THE EPIDEMIOLOGIC APPROACH

How does the epidemiologist proceed to identify the cause of a disease? Epidemiologic reasoning is a multi-step process. The first step is to determine whether an association exists between a factor (e.g., an environmental exposure) or a characteristic (e.g., an increased serum cholesterol level), and the development of the disease in question. We do this by studying the characteristics of groups and the characteristics of individuals.

If we find that there is indeed an association between an exposure and a disease, is it necessarily a causal relationship? No, not all associations are causal. The second step, therefore, is to try to derive appropriate inferences regarding a possible causal relationship from the patterns of the associations that have been found. These steps are discussed in detail in later chapters.

Epidemiology often begins with descriptive data. For example, Figure 1–6 shows rates of hepatitis B in the United States in 1993 by state. Clearly, there are marked regional variations in reported hepatitis B. The first questions to ask when we see such differences between two groups or two regions or over time are, Are they real? Are the data from each area of comparable quality? Before trying to interpret the data, we should be satisfied that the data are valid. If the differences are real, then we ask, Why have they occurred? Are there environmental differences between high-risk and low-risk areas or are there ethnic and biologic differences in the people who live in those areas? This is where epidemiology begins its investigation.

Many years ago it was observed that communities in which the level of fluoride in the drinking water differed also differed by the frequency of dental caries in the permanent teeth of their residents: Communities that had low natural fluoride levels had high levels of caries and communities

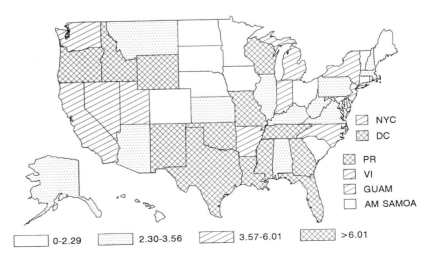

Figure 1–6. Hepatitis B: reported cases per 100,000 population, United States and territories, 1993. (Adapted from Centers for Disease Control and Prevention: Summary of notifiable diseases, United States: 1993. MMWR 42:34, 1994.)

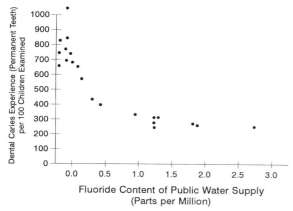

Figure 1–7. Relationship between amount of dental caries in permanent teeth and fluoride content in public water supply. (Adapted from Dean HT, Arnold FA, Jr, Elvove E: Domestic water and dental caries: V. Additional studies of the relation of fluoride in domestic waters to dental caries experience in 4,425 white children aged 12 to 14 years of 13 cities in 4 states. Pub Health Rep 57:1155–1179, 1942.)

that had higher levels of fluoride in their drinking water had low levels of caries (Fig. 1–7). This suggested that fluoride might be an effective preventive if it were artificially added to the drinking water supply. A trial was therefore carried out to test the hypothesis. Although ideally we would like to randomize a group of people either to fluoride or to no fluoride, this was not possible to do with drinking water because each community generally shares a common water supply. Consequently, two similar communities in upstate New York, Kingston and Newburgh, were chosen for the trial. The DMF index was used, which is a count of decayed, miss-

ing, and filled teeth. Baseline data were collected in both cities, and at the start of the study the DMF indices were comparable in each group in the two communities. The water in Newburgh was then fluoridated and the children were re-examined. Figure 1–8 shows that in each age group the DMF index in Newburgh had dropped significantly some 10 years or so later, whereas in Kingston there was no change. This is strongly suggestive evidence that fluoride was preventing caries.

It was possible to go one step further in trying to demonstrate a causal relationship of fluoride ingestion with low rates of caries. The issue of fluoridating water supplies has been extremely controversial, and in certain communities in which water has been fluoridated, there have been referenda to stop the fluoridation. It was therefore possible to look at the DMF index in Antigo, Wisconsin, a community that had had fluoride added to its water supply and then, after a referendum, had the fluoridation stopped. As seen in Figure 1–9, after the fluoride was removed, the DMF index rose. This provided yet a further piece of evidence that fluoride acted to prevent dental caries.

FROM OBSERVATIONAL DATA TO PREVENTIVE ACTION

Edward Jenner (Fig. 1–10) was born in 1749 and became very interested in the problem of smallpox. He observed, as had other people before him, that dairy maids, the young women whose occupation was milking the cows, developed a mild disease

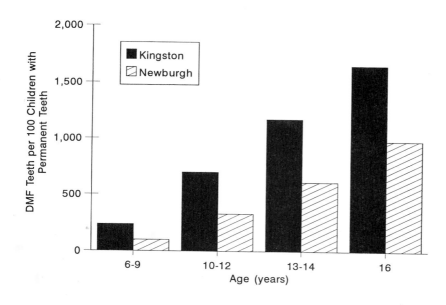

Figure 1–8. DMF indices after 10 years of fluoridation, 1954–1955. (Adapted from Ast DB, Schlesinger ER: The conclusion of a 10-year study of water fluoridation. Am J Pub Health 46:265–271, 1956. Copyright 1956 by the American Public Health Association. Adapted with permission.)

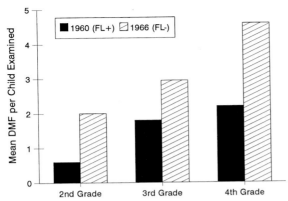

Figure 1–9. Effect of discontinuing fluoridation in Antigo, Wisconsin, November 1969. FL+, during fluoridation; FL−, after fluoridation was discontinued. (Adapted from Lemke CW, Doherty JM, Arra MC: Controlled fluoridation: The dental effects of discontinuation in Antigo, Wisconsin. J Am Dental Assoc 80:782–786, 1970. Reprinted by permission of ADA Publishing Co., Inc.)

called *cowpox*. Later, during smallpox outbreaks, the disease appeared not to develop in these young women. These data were observational, not based on any randomization. Jenner became convinced that cowpox would be a protection against smallpox and decided to test his hypothesis.

Figure 1–11 shows a painting of the first vaccination. A dairy maid, Sarah Nelmes, who has just had some cowpox material removed from her hand, is bandaging that hand. The cowpox material is being administered by Jenner to an 8-year-old "volunteer," James Phipps. Jenner was so convinced that cowpox would be protective that he exposed this

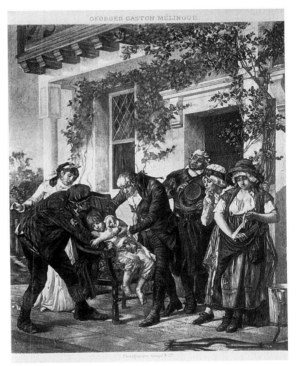

Figure 1–11. Painting of the first vaccination. (Roses DF: From Hunter and the great pox to Jenner and smallpox. Surg Gynecol Obstet 175:365–372, 1992. By permission of Surgery, Gynecology & Obstetrics, now known as the Journal of the American College of Surgeons.)

child to smallpox 6 weeks later. The child did not contract the disease. We shall not deal in this chapter with the ethical issues and implications of this experiment. (Clearly, Jenner did not have to justify his study before an institutional review board!) In any event, the results of the first vaccination and of what followed were the saving of literally millions of human beings throughout the world from disability and death caused by the scourge of smallpox. The important point is that Jenner knew nothing about viruses and nothing about the biology of the disease. He operated purely on observational data that provided him with the basis for a preventive intervention.

Figure 1–12 is a portrait of John Snow. Snow lived in the 19th century and was well known as the anesthesiologist who administered chloroform to Queen Victoria in childbirth. However, Snow's true love was the epidemiology of cholera, a disease that was a major problem in England in the middle of the 19th century. At that time the Registrar General was William Farr. The two men had a major disagreement about the cause of cholera. Farr adhered to what was called the *miasmatic theory of disease*. According to this theory, which was

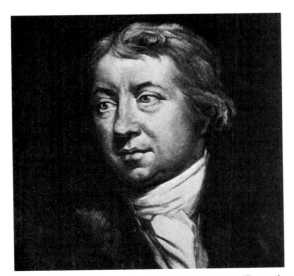

Figure 1–10. Photograph of Edward Jenner. (From the Wellcome Historical Medical Museum and Library, Mansell Collection, London.)

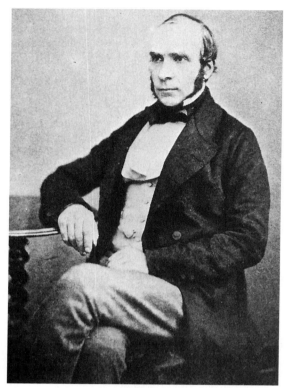

Figure 1–12. Photograph of John Snow. (From the Wellcome Historical Medical Museum and Library, London.)

commonly held at the time, disease was transmitted by a miasm, or cloud, that clung low on the surface of the earth. If this were so, we would expect that a person who lived at a lower altitude would be at greater risk of contracting a disease transmitted by this cloud.

Farr collected data to support his hypothesis (Table 1–1). The data are quite consistent with his

Table 1–1. Deaths from Cholera in 10,000 Inhabitants by Elevation of Residence Above Sea Level, London, 1848–1849

Elevation Above Sea Level (ft)	Deaths in 10,000 Inhabitants
<20	120
20–40	65
40–60	34
60–80	27
80–100	22
100–120	17
340–360	8

Data from Farr W: Vital Statistics: A Memorial Volume of Selections from the Reports and Writings of William Farr (edited for the Sanitary Institute of Great Britain by Noel A. Humphreys). London, The Sanitary Institute, 1885.

hypothesis: the lower the elevation the higher the mortality from cholera. John Snow did not agree; he believed that cholera was transmitted through contaminated water. In London at that time, a person obtained water by signing up with one of the water supply companies. The intake for the water companies was in a very polluted part of the Thames River. At one point, one of the companies, the Lambeth Company, shifted its water intake upstream in the Thames to a less polluted part of the river; the other companies did not move the location of their water intake. Snow reasoned, therefore, that mortality from cholera would be lower in people getting their water from the Lambeth Company than in those obtaining their water from other companies. He carried out what we call today "shoe leather epidemiology," going from house to house, counting all deaths from cholera in each house, and determining which company supplied water to each house.

Snow's findings are shown in Table 1–2. The table shows the number of houses, the number of deaths from cholera, and the deaths per 10,000 houses. Although this is not an ideal rate, because a house can contain different numbers of people, it is not a bad approximation. We see that in houses served by the Southwark and Vauxhall Company, which was getting its water from a polluted part of the Thames, the death rate was 315 deaths per 10,000 houses. In homes supplied by the Lambeth Company, the rate was only 37 deaths per 10,000 houses. Remember that in Snow's day the enterotoxic *Vibrio cholerae* was unknown. Nothing was known about the biology of the disease. Snow's conclusion that contaminated water was associated with cholera was based entirely on observational data.

The point is that although it is extremely important for us to maximize our knowledge of the biology and pathogenesis of disease, it is not always necessary to know every detail of the pathogenic mechanism to be able to prevent a disease. For example, we know that virtually every case of rheumatic fever and rheumatic heart disease follows a streptococcal infection. The *Streptococcus* is probably the bacterium that has been studied and analyzed most extensively, but we still do not know how and why it causes rheumatic fever. We do know that after a severe streptococcal infection, as seen in military recruits, 97 of every 100 individuals infected do not develop rheumatic fever. In civilian populations, such as in schoolchildren, in which the infection is less severe, only 3 of every 1,000 infected school-

Table 1–2. Deaths from Cholera per 10,000 Houses, by Source
of Water Supply, London, 1854

Water Supply	No. of Houses	Deaths from Cholera	Deaths per 10,000 Houses
Southwark and Vauxhall Co.	40,046	1,263	315
Lambeth Co.	26,107	98	38
Other districts in London	256,423	1,422	56

Data adapted from Snow J: On the mode of communication of cholera. *In* Snow on Cholera: A Reprint of Two Papers by John Snow, M.D. New York, The Commonwealth Fund, 1936.

children develop rheumatic fever and 997 do not.[3] Why does the disease not develop in those 97 and 997 if they are exposed to the same organism? We do not know. We do not know if it is a result of an undetected difference in the organism or due to a co-factor that may facilitate the adherence of *Streptococcus* to epithelial cells. What we do know is that even without fully understanding the chain of pathogenesis from infection with *Streptococcus* to rheumatic fever we can prevent virtually every case of rheumatic fever if we either prevent or promptly and adequately treat streptococcal infections. The absence of biologic knowledge regarding pathogenesis should not be a hindrance or an excuse for not implementing effective preventive services.

Consider cigarette smoking and lung cancer. We do not know what specific component in cigarettes causes cancer, but we do know that 75% to 80% of lung cancers are caused by smoking. That does not mean we should not be conducting laboratory research to try and better understand how cigarettes cause cancer. But again, in parallel with that research, we should be mounting effective community and public health programs based on the observational data available right now. Figure 1–13 shows mortality data for breast cancer and lung cancer in women in the United States. Breast cancer mortality

has remained relatively constant over the past several decades. However, mortality from lung cancer in women has been increasing steadily, and by 1990 it exceeded the mortality rate for breast cancer. Thus, we are faced with the tragic picture of a preventable form of cancer, lung cancer, that results from a personal habit, smoking, as the current leading cause of cancer death in American women. The scourge of smoking in women is thus one of the major unmet prevention challenges for practitioners in both public health and clinical medicine.

CONCLUSION

Prevention and therapy are all too often viewed as mutually exclusive activities, as is shown in Figure 1–14. It is clear, however, that prevention not only is integral to public health, but also is

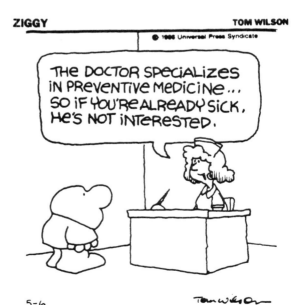

Figure 1–14. Prevention and therapy viewed as mutually exclusive activities. (From Wilson T: Ziggy cartoon. Universal Press Syndicate, 1986.)

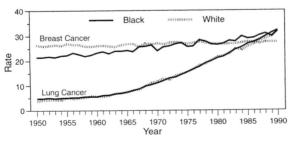

Figure 1–13. Age-adjusted lung and breast cancer death rates for women, by race, United States, 1950–1990. (From Centers for Disease Control and Prevention: Mortality trends for selected smoking-related cancers and breast cancer: United States, 1950–1990. MMWR 42:857–866, 1993.)

integral to clinical practice. The physician's role is to maintain health as well as to treat disease. But even treatment of disease has a major component of prevention. Whenever we treat illness we are preventing death, preventing complications in the patient, or preventing a constellation of effects on the patient's family. Thus, much of the dichotomy between therapy and prevention is an illusion. Therapy involves secondary and tertiary prevention, the latter denoting the prevention of complications such as disability. At times it also involves primary prevention. Thus, the entire spectrum of prevention should be viewed as integral to both public health and clinical practice. Epidemiology is an invaluable tool for providing the rational basis on which effective prevention programs can be planned and implemented and for conducting clinical investigations that contribute to the control of disease and to the amelioration of the human suffering associated with it.

References

1. Last JM: A Dictionary of Epidemiology, ed 2. New York, Oxford University Press, 1988.
2. Rose G: Sick individuals and sick populations. Int J Epidemiol 14:32–38, 1985.
3. Markowitz M, Gordis L: Rheumatic Fever, ed 2. Philadelphia, WB Saunders, 1972.

CHAPTER **2**

The Dynamics of Disease Transmission

> *I keep six honest serving men,*
> *(they taught me all I knew).*
> *Their names are what, why, and when*
> *and how and where and who.*
> ——Rudyard Kipling[1]

Human disease does not arise in a vacuum. It results from an interaction of the host (a person), the agent (e.g., a bacterium) and the environment (e.g., a contaminated water supply). Although some diseases are largely genetic in origin, virtually all disease results from an interaction of genetic and environmental factors, with the exact balance differing for different diseases. Many of the underlying principles governing the transmission of disease are most clearly demonstrated using communicable diseases as a model. Hence, this chapter primarily uses such diseases as examples in reviewing these principles. However, the concepts discussed are also applicable to diseases that do not appear to be of infectious origin.

Disease has been classically described as the result of an epidemiologic triad shown in Figure 2–1. According to this diagram, it is the product of an interaction of the human host, an infectious or other type of agent, and the environment that promotes the exposure. A vector, such as the mosquito or the deer tick, is often involved. For such an interaction to take place, the host must be susceptible. Human susceptibility is determined by a variety of factors including genetic background and nutritional and immunologic characteristics. The immune status of an individual is determined by many factors including prior experience both with natural infection and with immunization.

Diseases can be transmitted in a *direct* or *indirect* fashion. For example, a disease can be transmitted person-to-person (direct transmission) by means of direct contact or a disease can be transmitted indirectly through a contaminated water supply. Some of the modes of transmission are shown in Table 2–1.

Figure 2–2 is a classic photograph showing droplet dispersal after a sneeze. It vividly demonstrates the potential for an individual to infect a large

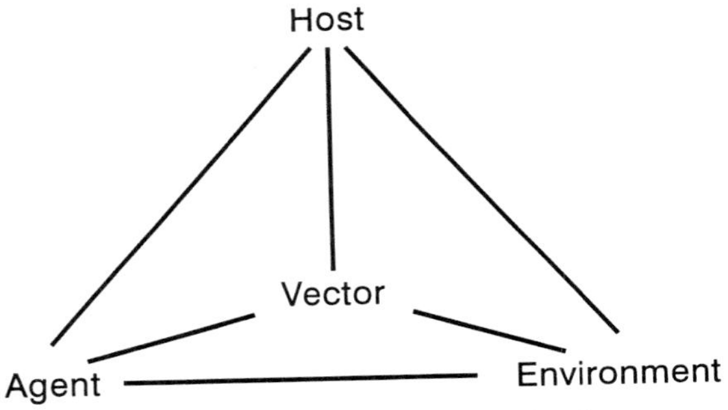

Figure 2–1. The epidemiologic triad of a disease.

Table 2–1. Modes of Disease Transmission

1. Horizontal
    a. Common vehicle
        1. Single exposure
        2. Multiple exposures
        3. Continuous exposure
    b. Contact (person-to-person)
    c. Vector
2. Vertical

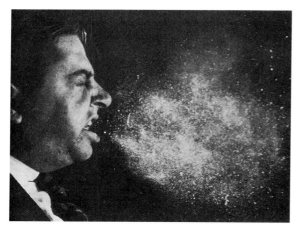

Figure 2–2. Droplet dispersal following a violent sneeze. (From Jennison MW: Aerobiology. Washington, DC, American Association for the Advancement of Science No. 17, 1947, p 102.)

number of people in a brief period of time. As Mims has pointed out:

An infected individual can transmit influenza or the common cold to a score of others in the course of an innocent hour in a crowded room. A venereal infection also, must spread progressively from person to person if it is to maintain itself in nature, but it would be a formidable task to transmit venereal infection on such a scale.[2]

Thus, different organisms spread in different ways, and the potential of a given organism for spreading and producing outbreaks depends on the characteristics of the organism, such as its rate of growth and the route by which it is transmitted from one person to another.

Figure 2–3 is a schematic diagram of the human body surfaces as sites of microbial infection and shedding.

The alimentary tract can be considered as an open tube that crosses the body, and the respiratory and urogenital systems can be seen as blind in-pouchings. Each offers an opportunity for infection. The skin is another important portal of entry for infectious agents, primarily through scratch or injury. Agents that often enter through the skin include streptococci or staphylococci and fungi such as tinea (ringworm). Two points should be made in this regard: First, the skin is not the exclusive portal of entry for many of these agents, and infections can be acquired through other routes as well. Second, the same routes as those described also serve

as points of entry for non-infectious disease-causing agents. Environmental toxins can be ingested, in-spired during respiration, or absorbed directly through the skin. With both infectious and non-infectious conditions, the clinical and epidemiologic characteristics of the condition often relate to the site of the exposure and the portal of entry.

CLINICAL AND SUBCLINICAL DISEASE

It is important to recognize the broad spectrum of disease severity. Figure 2–4 shows the iceberg concept of disease.

Just as most of an iceberg is underwater and hidden from view with only its tip visible, so it is with disease: only clinical illness is readily apparent (see Fig. 2–4, *right*). But infections without clinical illness are important, particularly in the web of disease transmission, although they are not visible clinically. In Figure 2–4, the corresponding biologic stages of pathogenesis and disease at the cellular level are seen on the *left*. The iceberg concept is important because it is not sufficient to count only the clinically apparent cases we see; for example, most cases of polio in prevaccine days were sub-clinical, but they were still capable of spreading the virus. One could therefore not hope to explain the epidemiology of polio without a recognition and assessment of the pool of inapparent cases.

Figure 2–5 shows the spectrum of severity for several diseases. Most cases of tuberculosis, for example, are inapparent. However, because inapparent cases can transmit the disease, such cases must be identified to control spread of the disease. In measles, many cases are of moderate severity and only a few are inapparent. At the other extreme, without intervention, rabies has no inapparent cases and most untreated cases are fatal. Thus we have a spectrum of severity patterns that varies with the disease. It appears to be related to the virulence of the organism (how good the organism is at produc-ing disease), and to the site in the body at which the organism multiplies. All these factors, as well as such host characteristics as the immune response, need to be appreciated to understand how disease spreads from one individual to another.

As clinical and biologic knowledge has increased over the years, so has our ability to distinguish different stages of disease. These include clinical and non-clinical disease:

CLINICAL DISEASE. Clinical disease is character-ized by signs and symptoms.

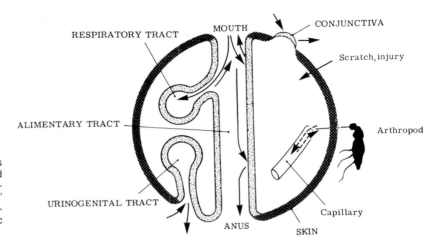

Figure 2–3. Body surfaces as sites of microbial infection and shedding. (From Mims CA, Dimmock NJ, Nash A, et al: Mims' Pathogenesis of Infectious Disease, ed 4. London, Academic Press, 1995, p 10.)

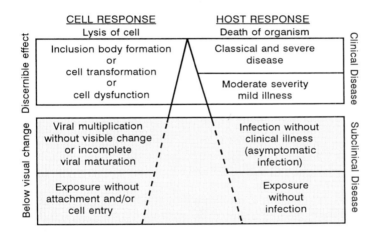

Figure 2–4. The "iceberg" concept of infectious diseases at the level of the cell and of the host. (Adapted from Evans AS (ed): Viral Infections of Humans: Epidemiology and Control, ed 3. New York, Plenum, 1991.)

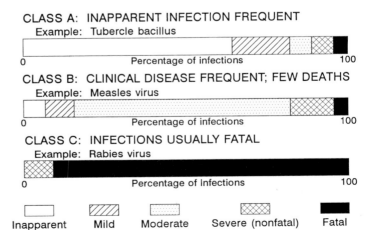

Figure 2–5. Distribution of clinical severity for three classes of infections (not drawn to scale). (Adapted from Mausner JS, Kramer S: Epidemiology: An Introductory Text. Philadelphia, WB Saunders, 1985, p 265.)

NONCLINICAL (INAPPARENT) DISEASE Nonclinical disease may include the following:

Preclinical Disease. Disease that is not yet clinically apparent, but in a stage that is destined to progress to clinical disease.

Subclinical Disease. Disease that is not clinically apparent and not destined to become clinically apparent. This type of disease is often diagnosed by serologic (antibody) response or culture of the organism.

Persistent (Chronic) Disease. A person fails to "shake off" the infection and it persists for years, at times for life. In recent years, an interesting phenomenon has been the manifestation of symptoms many years after an infection was thought to have been resolved. Some adults who recovered from poliomyelitis in childhood are now reporting severe fatigue and weakness; this has been called post-polio syndrome in adult life. These have thus become cases of clinical disease, albeit somewhat different from the initial illness.

Latent Disease. An infection with no active multiplication of the agent, as when viral nucleic acid is incorporated into the nucleus of a cell as a provirus. In contrast with persistent infection, only the genetic message is present in the host, not the viable organism.

CARRIER STATUS

In this situation the individual harbors the organism but is not infected as measured by serologic studies (no evidence of an antibody response) or by evidence of clinical illness. This person can still infect others, although the infectivity is often lower than with other infections. Carrier status may be of limited duration or it may be chronic, for months or years. One of the best-known examples of a long-term carrier was Typhoid Mary, who carried *Salmonella typhi* and died in 1938. Over a period of many years she worked as a cook in New York City, moving from household to household under different names. She was considered to have caused at least 10 typhoid fever outbreaks that included 51 cases and 3 deaths.

Disease transmission can also be characterized as *horizontal* or *vertical*. Horizontal transmission denotes transmission from one person to another, directly or indirectly. Vertical transmission denotes transmission from one generation to another, primarily genetic transmission. Although intrauterine transmission across the placenta can also be characterized as transmission from one generation to another, it may be more appropriately characterized as horizontal rather than vertical, as transmission across the placenta is from one host (the mother) to another (the fetus), in a manner more similar to that of any communicable disease than to a genetic disease.

The factors that can cause human disease include biologic, physical, and chemical factors as well as other types, such as stress, that may be harder to classify (Table 2–2).

ENDEMIC, EPIDEMIC, AND PANDEMIC. Three other terms need to be defined: *endemic, epidemic* and *pandemic. Endemic* is defined as the habitual presence of a disease within a given geographic area. It may also refer to the usual occurrence of a given disease within such an area. *Epidemic* is defined as the occurrence in a community or region of a group

Table 2–2. Factors That May Be Associated With Increased Risk of Human Disease

Host Characteristics	Type of Agents and Examples	Environmental Factors
Age	Biologic (bacteria, viruses)	Temperature
Sex	Chemical (poison, alcohol, smoke)	Humidity
Race	Physical (trauma, radiation, fire)	Altitude
Religion	Nutritional (lack, excess)	Crowding
Customs		Housing
Occupation		Neighborhood
Genetic profile		Water
Marital status		Milk
Family background		Food
Previous diseases		Radiation
Immune status		Air pollution
		Noise

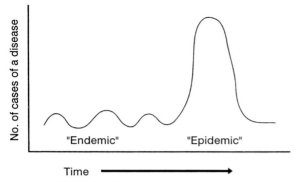

Figure 2–6. "Endemic" vs. "epidemic."

of illnesses of similar nature, clearly in excess of normal expectancy, and derived from a common or from a propagated source. *Pandemic* refers to a worldwide epidemic (Fig. 2–6).

How do we know when we have an excess over what is expected? Indeed, how do we know how much to expect? There is no precise answer to either question. Through ongoing surveillance we may determine what the usual or expected level may be. In regard to excess, sometimes an "interocular test" may be convincing: the difference is so clear it hits you between the eyes. For example, Figure 2–7 shows the number of deaths relating to a dense fog in London in December 1952; the excess above normal expectation is clearly seen on several days.

DISEASE OUTBREAKS. Let us assume that a food becomes contaminated with a microorganism. If an outbreak results in the group of people who have eaten the food, it would be called a *common vehicle*

exposure, because all the cases that developed were in persons exposed to the food in question. The food may be served only once — for example, at a catered luncheon — resulting in a *single exposure* to the people who eat it. Or the food may be served more than once, resulting in *multiple exposures* to people who eat it more than once. When a water supply is contaminated with sewage because of leaky pipes, the contamination can be either *periodic*, causing multiple exposures, as a result of changing pressures in the water supply system that may cause intermittent contamination, or *continuous*, in which a constant leak leads to a persistent contamination. The epidemiologic picture that is manifested depends on whether the exposure is single, multiple, or continuous.

For purposes of this discussion we will focus on the *single-exposure, common-vehicle outbreak* because the issues discussed are most clearly seen in this type of outbreak. What are the characteristics of such an outbreak? First, such outbreaks are explosive; there is a sudden and rapid increase in the number of cases of a disease in a population. Second, the cases are limited to people who share the common exposure. This is self-evident, because in the first wave of cases we would not expect the disease to develop in people who were not exposed unless there were another source of the disease in the community. Third, when such outbreaks are foodborne, it is generally rare for secondary cases to occur in persons who acquire the disease from a primary case. The reason for the relative rarity of secondary cases in this type of outbreak is not well understood.

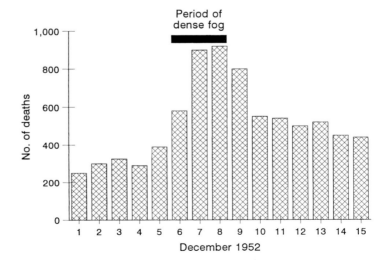

Figure 2–7. Deaths in greater London each day from Dec 1–15, 1952. (Data from Logan WPD: Mortality in the London fog incident, 1952. Lancet 1:336, 1953.)

DETERMINANTS OF DISEASE OUTBREAKS. The amount of disease in a population depends on a balance between the number of people in that population who are susceptible, and therefore at risk for the disease, and the number of people who are not susceptible, or immune, and therefore not at risk. They may be immune because they have had the disease previously or because they have been immunized. They may also be not susceptible on a genetic basis. Clearly, if the entire population is immune, no epidemic will develop. But the balance is usually struck somewhere in between, and when it moves toward susceptibility the likelihood of an outbreak increases. This has been observed particularly in formerly isolated populations who were exposed to disease. For example, in the 19th century, Panum observed that measles occurred in the Faroe islands in epidemic form when infected individuals entered an isolated and susceptible population.[3] Severe outbreaks of streptococcal sore throats developed when new susceptible recruits arrived at the Great Lakes Naval Station.[4]

HERD IMMUNITY. *Herd immunity* may be defined as the resistance of a group to an attack by a disease to which a large proportion of the members of the group are immune. If a large percent of the population is immune, the entire population is likely to be protected, not just those who are immune. Why does herd immunity occur? It happens because disease spreads from one person to another in any community. Once we reach a certain proportion of people who are immune in that community, the likelihood is small that an infected person will encounter a susceptible person to whom he can transmit the infection; more of his encounters will be with people who are immune. The presence of a large proportion of immune persons in the population lessens the likelihood that a person with the disease will come into contact with a susceptible individual.

Why is the concept of herd immunity so important? When we carry out immunization programs, it may not be necessary to achieve 100% immunization rates to immunize the population successfully. We can achieve highly effective protection by immunizing a large part of the population; the remaining part will be protected because of herd immunity.

In order for herd immunity to exist, certain conditions must be met (Table 2–3). If we have a reservoir in which the organism can exist outside the human host, herd immunity will not operate because other means of transmission are available. If immu-

Table 2–3. Some Requirements for Herd Immunity

1. Disease agent restricted to a single host species within which transmission occurs
2. Relatively direct transmission from one member of the host species to another
3. Infections must induce solid immunity
4. Outbreaks occur only in randomly mixing populations

nity is only partial, we will not build up a large subpopulation of immune people in the community.

What does this mean? Let us assume that 70% of a population is immune and 30% is susceptible. Herd immunity operates if the probability of an infected person encountering every *other individual* in the population (random mixing) is the same. But if a person is infected and all his interactions are with people who are susceptible (i.e., there is no random mixing of the population), he is likely to transmit the disease to other susceptible people. Herd immunity operates optimally when populations are constantly mixing together. This is a theoretical concept because, obviously, populations are never completely randomly mixed. All of us associate with family and friends, for example, more than we do with strangers. However, the degree to which herd immunity is achieved depends on the extent to which the population approaches a random mixing. Thus, we can interrupt the transmission of disease even if not everyone in the population is immune, so long as a critical percentage of the population is immune.

What percentage of a population must be immune in order for herd immunity to operate? This varies from disease to disease. For example, in the case of measles, which is highly communicable, it has been estimated that 94% of the population would have to be immune before the chain of transmission was interrupted.

INCUBATION PERIOD. This is defined as *the interval from receipt of infection to the time of onset of clinical illness.* If you become infected today, the disease with which you are infected may not develop for a number of days or weeks. During this time, the *incubation period,* you feel completely well and show no signs of the disease.

Why doesn't disease develop immediately on infection? What accounts for the incubation period? It may reflect the time needed for the organism to replicate sufficiently until the infecting organism reaches the critical mass needed for clinical disease to result. It probably also relates to the site in the body at which the organism replicates–whether it replicates superficially near the skin surface or deeper in the body. The dose of the infectious agent received at the time of infection may also influence the length of the incubation period. With a large dose, the incubation period may be shorter.

The incubation period is also of historical interest because it is related to what may have been the only medical advance associated with the Black Death in Europe. In 1374, when people were terribly frightened of the Black Death, the Venetian Republic appointed three officials who were responsible for inspecting all ships entering the port and for excluding the ships from the port if sick people were found on board. It was hoped that this would protect the community. In 1377, Ragusa detained travelers in an isolated area for 30 days (*trentini giorni*) after arrival to see if infection developed. This period was found to be insufficient and the period of detention was lengthened to 40 days (*quarante giorni*). This is the origin of the word *quarantine.*

How long would we want to isolate a person? We would want to isolate a person until he or she is no longer infectious to others. When a person is clinically ill, we generally have a clear sign of potential infectiousness. An important problem arises *before* he or she becomes clinically ill—that is, during the incubation period. If we knew when he or she became infected, and we knew the general length of the incubation period for the disease, we would want to isolate the infected person during this period to prevent the communication of the disease to others. In most situations, however, we do not know that a person has been infected, and we may not know until signs of clinical disease become manifest.

This leads to an important question: Is it worthwhile to quarantine—isolate—a patient, such as a child with chickenpox? The problem is that during at least part of the incubation period, when a person is still free of clinical illness, he or she is usually capable of transmitting the disease to others. Thus we have people who are not (yet) clinically ill, but who have been infected and are able to transmit the disease. For many of the common childhood diseases, by the time clinical disease develops in the child, he or she has already transmitted the disease to others. Therefore, isolating a person at the point at which he or she becomes clinically ill will not be effective.

Different diseases have different incubation periods. A precise incubation period does not exist for a given disease, but rather a range of incubation periods is characteristic for that disease. Figure 2–8 shows the range of incubation periods for several diseases. In large measure, the length of the incubation period is characteristic of the infective organism.

The incubation period of infectious diseases has its analogue in non-infectious diseases. Thus even when an individual is exposed to a carcinogen or other toxin, the disease is often manifest only after months or years. For example, mesotheliomas re-

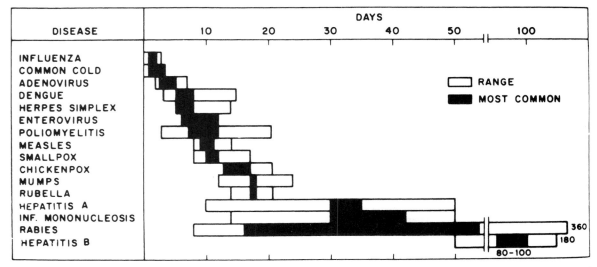

Figure 2–8. Incubation periods in viral diseases. (From Evans AS (ed): Viral Infections of Humans: Epidemiology and Control, ed 3. New York, Plenum, 1991.)

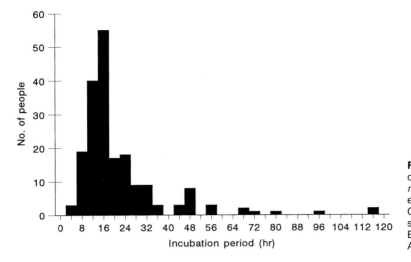

Figure 2–9. Incubation periods for 191 delegates affected by a *Salmonella typhimurium* outbreak at a medical conference in Wales, 1986. (Adapted from Glynn JR, Palmer SR: Incubation period, severity of disease, and infecting dose: Evidence from a *Salmonella* outbreak. Am J Epidemiol 136:1369–1377, 1992.)

sulting from asbestos exposure may occur 20 to 30 years after the exposure.

Figure 2–9 is a graphic representation of an outbreak of *Salmonella typhimurium* at a medical conference in Wales in 1986. Each bar represents the number of cases of disease developing at a certain point in time after the exposure; the number of hours since exposure are shown along the horizontal axis. Note that there was a rapid, explosive rise in the number of cases within the first 16 hours, which suggests a common-vehicle single-exposure epidemic. If a line were drawn connecting the tops of the bars, it would rise quickly and then taper off to the right. This curve is called the *epidemic curve*, which is defined as the distribution of the times of onset of the disease. In a single-exposure common-vehicle epidemic, the epidemic curve represents the distribution of the incubation periods. This should be intuitively apparent: If the infection took place at one point in time, the interval from that point to the onset of each case is the incubation period in that person.

The configuration of the curve in Figure 2–9 is the classic epidemic curve for a single-exposure common-vehicle outbreak. The reason for this configuration is not known. But it has an interesting property: if the curve is plotted against the logarithm of time rather than against time, the curve becomes a normal curve (Fig. 2–10). If plotted on log-normal graph paper, we obtain a straight line, and estimation of the median incubation period is facilitated.

The three critical variables in investigating an outbreak or epidemic are: (1) When did the exposure take place? (2) When did the disease begin? and (3) What was the incubation period for the disease? If we know any two of these, we can calculate the third.

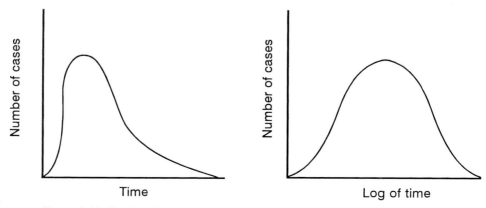

Figure 2–10. Number of cases plotted against time and against the logarithm of time.

An attack rate is defined as

$$\frac{\text{Number of people at risk who develop}}{\text{Total number of people at risk}}$$

It is similar to an incidence rate, which is also used for less acute diseases. The attack rate (or the incidence rate) is useful for comparing the risk of disease in groups with different exposures. The attack rate can be specific for a given exposure. For example, the attack rate in people who ate a certain food is called a *food-specific attack rate*. It is calculated by

$$\frac{\text{Number of people who ate a certain food}}{\text{Total number of people who ate that food}}$$

In general, *time* is not explicitly specified in an attack rate; given what is usually known about how long after an exposure most cases develop, the time period is implicit in the attack rate. Examples of calculating attack rates are seen in Table 2–5.

A person who acquires the disease from that exposure (e.g., from a contaminated food) is called a *primary case*. A person who acquires the disease from exposure to a primary case is called a *secondary case*. The *secondary attack rate* is therefore defined as the attack rate in susceptible people who have been exposed to a primary case. It is a good measure of person-to-person spread of disease after the disease has been introduced into a population, and it can be thought of as a ripple moving out from the primary case. We often calculate the secondary attack rate in family members of the index case. The secondary attack rate also has its application in non-infectious diseases when family members are examined to determine the extent to which a disease clusters among first-degree relatives of an index case, which may yield a clue regarding the contributions of genetic and environmental factors to the cause of a disease.

Exploring the Occurrence of Disease

The concepts outlined in this chapter form the basis for exploring the occurrence of disease. When a disease appears to have occurred at more than an endemic level, and we wish to investigate its occurrence, we ask:

Who was attacked by the disease?

When did the disease occur?

Where did the cases arise?

It is well known that disease risk is affected by all these factors.

WHO. The characteristics of the human host are clearly related to disease risk. Factors such as sex, age, and race have a major effect. As shown in Figure 2–11, rates of gonorrhea are higher in men, although the trends over time appear to be the same in both sexes. This graph raises the question of whether gonorrhea is actually more frequent in men or whether it is more readily recognized or reported in men. Pertussis is clearly related to age, being most common in children younger than 1 year (Fig. 2–12). Age and race together may play a role in disease occurrence. For example, as shown in Figure 2–13, age patterns for tuberculosis show that the peak risk of tuberculosis is higher in minorities than in whites and occurs at a much earlier age.

WHEN. Certain diseases occur with a certain periodicity. For example, aseptic meningitis peaks yearly (Fig. 2–14). A regular variation in reported cases is also seen with tuberculosis (Fig. 2–15). Often there is a seasonal pattern: for example, diarrheal disease is most common during the summer months and respiratory disease during the winter months. The question of *when* is also addressed by examining trends of disease incidence over time. For example, cases of acquired immunodeficiency syndrome (AIDS) are increasing each year, and there is considerable discussion regarding projections of future incidence.

WHERE. Disease is not randomly distributed in time or place. For example, Figure 2–16 shows the geographic distribution of Rocky Mountain spotted fever in the United States in 1989; there is a clear clustering of cases along the East Coast and in the south central part of the country. Geographic localization of a disease is seen in another example. In May 1993 there was an outbreak of respiratory illness in the southwestern United States (Fig. 2–17). Onset of the illness was associated with fever, myalgia, and variable respiratory symptoms followed by abrupt onset of acute respiratory distress. Case fatality was 62%. The illness was subsequently recognized as being due to a hantavirus, with the deer mouse serving as the rodent reservoir. Cases have since been reported in other areas of the United States. Interestingly, cases of disease that had been previously associated with hantavirus infection had been characterized by hemorrhagic features and renal involvement. The earliest retro-

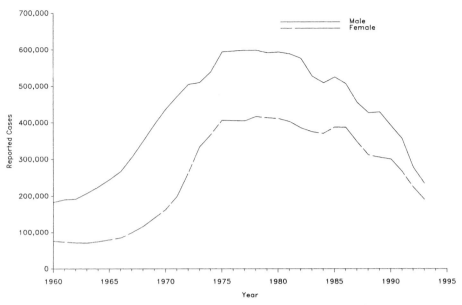

Figure 2–11. Gonorrhea—by sex, United States, 1960–1993. (From Centers for Disease Control and Prevention: Summary of notifiable diseases, United States: 1993. MMWR 42:28, 1994.)

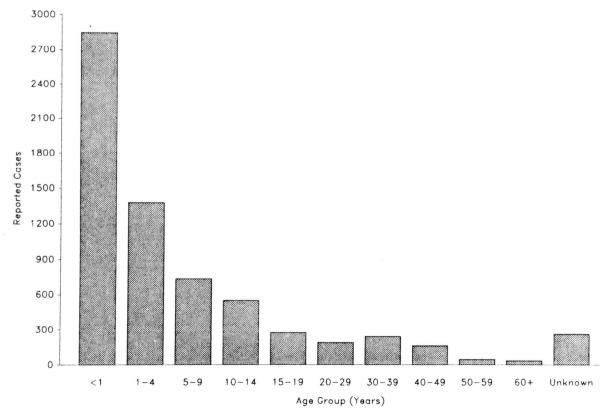

Figure 2–12. Pertussis (whooping cough)—by age, United States, 1993. (From Centers for Disease Control and Prevention: Summary of notifiable diseases, United States: 1993. MMWR 42:43, 1994.)

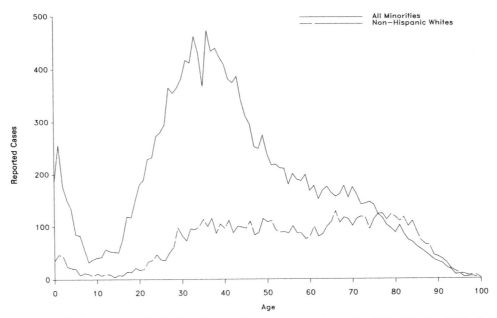

Figure 2–13. Tuberculosis: frequency distribution of cases by age, race, and ethnicity, United States, 1993. (From Centers for Disease Control and Prevention: Summary of notifiable diseases, United States: 1993. MMWR 42:60, 1994.)

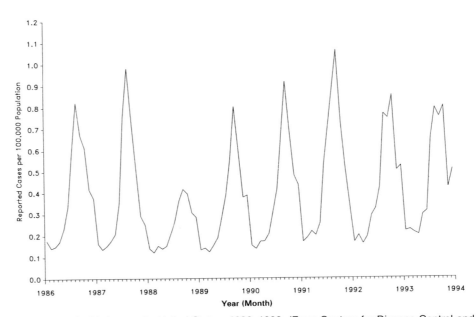

Figure 2–14. Aseptic meningitis by month, United States, 1986–1993. (From Centers for Disease Control and Prevention: Summary of notifiable diseases, United States: 1993. MMWR 42:22, 1994.)

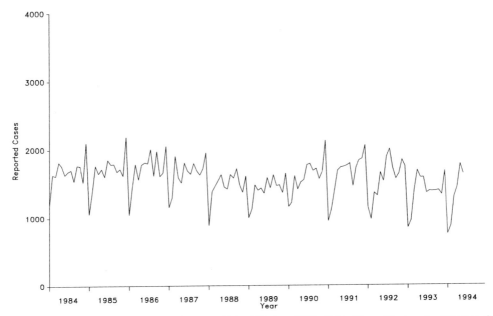

Figure 2–15. Tuberculosis by 4-week period of report, United States, 1984–1994. (From Centers for Disease Control and Prevention: Table III. MMWR 43:542, 1994.)

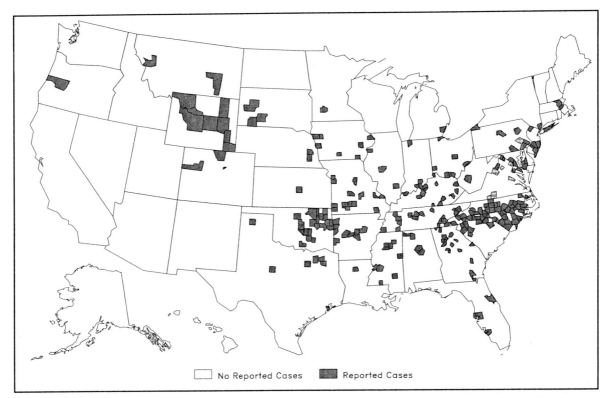

Figure 2–16. Rocky Mountain spotted fever: counties reporting cases, United States, 1993. (From Centers for Disease Control and Prevention: Summary of notifiable diseases, United States: 1993. MMWR 42:48, 1994.)

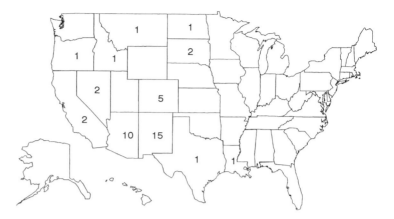

Figure 2–17. Number of cases of Hantavirus pulmonary syndrome, by state, United States, July 7, 1991–Oct 21, 1993. (Adapted from Centers for Disease Control and Prevention: Update: Hantavirus pulmonary syndrome, United States: 1993. MMWR 42:816–817, 1993.)

spectively confirmed case occurred in July 1991 (Fig. 2–18).

Another interesting geographic distribution is seen with Lyme disease. Surveillance for the disease began in 1982, and a fairly steady trend of increasing numbers of cases reported each year can be seen in Figure 2–19. The distribution of the cases in 1992 is seen in Figure 2–20. Most cases were reported from the northeastern, mid-Atlantic, north central, and Pacific coast regions. The 19 states in which established enzootic cycles of *Borrelia burgdorferi*, the causative agent, have been reported, accounted for 94% of the cases. The distribution of the disease closely parallels that of the deer tick vector.

OUTBREAK INVESTIGATION

The characteristics just discussed are the central issues in virtually all outbreak investigations. The

steps for investigating an outbreak follow this general pattern (Table 2–4).

CROSS-TABULATION

When confronted with several possible causal agents as is often the case in a foodborne disease outbreak, a very helpful method for determining which of the possible agents is likely to be the cause is called *cross-tabulation*. This is illustrated by an outbreak of foodborne streptococcal disease in a Florida prison reported some years ago by the Centers for Disease Control and Prevention.[5]

In August 1974, an outbreak of group A β-hemolytic streptococcal pharyngitis affected 325 of 690 inmates. In a questionnaire of 185 randomly selected inmates, 47% reported a sore throat between August 16th and 22nd. Based on a second questionnaire, food-specific attack rates

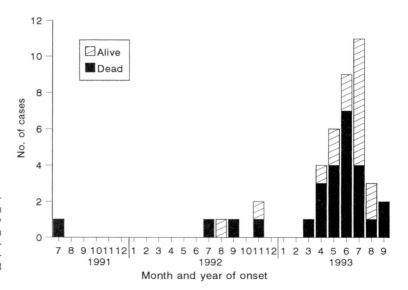

Figure 2–18. Number of cases of Hantavirus pulmonary syndrome, by month and year of onset, United States, July 7, 1991–Oct 21, 1993. (Adapted from Centers for Disease Control and Prevention: Update: Hantavirus pulmonary syndrome, United States: 1993. MMWR 42:816–817, 1993.)

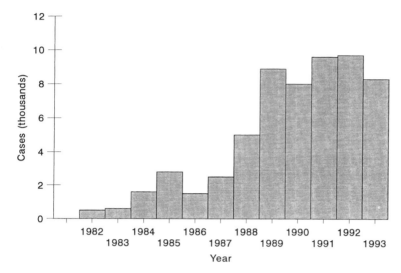

Figure 2–19. Reported cases of Lyme disease, by year, United States, 1982–1992. (Adapted from Centers for Disease Control and Prevention: Lyme disease, United States: 1993. MMWR 43:564, 1994.)

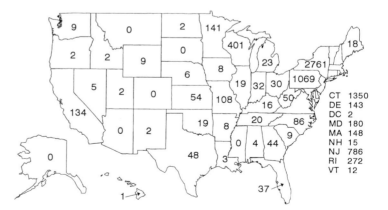

Figure 2–20. Reported cases of Lyme disease, United States, 1992. (Adapted from Centers for Disease Control and Prevention: Lyme disease, United States: 1993. MMWR 43:564, 1994.)

Table 2–4. Steps in Investigation
of an Acute Outbreak

Investigation of an acute outbreak may be primarily
deductive (i.e., reasoning from premises or propositions
proved antecedently) or inductive (i.e., reasoning from
particular facts to a general conclusion), or it may be a
combination of both.

Important considerations in the investigation of an acute
outbreak of infectious diseases include determining that
an outbreak has in fact occurred and defining the extent
of the population at risk, determining the measure of
spread and reservoir, and characterizing the agent.

Steps commonly used are as follows:

1. *Define the epidemic.*
   a. Define the "numerator" (cases).
      1. Clinical features: is the disease known?
      2. What are its serologic or cultural aspects?
      3. Are the causes partially understood?
   b. Define the "denominator": What is the population at
      risk of developing disease?
   c. Calculate the attack rates.

2. *Examine the distribution of cases by the following:*
   a. Time ⎫
   b. Place ⎬ Look for time-place interactions.
   c. Person: examine the risk in subgroups of the
      affected population according to personal
      characteristics: sex, age, residence, occupation
      (rank), social group, etc.

3. *Look for combinations (interactions) of relevant
   variables.*

4. *Develop hypotheses based on the following:*
   a. Existing knowledge (if any) of the disease
   b. Analogy to diseases of known etiology

5. *Test hypotheses.*
   a. Further analyze existing data (case-control studies).
   b. Collect additional data.

6. *Recommend control measures*
   a. Control of present outbreak
   b. Prevention of future similar outbreaks

for items served to 314 randomly selected inmates
showed a significant association between two
food items and risk of developing a sore throat:
egg salad and beverage at lunch on August 16th
(Table 2–5).

In Table 2–5, for each of the suspect exposures
(beverage and egg salad) the attack rate was calculated for those who ate (were exposed) and those
who did not eat (were not exposed). For both beverage and egg salad, attack rates are clearly higher
among those who ate (or drank) than among those
who did not. However, this table does not permit
us to determine whether the beverage or the egg
salad accounted for the outbreak.

In order to answer this question, we use the
technique of cross-tabulation. In Table 2–6 we
again examine the attack rates in those who ate egg
salad compared with those who did not, but this
time we do so separately for those who drank the
beverage and for those who did not.

Looking at the data by columns, we see that both
among those who ate egg salad and among those
who did not, drinking the beverage did not increase
the incidence of streptococcal illness (75.6% vs.
80% and 26.4% vs. 25%). However, looking at the
data in the table horizontally, we see that eating
egg salad significantly increased the attack rate of
the illness, both in those who drank the beverage
(75.6% vs. 26.4%) and in those who did not (80%
vs. 25%). Thus, the egg salad is clearly implicated.

This example demonstrates the use of cross-
tabulation in a foodborne outbreak of an infectious disease, but the method has broad applicability to any condition in which multiple etiologic
factors are suspected. It is discussed further in
Chapter 14.

SUMMARY

This chapter has reviewed some basic concepts
that underlie the epidemiologic approach to acute
communicable diseases. Many of these concepts
apply equally well to non-acute diseases that at
this time do not appear to be infectious in origin.
Moreover, for an increasing number of chronic diseases thought originally to be non-infectious, infection seems to play some role. Thus, hepatitis B
infection is a major cause of primary liver cancer.

Table 2–5. Food-Specific Attack Rates for Items Consumed
August 16, 1974, Dade County Jail, Miami

	Ate			Did Not Eat			
Item Consumed	**Sick**	**Total**	**% Sick (Attack rate)**	**Sick**	**Total**	**% Sick (Attack rate)**	**P**
Beverage	179	264	67.8	22	50	44.0	<.010
Egg salad sandwiches	176	226	77.9	27	73	37.0	<.001

From Centers for Disease Control and Prevention: Outbreak of foodborne streptococcal disease. MMWR 23:365, 1974.

Table 2–6. Cross-Table Analysis for Egg Salad and Beverage Consumed August 16, 1974, Dade County Jail, Miami

	Ate Egg Salad				Did Not Eat Egg Salad			
	Sick	Well	Total	% Sick (Attack rate)	Sick	Well	Total	% Sick (Attack rate)
Drank beverage	152	49	201	75.6	19	53	72	26.4
Did not drink beverage	12	3	15	80.0	7	21	28	25.0

From Centers for Disease Control and Prevention: Outbreak of foodborne streptococcal disease. MMWR 23:365, 1974.

Papillomaviruses have been implicated in cervical cancer, and Epstein-Barr virus has been implicated in Hodgkin's disease. The boundary between the epidemiology of infectious and non-infectious diseases has blurred in many areas. In addition, even for diseases that are not infectious in origin, the patterns of spread share many of the same dynamics, and the methodologic issues in studying them are similar. Many of these issues are discussed in detail in Section II.

References

1. Kipling R: Just-So Stories: The Elephant's Child, 1902, Reprinted by Everyman's Library Children's Classics, New York, Alfred A Knopf, 1992, p 79.
2. Mims CA: The Pathogenesis of Infectious Disease, ed 3. London, Academic Press, 1987.
3. Panum PL: Observations Made During the Epidemic of Measles on the Faore Islands in the Year 1846. Delta Omega Society, 1940.
4. Frank PF, Stollerman GH, Miller LF: Protection of a military population from rheumatic fever. JAMA 193:775, 1965.
5. Outbreak of foodborne streptococcal disease. Mortality and Morbidity Weekly Reports, 23:365, 1974.

Review Questions

1. *Endemic* means that a disease
   a. Occurs clearly in excess of normal expectancy
   b. Is habitually present in human populations
   c. Affects a large number of countries simultaneously
   d. Exhibits a seasonal pattern
   e. Is prevalent among animals

Questions 2 and 3 Are Based on the Information Given Below

The first table shows the total number of persons who ate each of two specified food items that were possibly infective with group A streptococci. The second table shows the number of sick persons (with acute sore throat) who ate each of the various specified combinations of the food items.

Total Number of Persons Who Ate Each Specified Combination of Food Items

	Ate Tuna	Did Not Eat Tuna
Ate egg salad	75	100
Did not eat egg salad	200	50

Total Number of Persons Who Ate Each Specified Combination of Food Items and Who Later Became Sick (With Acute Sore Throats)

	Ate Tuna	Did Not Eat Tuna
Ate egg salad	60	75
Did not eat egg salad	70	15

2. What is the sore throat attack rate in persons who ate both egg salad and tuna?
   a. 60/75
   b. 70/200
   c. 60/135
   d. 60/275
   e. None of the above

3. According to the results shown in the preceding tables, which of the following food items (or combination of food items) is (are) most likely to be the infective item(s):
   a. Tuna only
   b. Egg salad only
   c. Neither tuna nor egg salad
   d. Both tuna and egg salad
   e. Cannot be calculated from the data given

4. In the study of an outbreak of an infectious disease, plotting an epidemic curve is useful because:
   a. It helps determine what type of outbreak (e.g., single-source, person-to-person) has occurred
   b. It shows whether herd immunity has occurred
   c. It helps determine the median incubation period
   d. *a* and *c*
   e. *a, b,* and *c*

5. Which of the following is characteristic of a single exposure, common vehicle outbreak?
   a. Frequent secondary cases
   b. Increasing severity with increasing age
   c. Explosive
   d. Cases include both people who have been exposed and those who were not exposed
   e. All of the above

CHAPTER 3

Measuring the Occurrence of Disease

Many years ago, the physicist James Maxwell (1831–1879) said, ''We owe all the great advances in knowledge to those who endeavor to find out how much there is of anything.'' Lord Kelvin, an engineer, mathematician, and physicist (1824–1907) wrote: ''One's knowledge of science begins when he can measure what he is speaking about and express it in numbers.'' To examine the transmission of disease in human populations, we clearly need to be able to measure the frequency both of disease occurrence and of deaths from the disease. In this chapter we therefore turn to how we use *rates* to express the extent of morbidity and mortality resulting from a disease; in the next chapter, we turn to how we use screening and diagnostic tests to distinguish individuals who are ill from those who are not ill.

Let us begin this discussion by considering the development and course of a disease in an individual over a period of time.

Figure 3–1 shows a time frame for development of disease in an individual. As seen in this figure, an individual is healthy (i.e., without disease), and at some point the biologic onset of disease occurs. The person is often unaware of when the disease began. Later, symptoms develop and lead the patient to seek medical care. In certain situations, hospitalization may be required, either for diagno-

sis, for treatment, or for both. In any case, at some point a diagnosis is made and treatment is initiated. One of several outcomes can then result: cure, control of the disease, disability, or death.

What sources of information can be used to obtain information about the person's illness? For the period of the illness that necessitated hospitalization, medical and hospital records are useful. If hospitalization is not required, physicians' records may be the best source. And if we want information regarding the illness even before medical care was sought, we may have to obtain this information from the person himself, using a questionnaire or interview. Not shown in this figure are the records of health insurers, which at times can provide very useful information.

The source of data from which cases are identified clearly influences the rates that we calculate for expressing the frequency of disease. For example, hospital records will not include data regarding patients who obtained care only in physicians' offices. Consequently, when we see rates for the frequency of occurrence of a certain disease, we must identify the sources of the cases and how the cases were identified before we interpret the rates and compare them to rates reported in other populations and at other times.

Let us turn to the use of rates for expressing the

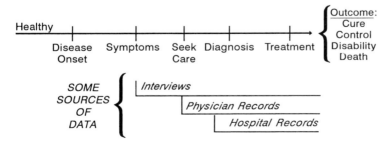

Figure 3–1. The natural history of disease and some sources of data.

extent of disease in a community or other population. *Measures of illness* or *morbidity* are discussed first, followed by discussion of *measures of mortality.*

MEASURES OF MORBIDITY

Incidence

The *incidence* of a disease is defined as the number of new cases of a disease that occur during a specified period of time in a population at risk for developing the disease.

Incidence per 1,000 =

$$\frac{\text{No. of \textit{new} cases of a disease occurring in the population during a specified period of time}}{\text{No. of persons at risk of developing the disease during that period of time}} \times 1,000$$

In this rate, the result has been multiplied by 1,000 so that we can express the incidence per 1,000 persons. The choice of 1,000 is completely arbitrary—we could have used 10,000, 1 million, or any other figure.

The critical element in the definition of incidence is *new* cases of disease. Incidence is a measure of events—the disease develops in a person who did not have the disease previously. Because incidence is a measure of events (i.e., transition from a non-diseased to a diseased state), incidence is a *measure of risk.* This risk can be looked at in any population group, such as a particular age group, males or females, an occupational group, or a group that has been exposed to a certain environmental agent, such as radiation or a chemical toxin.

The denominator of incidence represents the number of people who are at risk for developing the disease. For incidence to be meaningful, *any individual who is included in the denominator must have the potential to become part of the group that is counted in the numerator.* Thus, if we are calculating incidence for uterine cancer, the denominator must include only women, because men would not have the potential to become part of the group that is counted by the numerator—that is, men are not at risk for developing uterine cancer. Although this point seems obvious, it is not always so clear, and we shall return to this issue later in the discussion.

Another important issue in regard to the denominator is the issue of time. For incidence to be a measure of risk, we must specify a period of time and we must know that all of the individuals in the

group represented by the denominator have been followed up for that entire period. The choice of time period is arbitrary: We could calculate incidence in 1 week, incidence in 1 month, incidence in 1 year, incidence in 5 years, and so on. The important point is that whatever time period is used in the calculation must be clearly specified, and all individuals included in the calculation must have been observed (at risk) for the entire period. The incidence calculated using a period of time during which all of the individuals in the population are considered to be at risk for the outcome is called *cumulative incidence,* which is a measure of risk.

Often, however, every individual in the denominator has not been followed up for the full time period specified. For a variety of reasons, including loss to follow-up, different individuals may be observed for different lengths of time. In this case, we calculate an *incidence rate* (also called an *incidence density*), in which the denominator consists of the sum of the different times each individual was at risk. This is often expressed in terms of person-years, which is further discussed in Chapter 5.

Occasionally, time may be implicitly rather than explicitly specified. For example, in investigating a foodborne disease outbreak, we know that most cases occur within a few hours or a few days after the exposure. Thus, cases that develop months later are not considered to be part of the same outbreak. But in most situations in which current knowledge of the biology and natural history of the disease does not clearly define a time frame, time must be stated explicitly.

Although in most situations it is necessary to express incidence by specification of a denominator, the number of cases alone may be informative at times. For example, Figure 3–2 shows the number of expected and observed cases of tuberculosis reported in the United States from 1980 to 1992. (Note that the vertical axis is a logarithmic scale.) The smallest number of cases ever reported in a year in the United States (since reporting began) was in 1985. The number declined from 1980 to 1985 and the figure shows the number of cases that would have been expected had the decline continued. However, the decline suddenly stopped in 1985. From 1985 to 1992, reported tuberculosis cases increased by 20%; had the projected decline continued, approximately 51,700 fewer cases would have been expected. Much of the increase in tuberculosis seen here is associated with human immunodeficiency virus (HIV) infection. However, even before acquired immunodeficiency syndrome (AIDS)

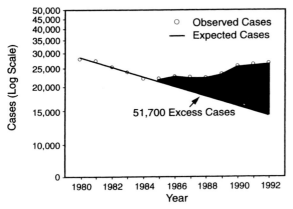

Figure 3–2. Expected and observed number of tuberculosis cases, United States, 1980–1992. (From Centers for Disease Control and Prevention: MMWR 42:696, 1993.)

Table 3–1. Examples of Point and Period Prevalence and Cumulative Incidence in Interview Studies of Asthma

Interview Question	Type of Measure
"Do you currently have asthma?"	Point prevalence
"Have you had asthma during the last (n) years?"	Period prevalence
"Have you ever had asthma?"	Cumulative or lifetime incidence

and HIV were recognized as major public health problems, tuberculosis had remained a serious but often-neglected problem, particularly in certain urban areas of the United States. We see that even a graph that plots numbers of cases can be very helpful when there is no reason to suspect a significant change in the denominator during a given time period.

Prevalence

Prevalence is defined as the number of affected persons present in the population at a specific time divided by the number of persons in the population at that time.

Prevalence per 1,000 =

$$\frac{\text{No. of cases of a disease present in the population at a specified time}}{\text{No. of persons in the population at that specified time}} \times 1,000$$

For example, if we are interested in knowing the prevalence of arthritis in a certain community on a certain date, we might visit every household in that community and, using interviews or physical examinations, determine how many people have arthritis on that day. This number becomes the numerator for the prevalence rate. The denominator is the population in the community on that date.

What is the difference between *incidence* and *prevalence*? Prevalence can be viewed as a slice through the population at a point in time at which it is determined who has the disease and who does not. But in so doing we are not determining *when* the disease developed. Some individuals may have developed arthritis yesterday, some last week, some last year, and some 10 or 20 years ago. *Thus, when*

we survey a community to estimate the prevalence of a disease, we generally do not take into account the duration of the disease. Because the numerator of prevalence thus includes a mix of people with different durations of disease, we do not have a measure of risk. If we wish to measure risk, we must use incidence, because in contrast to prevalence, it includes only new cases or events.

In the medical and public health literature, the word *prevalence* is often used in two ways:

POINT PREVALENCE. Prevalence of the disease at a point in time—the usage we have just discussed.

PERIOD PREVALENCE. How many people have had the disease at any time during a certain period, such as during a single calendar year. Some people may have developed the disease during that period, and others may have had the disease before and died during that period. The important point is that every person represented by the numerator had the disease at some time during the period specified.

The two types of prevalence, as well as cumulative incidence, are illustrated in Table 3–1 using questions regarding asthma.

Returning to point prevalence, practically speaking, it is close to impossible to survey an entire city on a single day. Therefore, although conceptually we are thinking in terms of a single point in time,

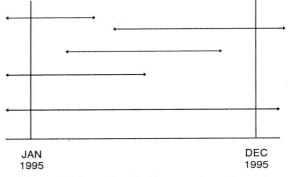

JAN 1995   DEC 1995

Figure 3–3. Example of incidence and prevalence: I.

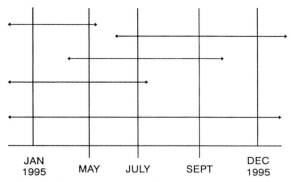

Figure 3–4. Example of incidence and prevalence: II.

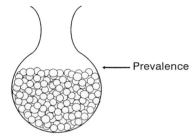

Figure 3–5. Relationship between incidence and prevalence: I.

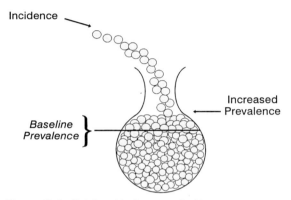

Figure 3–6. Relationship between incidence and prevalence: II.

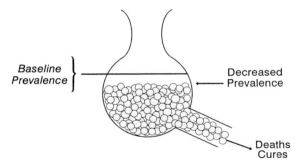

Figure 3–7. Relationship between incidence and prevalence: III.

in reality the survey would take much longer. When we see the word *prevalence* used without a modifier, it generally refers to point prevalence, and for the remainder of this chapter, we will use *prevalence* to mean point prevalence.

Let us consider incidence and prevalence. Figure 3–3 shows five cases of a disease in a community in 1995. The first case of the disease occurred in 1994 and the patient died in 1995. The second case developed in 1995 and continued into 1996. The third case was a person who became ill in 1995 and was cured in 1995. The fourth case occurred in 1994 and was cured in 1995. The fifth case occurred in 1994, and continued through 1995 and into 1996.

For purposes of this example we will consider only the cases (numerators) and will ignore the denominators. What is the numerator for incidence in 1995 in this example? We know that incidence counts only *new* cases, and because two of the five cases developed in 1995, the numerator for incidence will be 2.

What about the numerator for point prevalence? This depends on when we do our prevalence survey (Fig. 3–4). Thus, if we do the survey in May the numerator will be 4. If we do the survey in July the numerator will also be 4. If we do the survey in September the numerator will be 3, and if we do it in December the numerator will be 2. Thus, the prevalence will depend on the point during the year at which the survey is performed.

Figure 3–5 illustrates the relation between incidence and prevalence. A flask is shown that represents a community, and the liquid in the flask represents the prevalence of a disease in the community. How can we add to or increase the prevalence? As seen in Figure 3–6, we can do so through incidence—by the addition of new cases. What if we were able to drain liquid from the flask and lower the prevalence? How might this be accomplished? As seen in Figure 3–7, it could occur either through death or through cure. Clearly these two outcomes represent a major difference to a patient, but in regard to prevalence, cure and death have the same effect: they reduce the number of diseased persons in the population and thus lower prevalence. Therefore, what exists is the dynamic situation shown in Figure 3–8. A continual addition of new cases (incidence) is increasing the prevalence, while death and/or cure is decreasing the prevalence.

This effect of lowering prevalence through either

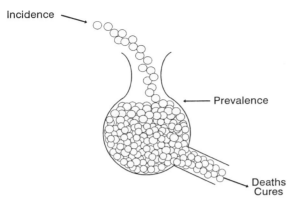

Figure 3–8. Relationship between incidence and prevalence: IV.

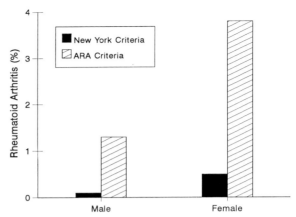

Figure 3–9. Percent of population with diagnosis of rheumatoid arthritis, New York criteria vs. American Rheumatism Association (ARA) criteria, Sudbury, Mass, 1964. (Adapted from O'Sullivan JB, Cathcart ES: The prevalence of rheumatoid arthritis: Follow-up evaluation of the effect of criteria on rates in Sudbury, Massachusetts. Ann Intern Med 76:573–577, 1972.)

death or cure underlies an important issue in public health and clinical medicine. For example, when insulin first became available, what happened to the prevalence of diabetes? The prevalence increased because diabetes was not cured, but was only controlled. Many people with diabetes who formerly would have died now survived, and the prevalence therefore increased. This seeming paradox is often the case with public health programs: A new measure is introduced that enhances survival or detects the disease in more people, and the net effect is an apparent increase in prevalence. It may be difficult to convince some people that a program is successful if the prevalence of the disease that is the target

of the program actually increases. But this clearly occurs when death is prevented and the disease is not cured.

We have said that prevalence is not a measure of risk. If so, why bother to estimate prevalence? Prevalence is an important and useful measure of the burden of disease in the community. For example, how many people with arthritis live in the community? This might help us determine how many clinics are needed, what types and amount of rehabilitation services are needed, and how many and what types of health professionals are needed. Prevalence is therefore valuable for planning health services, though even when we use prevalence we also want to make future projections and estimate the changes that are likely to take place in the disease burden in coming years. But if we want to look at the cause or etiology of disease, we must explore the relationship between an exposure and the risk of disease, and incidence rates must be used for this purpose.

Table 3–2 lists some possible sources of morbidity statistics. Each has its limitations, primarily because most of these sources are not established for research purposes. They may therefore be characterized by incomplete or ambiguous data and by selection biases in regard to who is ascertained.

Table 3–2. General Sources of Morbidity Statistics

1. Disease reporting—communicable diseases, cancer registries
2. Data accumulated as a by-product of insurance and prepaid medical care plans
   a. Group health and accident insurance
   b. Prepaid medical care plans
   c. State disability insurance plans
   d. Life insurance companies
   e. Hospital insurance plans—Blue Cross
   f. Railroad Retirement Board
3. Tax financed public assistance and medical care plans
   a. Public assistance, aid to the blind, aid to the disabled
   b. State or federal medical care plans
   c. Armed forces
   d. Veterans Administration
4. Hospitals and clinics
5. Absenteeism records—industry and schools
6. Pre-employment and periodic physical examinations in industry and schools
7. Case-finding programs
8. Selective service records
9. Morbidity surveys on population samples (e.g., National Health Survey, National Cancer Surveys)

Problems With Incidence and Prevalence Measurements

PROBLEMS WITH NUMERATORS. The first problem is defining who has the disease. One example demonstrates this problem: Rheumatoid arthritis (RA) is often a difficult disease to diagnose, and when such a diagnostic difficulty arises, expert groups are often convened to develop sets of diagnostic criteria. Two sets of diagnostic criteria for RA are those of the New York Rheumatism Association and the American Rheumatism Association (Table 3–3). Figure 3–9 shows the results of a survey conducted in Sudbury, Mass, using both sets of criteria. We see that the prevalence estimate is significantly affected by the set of criteria that is used.

The next issue relating to numerators is that of ascertaining which persons should be included in the numerator. How do we find the cases? We can use regularly available data or we can conduct a study specifically designed to gather data for estimating incidence or prevalence. In many such studies the data are obtained from interviews, and some of the problems with interview data are listed in Table 3–4.

PROBLEMS WITH HOSPITAL DATA. Data from hospital records are one of the most important sources of information in epidemiologic studies. However,

Table 3–4. Possible Sources of Error in Interview Surveys

1. The person with the disease may have no symptoms and may not be aware of the disease.
2. The person with the disease may have had symptoms but may not have had medical attention and therefore may not know the name of the disease.
3. The person with the disease may have had medical attention but the diagnosis may not have been made or conveyed to the person or the person may have misunderstood.
4. The respondent may not accurately recall an episode of illness or events and exposures related to the illness.
5. The respondent may be involved in litigation regarding the illness and may choose not to respond or may alter his or her response.
6. The respondent may provide the information but the interviewer may not record it or may record it incorrectly.
7. The interviewer may not ask the question he or she is supposed to ask or may ask it incorrectly.
8. The interviewer may be biased by knowing the hypothesis being tested and may probe more intensively in one group of respondents than in another.
9. Problems of selection bias may occur, possibly including significant non-response rates.

Table 3–3. Criteria for Rheumatoid Arthritis*

American Rheumatism Association Criteria	New York Criteria
1. Morning stiffness	1. History of episode of three painful limb joints†
2. Joint tenderness or pain on motion	2. Swelling, limitation, subluxation, or ankylosis of three limb joints (must include a hand, wrist, or foot *and* symmetry of one joint pair *and* must exclude distal interphalangeal joints, fifth proximal interphalangeal joints, first metatarsophalangeal joints, and hips)
3. Soft-tissue swelling of one joint	3. X-ray changes (erosions)
4. Soft-tissue swelling of a second joint (within 3 mo)	4. Serum positive for rheumatoid factors
5. Soft-tissue swelling of symmetrical joints (excludes distal interphalangeal joint)	
6. Subcutaneous nodules	
7. X-ray changes	
8. Serum positive for rheumatoid factors	

*A score of three or four points indicates "probable" rheumatoid arthritis; five or more points indicates "definite" rheumatoid arthritis.
†Count each joint group (e.g., proximal interphalangeal joints) as one joint, scoring each side separately.
From O'Sullivan JB, Cathcart ES: The prevalence of rheumatoid arthritis. Ann Intern Med 76:573, 1972.

Table 3–5 lists some of the problems that arise in using hospital data for research purposes. First, hospital admissions are selective. They may be selective on the basis of personal characteristics, severity of disease, associated medical conditions, and admissions policies that vary from hospital to hospital. Second, hospital records are not designed for research but rather for patient care. Records may be incomplete, illegible, or missing. The diagnostic quality of the records of hospitals, physicians, and clinical services may differ. Thus, if we want to aggregate patients from different hospitals, we may have problems of comparability. Third, if we wish to calculate rates, we have a problem defining denominators, because most hospitals do not have

Table 3–5. Some Limitations of Hospital Data

1. Hospital admissions are selective in relation to
   a. Personal characteristics
   b. Severity of disease
   c. Associated conditions
   d. Admission policies
2. Hospital records are not designed for research. They may be
   a. Incomplete, illegible, or missing
   b. Variable in diagnostic quality
3. Population(s) at risk (denominator) is (are) generally not defined

defined catchment areas that would require all persons in a given area who are hospitalized to be admitted to a particular hospital, and that none from outside the catchment area would be admitted to that hospital.

PROBLEMS WITH THE DENOMINATOR. Many factors affect the denominators used. Selective undercounting of certain groups in the population may occur. For example, young males in ethnic minority groups have been missed in many counts of the population. Frequently, we wish to determine whether a certain group has a higher-than-expected risk of disease so that appropriate preventive measures can be directed to that group. We are therefore interested in the rates of disease for different ethnic groups rather than just for the population as a whole. However, there are different ways to classify people by ethnic group, such as by language, country of origin, heritage, or parental ethnic group. When different studies use different definitions, comparison of the results is difficult. What is most important in any study is that the working definition be clearly stated so that the reader can judge whether the results are truly comparable.

In an earlier section we stated that for a rate to make sense, everyone in the group represented by the denominator must have the potential to enter the group that is represented by the numerator. The issue is not a simple one. For example, hysterectomy is one of the most commonly performed surgical procedures in the United States. This raises a question about uterine cancer rates. For if we include women who have had hysterectomies in the denominator, clearly they are not at risk for developing uterine cancer. Figure 3–10 shows uterine cancer rates from Alameda County, Calif; both uncorrected rates and rates corrected for hysterectomy are presented. We see that the corrected rates are higher. Why? Because in the corrected rates women who have had hysterectomies are removed from the denominator. Consequently, the denominator gets smaller and the rate increases. However, in this case the trend over time is not significantly changed whether we use corrected or uncorrected rates.

Relation Between Incidence and Prevalence

We have said that incidence is a measure of risk and that prevalence is not, because it does not take into account the duration of the disease. There is, however, an important relation between incidence and prevalence: In a steady-state situation, in which

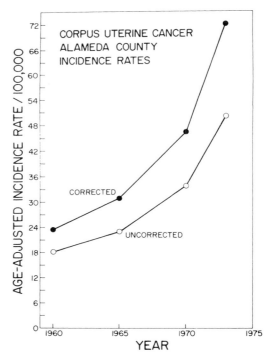

Figure 3–10. Age-adjusted uterine cancer incidence rates, corrected and uncorrected by hysterectomy status, Alameda County, California. (From Lyon JL, Gardner JW: The rising frequency of hysterectomy: Its effect on uterine cancer rates. Am J Epidemiol 105:439–443, 1977.)

the rates are not changing and in-migration equals out-migration, the following equation applies:

$$\text{Prevalence} = \text{Incidence} \times \text{Duration of Disease}$$

This is demonstrated in the following hypothetical example. Using chest x-rays, 2,000 persons are screened for tuberculosis: 1,000 are upper-income individuals from Hitown and 1,000 are lower-income individuals from Lotown (Table 3–6). X-ray findings are positive in 100 of the Hitown people and in 60 of the Lotown people. Can we therefore conclude that the risk of tuberculosis is higher in Hitown people than in Lotown people? Clearly, we cannot, for what we are measuring with a chest x-ray is the point prevalence of disease—we do not know how long any of the people with positive

Table 3–6. Hypothetical Example of Chest X-Ray Screening: I

Screened Population	No. With Positive X-Ray
1,000 Hitown	100
1,000 Lotown	60

Table 3–7. Hypothetical Example of Chest X-Ray Screening: II

Screened Population	No. With Positive X-Ray	Point Prevalence per 1,000 Population
1,000 Hitown	100	100
1,000 Lotown	60	60

x-rays have had their disease (Table 3–7). We could in fact consider a hypothetical scenario that might explain the higher prevalence in Hitown people that is not related to any higher risk in Hitown people (Table 3–8). We have said that prevalence = incidence × duration. Let us assume that Lotown people have a much higher risk (incidence) of tuberculosis than Hitown people—20 cases/year in Lotown people compared with 4 cases/year in Hitown people. But for a variety of reasons, such as poorer access to medical care and poor nutritional status, Lotown people survive with their disease, on average, for only 3 years, whereas Hitown people survive, on average, for 25 years. In this example, therefore, there is a higher prevalence in Hitown people than in Lotown people not because the risk of disease is higher in Hitown people, but because affected Hitown people survive longer; the prevalence of disease (incidence × duration) is therefore higher in Hitown people than in Lotown people.

Figure 3–11 shows the percent of all births in New Zealand that were extramarital from 1965 to 1978. Much concern was expressed because of the apparent steady rise in extramarital births. However, as seen in Figure 3–12 there had really been no increase in the *rate* of extramarital births; there had been a decline in total births that was largely accounted for by a decline in births to married women. The extramarital births, as a result, accounted for a greater percent of all births, even though the rate of extramarital births had not increased.

This example makes two points: First, a proportion is not a rate, and we shall return to this point in our discussion of mortality. Second, birth can be viewed as an event just as development of disease is an event, and appropriate rates can be computed. In discussing babies born with malformations, some people prefer to speak of the *prevalence* of malformations at birth rather than the *incidence* of malformations at birth, because the malformation was clearly present (but often unrecognized) even before birth. Furthermore, because some proportion of cases with malformations abort before birth, any estimate of the frequency of malformations at birth is probably a significant underestimate of the true incidence. Hence the term *prevalence at birth* is often used.

Figure 3–13 shows breast cancer incidence rates in women by age, and distribution of breast cancer in women by age. Ignore the bar graph for the moment and consider the line curve. The pattern is one of continually increasing incidence with age, with a change in the slope of the curve between ages 40 and 45 years, a change observed in many countries. It has suggested that something happens about the time of menopause, and that premenopausal and postmenopausal breast cancer may in fact be different diseases. Note that even in old age the incidence or risk of breast cancer continues to rise.

Now let us look at the histogram—the distribution of breast cancer cases by age. If the incidence is increasing so dramatically with age, why are only fewer than 5% of the cases occurring in the oldest age group of women? The answer is that there are very few women alive in that age group, so that even though they have the highest risk of breast cancer, the group is so small that they contribute only a small proportion of the total number of

Table 3–8. Hypothetical Example of Chest X-Ray Screening: III

Screened Population	Point Prevalence per 1,000	Incidence (Occurrences per yr)	Duration (yr)
Hitown	100	4	25
Lotown	60	20	3
	Prevalence = Incidence × Duration		

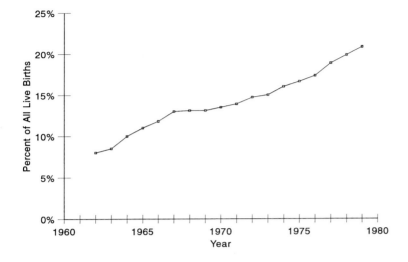

Figure 3–11. Ratios of births to unmarried women in New Zealand, 1965–1978, based on data from the Department of Statistics. (Adapted from Benfield J, Kjellstrom T: New Zealand ex-nuptial births and domestic purposes benefits in a different perspective. N Z Nurs J 74:28–31, 1981.)

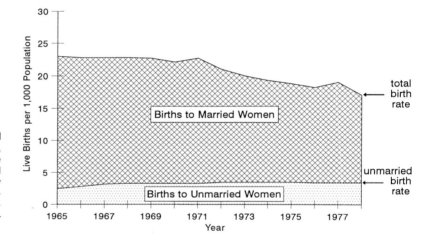

Figure 3–12. Births to married and unmarried women in New Zealand, 1965–1978, based on data from the Department of Statistics. (Adapted from Benfield J, Kjellstrom T: New Zealand ex-nuptial births and domestic purposes benefits in a different perspective. N Z Nurs J 74:28–31, 1981.)

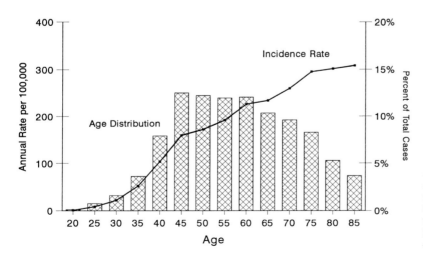

Figure 3–13. Breast cancer incidence rates in white women and distribution of cases by age. (Data from Cutler SJ, Young Jr JL: Third National Cancer Survey: Incidence Data. Nat Cancer Inst Monograph 41, 1975.)

breast cancer cases seen at all ages. The fact that so few cases of breast cancer are seen in this age group has contributed to a false public impression that the risk of breast cancer is low in this group and that mammography is therefore not important in the elderly. This is a serious misperception. The need to change public thinking on this issue is a major public health challenge. We therefore see the importance of recognizing the distinction between the distribution of disease or the proportion of cases, and the incidence rate or risk of the disease.

SPOT MAPS. One approach to examining geographic or spatial differences in incidence is to plot the cases on a map, with each point representing a case. Figure 3–14 shows a spot map for rheumatic fever in Baltimore in 1960–1964. Rheumatic fever was frequently observed in this period, and as seen on the map, the cases clustered in the inner city, consistent with the often-made observation that rheumatic fever is strongly associated with low socioeconomic status. It should be pointed out that such a clustering seen on a spot map does not demon-

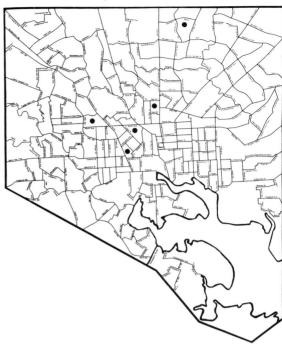

Figure 3–15. Spot map for rheumatic fever patients, ages 5 to 19 years, hospitalized for first attacks in Baltimore, 1977–1981. (Reproduced with permission. From Gordis L: The virtual disappearance of rheumatic fever in the United States: Lessons in the rise and fall of disease. Circulation 72:1155–1162, 1985. Copyright 1985, American Heart Association.)

strate a higher incidence in the area of the cluster. For if the population also clusters in this area, the rate in the area of the cluster may be no different than that elsewhere in the city. However, a spot map may offer important clues to disease etiology that can then be pursued with more rigorous studies.

Figure 3–15 shows such a spot map for 1977–1981. By 1977–1981 the disease had become almost nonexistent in Baltimore, despite the absence of any concerted program aimed at disease eradication.

Clustering, the phenomenon shown by spot maps, is often reported. Residents of a community may report apparent clusters of cancer deaths in children. For example, in Woburn, Mass, a cluster of cases of childhood leukemia was reported and attributed to industrial contamination.[1] This cluster led to action in the courts.[2] However, many apparent clusters are due only to chance, and an important epidemiologic challenge is to investigate such groups of cases and rule out an environmental etiology for what appears to be a greater-than-expected proximity of cases of a disease in time and space.

SUMMARY. In this section we have seen that a

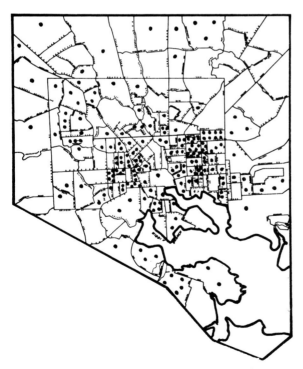

Figure 3–14. Residence distribution of rheumatic fever patients ages 5 to 19 years hospitalized for first attacks, Baltimore, 1960–1964. (Reprinted from Gordis L, Lilienfeld A, Rodriguez R: Studies in the epidemiology and preventability of rheumatic fever: I. Demographic factors and the incidence of acute attacks. J Chron Dis 21:645–654, 1969. Copyright 1969, with kind permission from Elsevier Science Ltd.)

rate involves specification of a numerator and of a denominator of people at risk and of time—either explicitly or implicitly. We now turn to measures of mortality.

MEASURES OF MORTALITY

Figure 3–16 shows the number of cancer deaths up to the year 2000 in the United States. Clearly, the number of people dying from cancer will be increasing significantly through the year 2000, but from this graph we cannot say that the *risk* of dying from cancer will be increasing, because the only data we have is numbers of deaths (numerators); we do not have denominators (populations at risk). If, for example, the United States population is increasing at the same rate, the risk of dying from cancer does not change.

For this reason, if we wish to address risk of dying, we must deal with rates. Figure 3–17 shows mortality rates for several types of cancer in males from 1930 to 1985. The most dramatic increase is in deaths from lung cancer—clearly of epidemic proportions and, tragically, a preventable cause of death. Other cancers are also of interest. Stomach cancer has declined dramatically, although the precise explanation is not known. It has been suggested that the decline may be due to the increased availability of refrigeration, which decreased the need for smoking foods and thereby decreased human exposure to carcinogens produced in the smoking process or perhaps to improved hygiene, which may have reduced the incidence of *Helicobacter pylori* infections.

Figure 3–18 shows a similar presentation for cancer mortality in women.

From 1930 to 1985, breast cancer mortality remained at essentially the same level. Can we therefore conclude that therapy for breast cancer has been ineffective? No, we cannot. It is possible that in women with breast cancer the risk of dying of the disease could have decreased during a period in which the incidence of the disease might have increased; thus, the two factors could have effectively canceled each other out, and mortality from breast cancer would have shown no change. Nevertheless, it still gives one pause to realize that despite the large number of new therapies for breast cancer introduced during the past decades, no decline in mortality from breast cancer has been observed. It would be desirable to study changes in the incidence of breast cancer. Such a study is difficult, because with aggressive public education campaigns encouraging women to have mammography and to do breast self-examination, many breast cancers may be detected today that might have gone undetected years ago. Nevertheless, available evidence suggests that the incidence of breast cancer in women has increased in recent years.

Uterine cancer mortality has declined, perhaps because of earlier detection. Lung cancer has increased and has exceeded breast cancer as a cause of death in women. Lung cancer is therefore the leading cause of cancer death in women; it is a tragedy that a preventable cause of cancer, precipitated by a voluntarily adopted lifestyle habit, has become the main cause of cancer death in women.

Mortality Rates

How is mortality expressed in quantitative terms? Let us examine some types of mortality rates. The

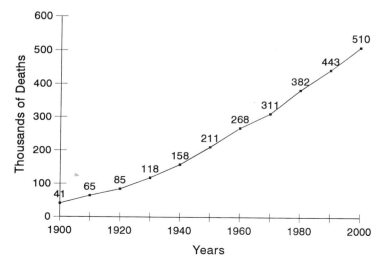

Figure 3–16. Forecast of cancer deaths if present trends continue. (Data from the American Cancer Society.)

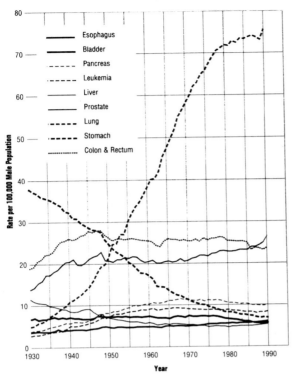

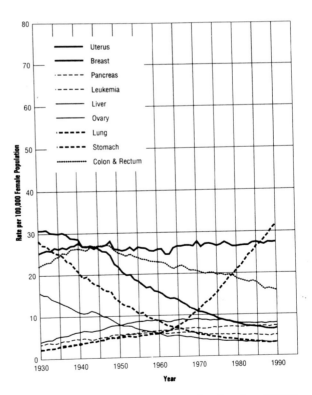

Figure 3–17. Cancer death rates for males, United States, 1930–1990 (age-adjusted to the 1970 U.S. standard population). (From Boring C, Squires TS, Tong T, Montgomery S: Cancer statistics, 1994. CA Cancer J Clin 44:7–26, 1994.)

first is the annual death rate or mortality rate from all causes:

Annual mortality rate for all causes
(per 1,000 population) =

$$\frac{\text{Total no. of deaths from all causes in 1 year}}{\text{No. of persons in the population at midyear}} \times 1{,}000$$

Note that because the population changes over time, the number of persons in the population at midyear is generally used as an approximation.

The same principles mentioned in the discussion of morbidity apply to mortality: For a rate to make sense, anyone in the group represented by the denominator must have the potential to enter the group represented by the numerator.

We may not always be interested in a rate for the entire population; perhaps we are interested only in a certain age group, in one sex, or in one ethnic group. Thus, if we are interested in mortality in children younger than 10 years, we can calculate a rate specifically for that group:

Annual mortality rate from all causes for children under age 10 years (per 1,000 population) =

$$\frac{\begin{array}{c}\text{No. of deaths from all causes in 1 year}\\ \text{in children under age 10 years}\end{array}}{\begin{array}{c}\text{No. of children in the population under}\\ \text{age 10 years at midyear}\end{array}} \times 1{,}000$$

Note that in putting a restriction on age, for example, the same restriction must apply to *both* the numerator and denominator, so that every person in the denominator group will be at risk for entering the numerator group. When a restriction is placed on a rate, it is called a *specific rate*. This then, is an *age-specific mortality rate*.

We could also place a restriction on a rate by specifying a diagnosis, and thus limit the rate to deaths from a certain disease—that is, a *disease-specific* or a *cause-specific rate*. For example, if we are interested in mortality from lung cancer, we would calculate it in the following manner:

Figure 3–18. Cancer death rates for females, United States, 1930–1990 (age-adjusted to the 1970 U.S. standard population). (From Boring C, Squires TS, Tong T, Montgomery S: Cancer statistics, 1994. CA Cancer J Clin 44:7–26, 1994.)

Annual mortality rate from lung cancer
(per 1,000 population) =

$$\frac{\text{No. of deaths from lung cancer per year}}{\text{No. of persons in the population at midyear}} \times 1,000$$

We can also place restrictions on more than one characteristic simultaneously—for example, age and cause of death–as follows:

Annual mortality rate from leukemia for children under age 10 years (per 1,000 population) =

$$\frac{\begin{array}{c}\text{No. of deaths from leukemia in one year}\\\text{in children under age 10 years}\end{array}}{\begin{array}{c}\text{No. of children in the population under}\\\text{age 10 years at midyear}\end{array}} \times 1,000$$

Time must also be specified in any mortality rate. Mortality can be calculated over 1 year, 5 years, or longer. The time period selected is arbitrary, but it is important that it be specified precisely.

Case-Fatality Rates

We must distinguish between a *mortality rate* and a *case-fatality rate*. A case-fatality rate is calculated as follows:

Case fatality rate (percent) =

$$\frac{\begin{array}{c}\text{No. of individuals dying during}\\\text{a specified period of time after}\\\text{disease onset or diagnosis}\end{array}}{\begin{array}{c}\text{No. of individuals with the}\\\text{specified disease}\end{array}} \times 100$$

In other words, what percent of *people diagnosed as having a certain disease* die within a certain time after diagnosis? What is the difference between case-fatality and mortality rate? In mortality, the denominator represents the entire population at risk of dying from the disease, including both those who have the disease and those who do not have the disease (but who are at risk of developing the disease). In case-fatality, however, the denominator is limited to those who already have the disease. Thus, case-fatality is a measure of the severity of the disease. It can also be used to measure any benefits of a new therapy: As therapy improves, case-fatality would be expected to decline.

The numerator of a case-fatality rate should ideally be restricted to deaths *from that disease*. However, it is not always easy to distinguish between deaths from that disease and deaths from other causes. For example, an alcoholic person may die in a car accident; the death may or may not be related to alcohol intake.

Let us look at a hypothetical example to clarify the difference between mortality and case-fatality (Table 3–9).

Assume that in a population of 100,000 persons, 20 have disease X. In 1 year 18 people die from that disease. The mortality is very low (.018%) because the disease is rare; however, once a person has the disease, the chances of his dying are great (90%).

Proportionate Mortality

Another measure of mortality is proportionate mortality, which is not a rate. The proportionate mortality from cardiovascular disease in the United States in 1995 is defined as follows:

Proportionate mortality from cardiovascular diseases in the U.S. in 1995 (percent) =

$$\frac{\begin{array}{c}\text{No. of deaths from cardiovascular}\\\text{diseases in the U.S. in 1995}\end{array}}{\text{Total deaths in the U.S. in 1995}} \times 100$$

In other words, of all deaths in the United States, what proportion were due to cardiovascular disease? Figure 3–19 shows proportionate mortality from heart disease by age group. In each age group the full bar represents all deaths (100%), and those from heart disease are indicated by the shaded portion. We see that the proportion of deaths due to heart disease increases with age. However, this does not tell us that the *risk* of death from heart disease is also increasing. This is demonstrated in the following examples.

Table 3–10 shows all deaths and deaths from heart disease in two communities, A and B. All-cause mortality in community A is twice that in community B. When we look at proportionate mortality we find that 10% of the deaths in community A and 20% of the deaths in community B are due to heart disease. Does this tell us that the risk of dying from heart disease is twice as high in commu-

Table 3–9. Comparison of a Mortality Rate and a Case-Fatality Rate

---

Assume a population of 100,000 people of whom 20 are sick with disease "X," and in 1 year, 18 die from disease "X."

The mortality rate in that year from disease "X" =

$$\frac{18}{100,000} = .00018 = .018\%$$

The case-fatality rate from disease "X" =

$$\frac{18}{20} = .9 = 90\%$$

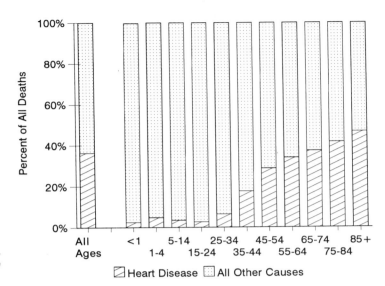

Figure 3–19. Deaths from heart disease as a percent of deaths from all causes, by age group, United States, 1986.

nity B than in A? The answer is no. For when the mortality rates from heart disease are calculated (10% of 30/1,000 and 20% of 15/1,000), we find that the mortality rates are identical.

As seen in the example in Table 3–11, if the all-cause mortality rates differ, cause-specific mortality rates can differ significantly even when the proportionate mortality is the same. Thus, proportionate mortality can give us a quick look at the major causes of death but cannot tell us the risk of dying from a disease; we need a mortality rate for that.

Years of Potential Life Lost

In recent years, another mortality index, years of potential life lost (YPLL), has been increasingly used. YPLL recognizes that death occurring in the same person at a younger age clearly involves a greater loss of future productive years than were it to occur at an older age. Figure 3–20 shows YPLL before age 65 years for children younger than 20

years. We see that the YPLL from injuries exceeds the combined effect of YPLL from congenital malformations and prematurity combined. Thus, if we want to have an impact on YPLL in children, we should address causes of injuries, half of which are related to motor vehicles.

Table 3–12 shows a ranking of causes of death in the United States for 1989 and 1990 by YPLL together with cause-specific mortality rates. By cause-specific mortality, HIV infection ranked eleventh, but by YPLL it ranked seventh—a reflection of the fact that a large proportion of HIV-related deaths are in young persons.

Why Look at Mortality?

Mortality is clearly an index of the severity of a problem from both clinical and public health standpoints, but mortality can also be used as an index of the risk of disease, as was shown in Figures 3–17 and 3–18. However, when a disease is

Table 3–10. Comparison of Mortality Rate and Proportionate Mortality: I. Deaths From Heart Disease in Two Communities, "A" and "B"

	Community A	Community B
Mortality rate from all causes	30/1,000	15/1,000
Proportionate mortality from heart disease	10%	20%
Mortality rate from heart disease	3/1,000	3/1,000

Table 3–11. Comparison of Mortality Rate and Proportionate Mortality: II. Deaths From Heart Disease in Two Communities, "A" and "B"

	Community A	Community B
Mortality rate from all causes	20/1,000	10/1,000
Proportionate mortality from heart disease	30%	30%
Mortality rate from heart disease	6/1,000	3/1,000

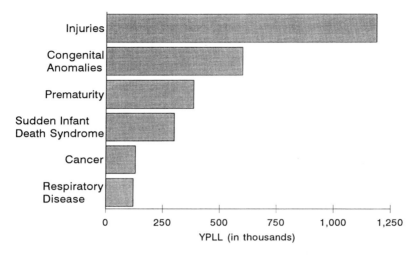

Figure 3–20. Years of potential life lost (YPLL) before age 65 years among children younger than 20 years from injuries and other diseases, United States, 1986. (Adapted from Centers for Disease Control and Prevention: Fatal injuries to children: United States, 1986. MMWR 39:442–451, 1990.)

mild and not fatal, mortality is not a good index of incidence. A mortality rate is a good reflection of incidence rate under two conditions: First, when the case-fatality rate is high (as in untreated rabies), and second, when the duration of disease (survival) is short. Under these conditions, mortality is a good measure of incidence and thus a measure of the risk of disease. For example, cancer of the pancreas is a highly lethal disease: death generally occurs within a few months of diagnosis, and long-term survival is rare. Thus mortality from pancreatic cancer is a good surrogate for incidence of the disease.

Figure 3–21 shows trends in mortality rates for the leading causes of death in men aged 25 to 44 years. The trends for women are seen in Figure 3–22. As indicated by the curves for mortality from AIDS, this disease is of epidemic proportions. Thus, at the time this graph was drawn, AIDS was the second leading cause of death in 25- to 44-year-old men, and it was the leading medical cause of death in men in this age group. In women, it was rapidly rising and was virtually the fourth leading cause of death in this age group. For diseases that are highly lethal, mortality can approximate incidence and can therefore provide strong evidence for emerging and increasing clinical and public health problems.

A comparison of mortality and incidence is seen in Figures 3–23 and 3–24. Figure 3–23 shows ectopic pregnancy rates by year in the United States

Table 3–12. Estimated Years of Potential Life Lost (YPLL) Before Age 65 Years and Mortality Rates per 100,000 Persons, By Cause of Death, United States, 1989 and 1990

Cause of Death (ICD–9 Codes)	YPLL for Persons Dying in 1989	YPLL for Persons Dying in 1990	Cause-Specific Crude Death Rate, 1990
All causes (total)	12,339,045	12,083,228	861.9
Unintentional injuries (E800–E949)	2,235,335	2,147,094	37.3
Malignant neoplasms (140–208)	1,832,039	1,839,900	201.7
Suicide/homicide (E950–E978)	1,402,524	1,520,780	22.5
Diseases of the heart (390–398, 402, 404–429)	1,411,399	1,349,027	289.0
Congenital anomalies (740–759)	660,346	644,651	5.3
Human immunodeficiency virus infection (042–044)	585,992	644,245	9.6
Prematurity (765, 769)	487,749	415,638	2.5
Sudden infant death syndrome (798)	363,393	347,713	2.2
Cerebrovascular disease (430–238)	237,898	244,366	57.9
Chronic liver disease and cirrhosis (571)	233,472	212,707	10.2
Pneumonia/influenza (480–487)	184,832	165,534	31.3
Diabetes mellitus (250)	145,501	143,250	19.5
Chronic obstructive pulmonary disease (490–496)	135,507	127,464	35.5

From Centers for Disease Control and Prevention: MMWR 41:314, 1992.

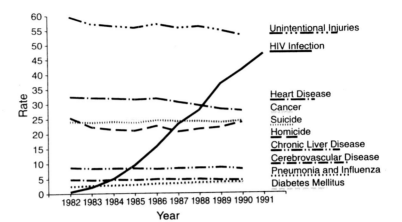

Figure 3–21. Death rates (per 100,000) for leading causes of death for men aged 25–44 years, by year, United States, 1982–1990. (From Centers for Disease Control and Prevention: MMWR 42:483, 1993.)

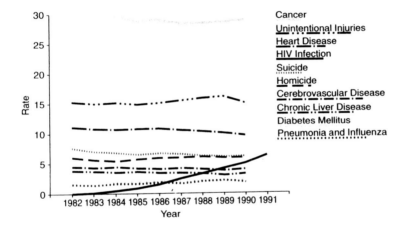

Figure 3–22. Death rates (per 100,000) for leading causes of death for women aged 25 to 44 years, by year, United States, 1982–1990. (From Centers for Disease Control and Prevention: MMWR 42:483, 1993.)

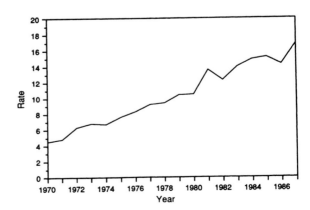

Figure 3–23. Ectopic pregnancy rates (per 1,000 reported pregnancies), by year, United States, 1970–1987. (From Centers for Disease Control and Prevention: MMWR 39:401, 1990.)

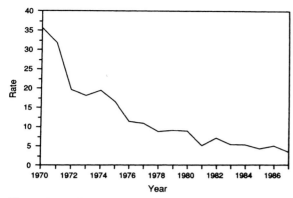

Figure 3–24. Ectopic pregnancy death rates (per 10,000 ectopic pregnancies), by year, United States, 1970–1987. (From Centers for Disease Control and Prevention: MMWR 39:403, 1990.)

from 1970 to 1987. During this period, the rate per 1,000 reported pregnancies increased almost fourfold. This increase has been attributed to improved diagnosis and to increased frequency of pelvic inflammatory disease resulting from sexually transmitted diseases. As also seen in Figure 3–24, however, death rates from ectopic pregnancy decreased markedly during the same time period, perhaps as a result of earlier detection and increasingly prompt medical and surgical intervention.

Problems With Mortality Data

Most of our information about deaths comes from death certificates. A death certificate is shown in Figure 3–25. By international agreement, deaths are coded according to the *underlying* cause. Underlying cause of death is defined as "the disease or injury which initiated the train of morbid events leading directly or indirectly to death or the circumstances of the accident or violence which produced the fatal injury."[3] Thus, the death certificate from which Figure 3–26 is taken would be coded as a death from chronic ischemic heart disease, the underlying cause, which is always found on the lowest used line in part I of item 23 of the certificate. The underlying cause of death therefore "excludes information pertaining to the immediate cause of death, contributory causes and those causes that intervene between the underlying and immediate causes of death."[4] As pointed out by Savage and co-workers,[5] the total contribution of a given cause of death may not be reflected in the mortality data as generally reported; this may apply to a greater extent in some diseases than in others.

Countries and regions vary greatly in the quality of the data on their death certificates. Studies of validity of death certificates compared to hospital and autopsy records generally find higher validity for certain diseases, such as cancers, than for others.

Deaths are coded according to the International Classification of Diseases (ICD), now in its 10th revision. Because coding categories and regulations change from one revision to another, any study of time trends in mortality that spans more than one revision must examine the possibility that observed changes could be due entirely or in part to changes in the ICD. In 1949, mortality rates from diabetes showed a dramatic decline in both males and females (Fig. 3–27). However, any euphoria that might have been engendered by these data was short-lived; analysis of this drop indicated that it occurred at a time of change from the 7th revision to the 8th revision of the ICD. Prior to 1949, policy had been for any death certificate that included a mention of diabetes anywhere to be coded as a death from diabetes. After 1949, only death certificates on which the underlying cause of death was listed as diabetes were coded as a death from diabetes. Hence, the decline seen in Figure 3–27 was artifactual. Whenever we see a time trend of an increase or decrease in mortality, the first question we must ask is, Is it real? Specifically, when we look at trends in mortality over time, we must ask whether any changes took place in how death certificates were coded during the period being examined that could have contributed to any changes observed in mortality during that period.

Changes in disease definition can also have a significant effect on the number of cases of the disease that are reported or that are reported and subsequently classified as meeting the diagnostic criteria for the disease. At the beginning of 1993 a new definition of AIDS was introduced; as shown in Figure 3–28, this resulted in a rapid rise in the number of reported cases. With the new definition, the number of reported cases has continued to be higher than it had been previously, even after the initial peak, and the increase is likely to be an artifact of the revised case definition.

In a lighter vein, Table 3–13 lists some causes of death that were listed on death certificates earlier in this century.

In discussing morbidity, we said that everyone in the group represented by the denominator must be at risk to enter the group represented by the numerator, and we looked at uterine cancer incidence rates as an example. Figure 3–29 shows a similar set of

1 - FOR STATE REGISTRAR

STATE OF MARYLAND / DEPARTMENT OF HEALTH AND MENTAL HYGIENE
CERTIFICATE OF DEATH

REG. NO.

TO BE COMPLETED BY FUNERAL DIRECTOR

1. DECEDENT'S NAME *(First, Middle, Last)*
2. DATE OF DEATH — MONTH DAY YEAR
3. TIME OF DEATH — M

4. SOCIAL SECURITY NUMBER
5. SEX — 1 ☐ M 2 ☐ F
6. AGE *(In yrs. last birthday)* YRS. — IF UNDER 1 YEAR: MONTHS DAYS — IF UNDER 24 HRS.: HOURS MIN.
7. DATE OF BIRTH *(Month, Day, Year)*
8. BIRTHPLACE *(State or Foreign Country)*

9a. FACILITY NAME *(If not institution, give street and number)*
9b. CITY, TOWN OR LOCATION OF DEATH
9c. COUNTY OF DEATH

RESIDENCE OF DECEDENT

10a. STATE
10b. COUNTY
10c. CITY, TOWN OR LOCATION
10d. INSIDE CITY LIMITS? 1 ☐ YES 2 ☐ NO

10e. STREET AND NUMBER
10f. ZIP CODE
10g. CITIZEN OF WHAT COUNTRY?

11. MARITAL STATUS — 1 ☐ Never Married 2 ☐ Married 3 ☐ Widowed 4 ☐ Divorced
12. WAS DECEDENT EVER IN U.S. ARMED FORCES? 1 ☐ YES 2 ☐ NO — IF YES, GIVE WAR OR DATES
13. WAS DECEDENT OF HISPANIC ORIGIN? (Specify Yes or No— If yes, specify Cuban, Mexican, Puerto Rican, etc.) 1 ☐ YES 2 ☐ NO Specify:
14. RACE — American Indian, Black, White, etc. Specify:

15. DECEDENT'S EDUCATION *(Specify only highest grade completed)* — Elementary/Secondary (0-12) — College (1-4 or 5 +)
16a. DECEDENT'S USUAL OCCUPATION *(Give kind of work done during most of working life. Do NOT use retired.)*
16b. KIND OF BUSINESS/INDUSTRY

17. FATHER'S NAME *(First, Middle, Last)*
18. MOTHER'S NAME *(First, Middle, Maiden Surname)*

19a. INFORMANT'S NAME *(Type/Print)*
19b. MAILING ADDRESS *(Street and Number or Rural Route Number, City or Town, State, Zip Code)*

20a. METHOD OF DISPOSITION — 1 ☐ Burial 2 ☐ Cremation 3 ☐ Removal from State 4 ☐ Donation 5 ☐ Other (Specify) _____
20b. PLACE AND DATE OF DISPOSITION *(Name of cemetery, crematory or other place)* — DATE
20c. LOCATION — City or Town, State

21. SIGNATURE OF FUNERAL SERVICE LICENSEE ▶
22. NAME AND ADDRESS OF FACILITY

TO BE COMPLETED BY PHYSICIAN: MEDICAL CERTIFICATION

23. PART I. Enter the diseases, or complications that caused the death. Do not enter the mode of dying, such as cardiac or respiratory arrest, shock, or heart failure. List only one cause on each line.

Approximate Interval Between Onset and Death

IMMEDIATE CAUSE (Final disease or condition resulting in death) ➤
a. _____
DUE TO (OR AS A CONSEQUENCE OF):

Sequentially list conditions, if any, leading to immediate cause. Enter UNDERLYING CAUSE (Disease or injury that initiated events resulting in death) LAST
b. _____
DUE TO (OR AS A CONSEQUENCE OF):
c. _____
DUE TO (OR AS A CONSEQUENCE OF):
d. _____

PART II. Other significant conditions contributing to death but not resulting in the underlying cause given in Part I.
24a. WAS AN AUTOPSY PERFORMED? 1 ☐ YES 2 ☐ NO
24b. WERE AUTOPSY FINDINGS AVAILABLE PRIOR TO COMPLETION OF CAUSE OF DEATH? 1 ☐ YES 2 ☐ NO

DID TOBACCO USE CONTRIBUTE TO CAUSE OF DEATH YES ☐ NO ☐ UNCERTAIN ☐

25. WAS CASE REFERRED TO MEDICAL EXAMINER? 1 ☐ YES 2 ☐ NO
26. PLACE OF DEATH (Check only one) — HOSPITAL: 1 ☐ Inpatient 2 ☐ ER/Outpatient 3 ☐ DOA — OTHER: 4 ☐ Nursing Home 5 ☐ Residence 6 ☐ Other (Specify)

27. MANNER OF DEATH — 1 ☐ Natural 2 ☐ Accident 3 ☐ Suicide 4 ☐ Homicide 5 ☐ Pending Investigation 6 ☐ Could not be determined
28a. DATE OF INJURY *(Month, Day, Year)*
28b. TIME OF INJURY M
28c. INJURY AT WORK? 1 ☐ YES 2 ☐ NO
28d. DESCRIBE HOW INJURY OCCURED

28e. PLACE OF INJURY — At home, farm, street, factory, office building, etc. (Specify)
28f. LOCATION *(Street and Number or Rural Route Number, City or Town, State)*

29a. CERTIFIER *(Check only one)* — 1 ☐ CERTIFYING PHYSICIAN: To the best of my knowledge, death occurred at the time, date and place, and due to the cause(s) and manner as stated.
2 ☐ MEDICAL EXAMINER: On the basis of examination and/or investigation, in my opinion, death occured at the time, date and place, and due to the cause(s) and manner as stated.

29b. SIGNATURE AND TITLE OF CERTIFIER
29c. LICENSE NUMBER
29d. DATE SIGNED *(Month, Day, Year)* ▶

30. NAME AND ADDRESS OF PERSON WHO COMPLETED CAUSE OF DEATH (ITEM 27) *(Type, Print)*

31. DATE FILED *(Month, Day, Year)*
32. REGISTRAR'S SIGNATURE

DHMH-16 Rev 1/89

Figure 3–25. Death certificate for the state of Maryland. (Courtesy of the State of Maryland Department of Health and Mental Hygiene.)

23. PART I. Enter the diseases, or complications that caused the death. Do not enter the mode of dying, such as cardiac or respiratory arrest, shock, or heart failure. List only one cause on each line.		Approximate Interval Between Onset and Death
IMMEDIATE CAUSE (Final disease or condition resulting in death) ➡	a. **Rupture of myocardium** DUE TO (OR AS A CONSEQUENCE OF):	**Mins.**
Sequentially list conditions, if any, leading to immediate cause. Enter UNDERLYING CAUSE (Disease or Injury that initiated events resulting in death) LAST	b. **Acute myocardial infarction** DUE TO (OR AS A CONSEQUENCE OF):	**6 days**
	c. **Chronic ischemic heart disease** DUE TO (OR AS A CONSEQUENCE OF):	**5 years**
	d. _____	

PART II. Other significant conditions contributing to death but not resulting in the underlying cause given in Part I. **Diabetes, Chronic obstructive pulmonary disease, smoking**	24a. WAS AN AUTOPSY PERFORMED? 1 ☒ YES 2 ☐ NO	24b. WERE AUTOPSY FINDINGS AVAILABLE PRIOR TO COMPLETION OF CAUSE OF DEATH? 1 ☒ YES 2 ☐ NO
DID TOBACCO USE CONTRIBUTE TO CAUSE OF DEATH YES ☒ NO ☐ UNCERTAIN ☐		

Figure 3–26. Example of a completed cause of death section on a death certificate, including immediate and underlying causes and other significant conditions.

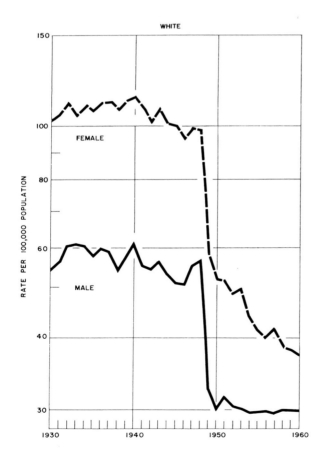

Figure 3–27. Drop in death rates for diabetes among 55- to 64-year-old men and women, United States, 1930–1960, due to changes in ICD coding. (From US Public Health Service publication No. 1000, series 3, No. 1. Washington, DC, US Government Printing Office, 1964.)

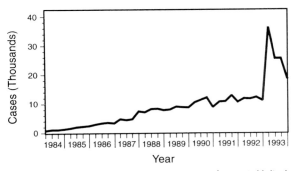

Figure 3–28. AIDS cases by quarter year of report, United States, 1984–1993. (From Centers for Disease Control and Prevention: MMWR 43:827, 1994.)

observations for uterine cancer mortality rates. The same principle regarding numerator and denominator applies to mortality rates as well.

COMPARING MORTALITY IN DIFFERENT POPULATIONS

An important use of mortality data is to compare two or more populations, or one population in different time periods. Such populations may differ in regard to many characteristics that affect mortality, of which age distribution is the most important.

Table 3–13. Some Causes of Death That Have Been Reported on Death Certificates

"A mother died in infancy"
"Deceased had never been fatally sick"
"Died suddenly, nothing serious"
"Went to bed feeling well, but woke up dead"
"Died suddenly without the aid of a physician"

Therefore, methods have been developed for comparing mortality in such populations while effectively holding constant such characteristics as age.

Table 3–14 shows data that exemplify the problem. Mortality for whites and blacks in Baltimore in 1965 is given. The data may seem surprising because we would expect rates to have been higher for blacks, given problems of living conditions and access to medical care, particularly at that time. When we look at Table 3–15, we see the data from Table 3–14 on the left, but now we have added data for each age-specific stratum (layer) of the population. Interestingly, although, mortality is higher in blacks than in whites in each age-specific group, the overall mortality (also called crude or unadjusted mortality) is higher in whites than in blacks. Why is this so? This is a reflection of the fact that in both whites and blacks, mortality in-

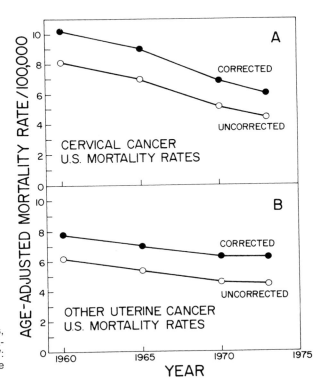

Figure 3–29. Age-adjusted uterine cancer mortality rates, corrected and uncorrected by hysterectomy status, Alameda County, California. (From Lyon JL, Gardner JW: The rising frequency of hysterectomy: Its effect on uterine cancer rates. Am J Epidemiol 105:439–443, 1977.)

Table 3–14. Crude Mortality Rates by Race, Baltimore City, 1965

Race	Mortality per 1,000 Population
White	14.3
Black	10.2

creases markedly in the oldest age groups; older age is the major contributor to mortality. But the white population in this example is older than the black population, and in 1965 there were few blacks in the oldest age groups. Thus, in whites the overall mortality is heavily weighted by high rates in the oldest age groups; because there are so few blacks in those age groups, the same effect is not seen in the black population. Clearly, the crude mortality reflects both differences in the force of mortality and differences in the age composition of the population. Let us look at two approaches for dealing with this problem.

Direct Age Adjustment

Table 3–16 shows mortality in a population in two time periods. The mortality rate is considerably higher in the later period. These data are supplemented with age-specific data in Table 3–17. Here we see three age groups, and mortality for the later period is lower in each group. How then is it possible to account for the higher overall mortality in the later period in this example?

The answer lies in the changing age structure of the population. Mortality is highest in oldest age groups, and during the later period the size of the oldest group has doubled while the number of young people has substantially declined. We would like to eliminate this age difference and in effect ask: If the age composition of the populations were the same, would there be any differences in mortality from the early to the later period?

One way to address this is shown in Table 3–18. A hypothetical "standard" population is created to which we apply both the age-specific mortality rates from the early period and the age-specific mortality rates from the later period. By using a single standard population we eliminate any possibility that observed differences could be a result of age differences in the population. (In this example, we have created a standard by adding the populations from the early and the later periods, but any population could have been used.)

By applying each age-specific mortality rate to the population in each age group of the standard population, we derive the expected number of deaths that would have occurred had those rates been applied. We can then calculate the total deaths expected in the standard population had the age-specific rates of the early period applied and the total deaths expected in the standard population had the age-specific rates of the later period applied. Dividing each of these two total expected numbers of deaths by the standard population, we can calculate an expected mortality rate in the standard population if it had had the mortality experience of the early period and the expected mortality rate for the standard population if it had had the mortality experience for the later period. These are called *age-adjusted rates,* and they appropriately reflect the decline seen in the age-specific rates. Differences in age-composition of the population are no longer a factor.

Although age-adjusted rates can be very useful in making comparisons, the first step should always be to carefully examine the age-specific rates for any interesting differences or changes. These may be hidden by the age-adjusted rates, and they may be lost if we proceed immediately to age adjustment.

In this example the rates have been adjusted for age, but they could be adjusted for any characteristic such as sex, socioeconomic status, or race, and techniques are available to adjust for multiple variables simultaneously.

Table 3–15. Death Rates by Age and Race, Baltimore City, 1965

Race	All Ages	Death Rates by Age per 1,000 Population					
		<1 yr	*1–4 yr*	*5–17 yr*	*18–44 yr*	*45–64 yr*	*≥65 yr*
White	14.3	23.9	0.7	0.4	2.5	15.2	69.3
Black	10.2	31.3	1.6	0.6	4.8	22.6	75.9

From Department of Biostatistics: Annual Vital Statistics Report for Maryland, 1965. Baltimore, Maryland State Department of Health, 1965.

Table 3–16. An Example of Age Adjustment: I. Comparison of Total Death Rates in a Population at Two Different Time Periods

	Early Period			Later Period		
	Population	No. of Deaths	Death Rate per 100,000	Population	No. of Deaths	Death Rate per 100,000
	900,000	862	96	900,000	1,130	126

Table 3–17. An Example of Age Adjustment: II. Comparison of Age-Specific Death Rates in Two Different Time Periods

Age Group (yr)	Early Period			Later Period		
	Population	No. of Deaths	Death Rate per 100,000	Population	No. of Deaths	Death Rate per 100,000
All ages	900,000	862	96	900,000	1,130	126
30–49	500,000	60	12	300,000	30	10
50–69	300,000	396	132	400,000	400	100
70 +	100,000	406	406	200,000	700	350

Table 3–18. An Example of Age Adjustment: III. Carrying Out an Age Adjustment Using the Total of the Two Populations as the Standard

Age Group (yr)	Standard Population	"Early" Rate per 100,000	Expected No. of Deaths Using "Early" Rate	"Later" Rate per 100,000	Expected No. of Deaths Using "Later" Rate
All	1,800,000				
30–49	800,000	12	96	10	80
50–69	700,000	132	924	100	700
70 +	300,000	406	1,218	350	1,050
Total no. of deaths expected			2,238		1,830

In the standard population age-adjusted rates:

$$\text{"Early"} = \frac{2238}{1,800,000} = 124.3$$

$$\text{"Later"} = \frac{1830}{1,800,000} = 101.7$$

Standardized Mortality Ratios

Another approach to adjustment is to calculate the standardized mortality ratio (SMR), which is defined as follows:

$$\frac{\text{Observed no. of deaths per year}}{\text{Expected no. of deaths per year}}$$

Let us look at the example in Table 3–19. In a population of 534,533 white male miners, 436 deaths from tuberculosis (TBC) occurred in 1950. Is this mortality experience from TBC greater than, less than, or about the same as that expected in white males of the same ages in the general population? For each age-specific group of white miners, we take the age-specific mortality rate from the general population (expected) and ask, How many deaths would we expect in these white miners if they had the same mortality experience as white men in the same age group in the general population? These data are listed in column 3. Column 4 shows the actual number of deaths observed in the miners.

The SMR is calculated by totaling the observed number of deaths (436) and dividing it by the expected number of deaths (181.09), which yields a result of 2.41. Multiplication by 100 is often done to yield results without decimals. If this were done in this case, the SMR would be 241. An SMR of 100 indicates that the observed number of deaths is the same as the expected number of deaths. An SMR over 100 indicates that the observed exceeds the expected, and an SMR below 100 indicates that the observed is less than expected.

The SMR is commonly used in occupational studies: Do people working in a certain industry have a higher mortality than do people of the same age in the general population? Is an additional risk associated with that occupation?

The Cohort Effect

Table 3–20 shows age-specific death rates per 100,000 persons from tuberculosis in Massachusetts from 1880 to 1930. For purposes of this discussion, we will ignore children ages 0 to 4 years, because tuberculosis in this age group is a somewhat different phenomenon. If, for example, we then read *down* the column in the table (the data for a given calendar year) for 1910, it appears that tuberculosis mortality peaks when people reach their 30s or 40s and then declines with advancing age. This view of the data, by year, is called a *cross-sectional view*.

Actually, however, the picture of tuberculosis risk is somewhat different (Table 3–21). A person who was 10 to 19 years in 1880 was 20 to 29 years in 1890, and 30 to 39 years in 1900. In other words, persons who were born in a certain year are moving through time together. We can now examine the mortality over time of the same cohort (i.e., a group of people who share the same experience), born in the same 10-year period. Looking at people who were 0 to 9 years in 1880 and following them over time, as indicated by the boxes in the table, it is

Table 3–19. Computation of an SMR for Tuberculosis, All Forms (TBC), for White Miners Ages 20 to 59 Years, United States, 1950

Age (yr)	Estimated Population of White Miners (1)	Death Rate (per 100,000) for TBC in Males in the General Population (2)	Expected Deaths From TBC in White Miners if They Had the Same Risk as the General Population (3) = (1)×(2)	Observed Deaths from TBC in White Miners (4)
20–24	74,598	12.26	9.14	10
25–29	85,077	16.12	13.71	20
30–34	80,845	21.54	17.41	22
35–44	148,870	33.96	50.55	98
45–54	102,649	56.82	58.32	174
55–59	42,494	75.23	31.96	112
Totals			181.09	436

$$\text{SMR} = \frac{\text{Observed deaths for an occupation} - \text{cause} - \text{race group}}{\text{Expected deaths for an occupation} - \text{cause} - \text{race group}} \times 100$$

$$\text{SMR (for 20–59-yr-olds)} = \frac{436}{181.09} \times 100 = 241$$

Adapted from Vital statistics: Special reports. Washington, DC, Department of Health, Education, and Welfare, vol 53(5), 1963.

Table 3–20. Age-Specific Death Rates per 100,000 From Tuberculosis (All Forms), Males, Massachusetts, 1880–1930

Age (yr)	Year					
	1880	*1890*	*1900*	*1910*	*1920*	*1930*
0–4	760	578	309	309	108	41
5–9	43	49	31	21	24	11
10–19	126	115	90	63	49	21
20–29	444	361	288	207	149	81
30–39	378	368	296	253	164	115
40–49	364	336	253	253	175	118
50–59	366	325	267	252	171	127
60–69	475	346	304	246	172	95
70+	672	396	343	163	127	95

Data from Frost WH: The age selection of mortality from tuberculosis in successive decades. J Hyg 30:91–96, 1939.

apparent that peak mortality actually occurred at a younger age than it would seem to have from the cross-sectional view of the data. When we examine changes in mortality over time, we should always ask whether any apparent changes that are observed could be the result of such a cohort effect.

Interpreting Observed Changes in Mortality

If we find a difference in mortality over time or between populations—either an increase or a decrease–it may be an artifactual or real. If it is an artifact, the artifact could result from problems with either the numerator or denominator (Table 3–22). However, if we conclude that the change is real, what could be the possible explanation? Some possibilities are seen in Table 3–23.

QUALITY OF LIFE

Most diseases have a major impact on the afflicted individual above and beyond mortality. Dis-

eases that may not be lethal may be associated with considerable suffering and disability. For this reason, it is also important to consider the impact of a disease as measured by its effect on a person's quality of life, even though such measures are not, in fact, measures of disease occurrence. For example, it is possible to examine the extent to which patients with arthritis are compromised by the illness in carrying out activities of daily living. Although considerable controversy exists about which quality-of-life measures are most appropriate and valid, there is general agreement that such measures can be reasonably used to plan short-term treatment programs for groups of patients. Such patients can be evaluated over a period of months to determine the effects of the treatment on their self-reported quality of life. Quality-of-life measures have also been used for establishing priorities for scarce health care resources. Although prioritization of health care resources is often primarily based on mortality data, because many diseases are chronic and non–life-threatening, quality of life must also

Table 3–21. Age-Specific Death Rates per 100,000 From Tuberculosis (All Forms), Males, Massachusetts, 1880–1930

Age (yr)	Year					
	1880	*1890*	*1900*	*1910*	*1920*	*1930*
0–4	760	578	309	309	108	41
5–9	43	49	31	21	24	11
10–19	126	115	90	63	49	21
20–29	444	361	288	207	149	81
30–39	378	368	296	253	164	115
40–49	364	336	253	253	175	118
50–59	366	325	267	252	171	127
60–69	475	346	304	246	172	95
70+	672	396	343	163	127	95

Data from Frost WH: The age selection of mortality from tuberculosis in successive decades. J Hyg 30:91–96, 1939.

Table 3–22. Possible Explanations of Trends or Differences in Mortality: I. Artifactual

1. Numerator	Errors in diagnosis
	Errors in age
	Changes in coding rules
	Changes in classification
2. Denominator	Errors in counting population
	Errors in classifying by demographic characteristics (e.g., age, race, gender)
	Differences in percentages of populations at risk

Table 3–23. Possible Explanations of Trends or Differences in Mortality: II. Real

Changes in survivorship without change in incidence
Change in incidence
Changes in age composition of the populations(s)
Combination of the above factors

be taken into account for this purpose. Patients may place different weights on different quality-of-life measures depending on differences in cultural background, education, and, for example, religious values. As a result, measuring quality of life and developing valid indices that are useful for obtaining comparative data in different patients and in different populations remain a major challenge.

CONCLUSION

This chapter has reviewed some approaches to quantitatively measuring and expressing human morbidity and mortality. The next question relates to the numerators of the morbidity rates: How do we identify people who have a disease and distinguish them from those who do not, and how do we evaluate the quality of the diagnostic and screening tests that are used to separate these individuals and populations? These questions are addressed in the next chapter.

References

1. Lagakos SW, Wessen BJ, Zelen M: An analysis of contaminated well water and health effects in Woburn, Massachusetts. J Am Stat Assoc 81:583–614, 1986.
2. Harr J: A Civil Action. New York, Random House, 1995.
3. National Center for Health Statistics: Instructions for Classifying the Underlying Cause of Death, 1983. Hyattsville, Md.
4. Chamblee RF, Evans MC: TRANSAX: The NCHS System for Producing Multiple Cause-of-Death Statistics, 1968–1978. Vital and Health Statistics, series 1, No. 20, DHHS publication No.(PHS) 86–1322. Washington, DC, Bureau of Vital and Health Statistics, June 1986.
5. Savage G, Rohde FC, Grant B, Dufour MC: Liver Cirrhosis Mortality in the United States, 1970–90: Surveillance Report No. 29. Bethesda, Md, Department of Health and Human Services, December 1993.

Review Questions

Questions 1 and 2 Are Based on the Information Given Below:

In an Asian country with a population of 6 million people, 60,000 deaths occurred during the year ending Dec 31, 1995. These included 30,000 deaths from cholera in 100,000 people who were sick with cholera

1. What was the cause-specific mortality rate from cholera in 1995? _____

2. What was the case-fatality rate from cholera in 1995? _____

Questions 3 and 4 Are Based on the Information Given Below:

Annual Incidence Rates Of Cerebrovascular Disease Per 10,000 in Four Countries

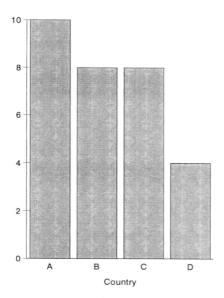

Country

Country	No. of Persons in Population	1-Year Case-Fatality Rate for Cerebrovascular Disease (%)
A	50,000	50
B	100,000	25
C	250,000	20
D	250,000	10

3. Which country has the largest annual number of new cerebrovascular disease cases?
   A
   B
   C
   D

4. Which country has the largest annual number of cerebrovascular disease deaths among new cases?
   A
   B
   C
   D

5. At an initial examination in Oxford, Mass, migraine headache was found in 5 of 1,000 men aged 30 to 35 years and in 10 of 1,000 women aged 30 to 35 years. The inference that women have a two times greater risk of developing migraine headache than do men in this age group is:
   a. Correct
   b. Incorrect, because a ratio has been used to compare male and female rates
   c. Incorrect, because of failure to recognize the cohort effect of age in the two groups
   d. Incorrect, because no data for a comparison or control group are given
   e. Incorrect, because of failure to distinguish between incidence and prevalence

6. Age-adjusted death rates are used to:
   a. Correct death rates for errors in the statement of age
   b. Determine the actual number of deaths that have occurred in specified age groups in a population
   c. Correct death rates for missing age information
   d. Compare deaths in persons of the same age group
   e. Eliminate the effects of differences in the age distributions of populations in comparing death rates

7. The incidence rate of a disease is five times greater in women than in men, but the prevalence rates show no sex difference. The best explanation is that:
   a. The crude all-cause mortality rate is greater in women
   b. The case-fatality rate for this disease is greater for women
   c. The case-fatality rate for this disease is lower in women
   d. The duration of this disease is shorter in men
   e. Risk factors for developing the disease are more common in women

8. The mortality rate due to disease X in city A is 75/100,000 in persons aged 65 to 69 years old. The mortality rate due to the same disease in city B is 150/100,000 in persons aged 65 to 69 years old. The inference that disease X is two times more prevalent in persons 65 to 69 years old in city B than it is in persons 65 to 69 years old in city A is:
   a. Correct
   b. Incorrect, because of failure to distinguish between prevalence and mortality
   c. Incorrect, because of failure to adjust for differences in age distributions
   d. Incorrect, because of failure to distinguish between period and point prevalence
   e. Incorrect, because a proportion is used when a rate is required to support the inference

Question 9 Is Based on the Information Given Below:

Annual Cancer Deaths in White Male Workers in Two Industries

	Industry A		Industry B	
	No. of Deaths	% of All Cancer Deaths	No. of Deaths	% of All Cancer Deaths
Respiratory system	180	33	248	45
Digestive system	160	29	160	29
Genitourinary	80	15	82	15
All other sites	130	23	60	11
Total	550	100	550	100

Based on the preceding information, it was concluded that workers in industry B are at higher risk of death from respiratory system cancer than workers in industry A. (Assume that the age distributions of the workers in the two industries are nearly identical.)

9. Which of the following statements is true?
   a. The conclusion reached is correct
   b. The conclusion reached may be incorrect because proportionate mortality rates were used when age-specific mortality rates were needed
   c. The conclusion reached may be incorrect because there was no comparison group
   d. The conclusion reached may be incorrect because proportional mortality was used when cause-specific mortality rates were needed
   e. None of the above

10. The following are standardized mortality ratios for lung cancer in England:

	Standardized Mortality Ratio	
Occupation	*1949–1960*	*1968–1979*
Carpenters	209	135
Bricklayers	142	118

Based on these SMRs *alone,* one may conclude that:

a. The number of deaths from lung cancer in carpenters in 1949–1960 was greater than the number of deaths from lung cancer in bricklayers during the same period

b. The proportionate mortality from lung cancer in bricklayers in 1949–1960 was greater than the proportionate mortality from lung cancer in the same occupational group in 1968–1979

c. The age-adjusted rate of lung cancer deaths in bricklayers was greater in 1949–1960 than it was in 1968–1979

d. The rate of death from lung cancer in carpenters in 1968–1979 was greater than would have been expected for a group of men of similar ages in all occupations

e. The proportionate mortality rate from lung cancer in carpenters in 1968–1979 was 1.35 times greater than would have been expected for a group of men of similar ages in all occupations.

Questions 11 and 12 Are Based on the Information Given Below:

	Community X		Community Y	
Age	No. of People	No. of Deaths From Disease Z	No. of People	No. of Deaths From Disease Z
Young	8,000	69	5,000	48
Old	11,000	115	3,000	60

Calculate the age-adjusted death rate for disease Z in communities X and Y by the direct method, using the total of both communities as the standard population.

11. The age-adjusted death rate from disease Z for community X is _____

12. The proportionate mortality from disease Z for community Y is:
a. 9.6/1,000
b. 13.5/1,000
c. 20.0/1,000
d. 10.8/1,000
e. None of the above

CHAPTER 4

Assessing the Validity and Reliability of Diagnostic and Screening Tests

To understand how a disease is transmitted and develops and to provide appropriate and effective health care, it is necessary to distinguish between people in the population who have the disease and those who do not. This is an important challenge both in the clinical arena, where patient care is the issue, and in the public health arena, where secondary prevention programs that involve early disease detection and intervention are being considered and where etiologic studies are being conducted to provide a basis for primary prevention. Thus, the quality of screening and diagnostic tests is the issue. Regardless of whether the test is a physical examination, chest x-ray, electrocardiogram, or blood or urine assay, the same issue arises: How good is the test in separating populations of people with and without the disease in question? This chapter addresses the question of how we assess the quality of newly available screening and diagnostic tests in order to make reasonable decisions regarding their utilization and interpretation.

BIOLOGIC VARIATION OF HUMAN POPULATIONS

In using a test to distinguish between individuals with normal and abnormal results, it is important to understand how characteristics are distributed in human populations.

Figure 4–1 shows the distribution of tuberculin test results in a population—the size of the induration (area of hardness at the site of the injection) in millimeters is shown on the horizontal axis and the number of individuals is indicated on the vertical . A large group centers on the value of 0 no induration—and another group centers near 20 mm of induration. This type of distribution, in which there are two peaks, is called a *bimodal curve.* The bimodal distribution permits the separation of individuals who had no prior experience with tuberculosis (people with no induration, seen on the left) from those who had prior experience with tuberculosis (those with about 20 mm of induration, seen on the right). Although some individuals fall into the "gray zone" in the center, and may belong to either curve, most of the population can be easily distinguished using the two curves. Thus, when a characteristic has a bimodal distribution, it is relatively easy to separate most of the population into two groups (e.g., ill and not ill, having a certain condition or abnormality and not having that condition or abnormality).

In general, however, most human characteristics are not distributed bimodally. Figure 4–2 shows the distribution of systolic blood pressures in a particular group. In this figure there is no bimodal curve; what we see is a *unimodal curve*—a single peak. Therefore, if we want to separate those in the group who are hypertensive from those who are not hypertensive, a cut-off level of blood pressure must be set above which people are designated hypertensive and below which they are designated normotensive. No obvious level of blood pressure distinguishes normotensive from hypertensive individuals. Although we could choose a cut-off for hypertension based on statistical considerations, we would ideally like to choose a cut-off on the basis of biologic information; that is, we would want to know that a pressure above the chosen cut-off level is associated with increased risk of subsequent disease, such as stroke, myocardial infarction, or subsequent mortality. Unfortunately, for many human characteristics,

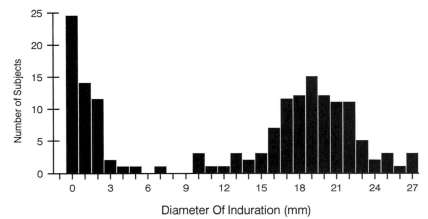

Figure 4–1. Distribution of tuberculin reactions. (Adapted from Edwards LB, Palmer CE, Magnus K: BCG Vaccination: Studies by the WHO Tuberculosis Research Office, Copenhagen, WHO Monograph No. 12. WHO, Geneva, 1953.)

we do not have such information to serve as a guide in setting this level.

In either distribution—unimodal or bimodal—it is relatively easy to distinguish the extreme values of abnormal and normal. Uncertainty remains, however, about cases that fall into the gray zone in either type of curve.

VALIDITY OF SCREENING TESTS

The *validity* of a test is defined as the ability of a test to distinguish between who has a disease and who does not. Validity has two components: sensitivity and specificity. The *sensitivity* of the test is defined as the ability of the test to identify correctly those who *have* the disease. The *specificity* of the test is defined as the ability of the test to identify correctly those who *do not have* the disease.

Tests With Dichotomous Results (Positive or Negative)

Suppose we have a hypothetical population of 1,000 people of whom 100 have a certain disease and 900 do not. A test is available that can yield either positive or negative results. We want to use this test to try to separate persons who have the disease from those who do not. The results obtained by applying the test to this population of 1,000 people are shown in Table 4–1.

How good was the test? First, how good was the test in correctly identifying those who had the disease? Table 4–1 indicates that of the 100 people with the disease, 80 were correctly identified as "positive" by the test, and a positive identification was missed in 20. Thus, the *sensitivity* of the test, which is defined as the proportion of diseased people who were correctly identified as such by the test, is 80/100 or 80%.

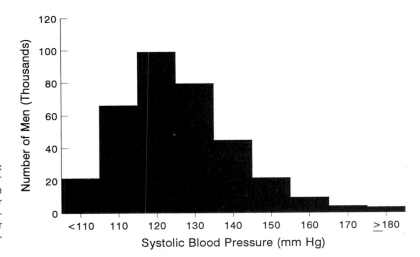

Figure 4–2. Distribution of systolic blood pressure for men screened for the Multiple Risk Factor Intervention Trial. (Data from Stamler J, Stamler R, Neaton JD: Blood pressure, systolic and diastolic, and cardiovascular risks: U.S. population data. Arch Intern Med 153:598–615, 1993.)

Table 4–1. Concept of the Sensitivity and Specificity of Screening Examinations

Example: Assume a population of 1,000 people of whom 100 have a disease and 900 do not have the disease

Screening Test to Identify the 100 People with the Disease

Results of Screening	True Characteristics in the Population		Total
	Disease	*No Disease*	
Positive	80	100	180
Negative	20	800	820
Total	100	900	1,000

$$\text{Sensitivity} = \frac{80}{100} = 80\%$$

$$\text{Specificity} = \frac{800}{900} = 89\%$$

Second, how good was the test in correctly identifying those who did *not* have the disease? Looking again at Table 4–1, of the 900 people who did not have the disease, the test correctly identified 800 as "negative." The *specificity* of the test, which is defined as the proportion of non-diseased people who are correctly called negative by the test, is therefore 800/900 or 89%.

Note that in order to calculate the sensitivity and specificity of a test, we must know who "really" has the disease and who does not from another source than the test we are using. We are in fact comparing our test results with some "gold standard"—an external source of "truth" regarding the disease status of each individual in the population. Sometimes this truth may be the result of another test that has been in use, and sometimes it is the result of a more definitive, and often more invasive, test (e.g., cardiac catheterization or tissue biopsy). However, in real life, when we use a test to identify diseased and non-diseased persons in a population, we clearly do not know who has the disease and who does not. (If this were already established, testing would be pointless.) But in order to quantitatively assess the sensitivity and specificity of a test, we must have another source of truth with which to compare the test results.

Table 4–2 compares the results of a dichotomous test (results either positive or negative) with the actual disease status. Ideally, we would like all of the tested subjects to fall into the two cells shown in the upper left and lower right of the table: people with the disease who are correctly called "positive" by the test *(true positives)* and people without the disease who are correctly called "negative" by the test *(true negatives)*. Unfortunately, such is rarely if ever the case. Some people who do not have the disease are erroneously called "positive" by the test *(false positives)*, and some people with the disease are erroneously called "negative" *(false negatives)*.

Why are these issues important? When we conduct a screening program, we often end up with a large group of people who screened positive, including both people who really have the disease (true positives) and people who do not have the disease (false positives). The issue of *false positives* is important because all people who screened positive are brought back in for more sophisticated and more expensive tests. Of the several problems that result, the first is a burden on the health care system.

Table 4–2. Comparison of the Results of a Dichotomous Test with Actual Disease Status

Test Results	Population	
	With Disease	*Without Disease*
Positive	Have disease and have positive test = true positive (TP)	No disease but have positive test = false positive (FP)
Negative	Have disease but have negative test = false negative (FN)	No disease and have negative test = true negative (TN)

$$\text{Sensitivity} = \frac{TP}{TP + FN} \qquad \text{Specificity} = \frac{TN}{TN + FP}$$

Another is the anxiety and worry induced in persons who have been told that they have tested positive. Considerable evidence indicates that many people who are labeled ''positive'' by a screening test never have that label completely erased, even if the results of a subsequent evaluation are negative. For example, children labeled ''positive'' in a screening program for heart disease were handled as handicapped by parents and school personnel even after being told that subsequent tests were negative. In addition, such individuals may be limited in regard to employment and insurability by erroneous interpretation of positive screening test results, even if subsequent tests fail to substantiate any positive finding.

Why is the problem of *false negatives* important? If a person has the disease but is erroneously informed that the test result is negative, and if the disease is a serious one for which effective intervention is available, the problem is indeed serious. For example, if the disease is a type of cancer that is curable only in its early stages, a false-negative result could represent a virtual death sentence. Thus, the importance of false-negative results depends on the nature and severity of the disease being screened for, the effectiveness of available intervention measures, and whether the effectiveness is greater if the intervention is administered early in the natural history of the disease.

Tests of Continuous Variables

So far we have discussed a test with only two possible results: positive or negative. But we often test for a continuous variable, such as blood pressure or blood glucose level, for which there is no ''positive'' or ''negative'' result. A decision must therefore be made in establishing a cut-off level above which a test result is considered positive and below which a result is considered negative. Let us consider the diagrams shown in Figure 4–3.

Figure 4–3A shows a population of 20 diabetics and 20 non-diabetics who are being screened using a blood sugar test whose scale is shown along the vertical axis from high to low. The diabetics are represented by black circles and the non-diabetics by cross-hatched circles. We see that although blood sugar levels tend to be higher in diabetics than in non-diabetics, no level clearly separates the two groups; there is some overlap of diabetics and non-diabetics at every blood sugar level. Nevertheless, we must select a cut-off point so that those whose results fall above the cut-off can be called

''positive,'' and can be called back for further testing, and those whose results fall below that point are called ''negative,'' and are not called back for further testing.

Suppose a relatively high cut-off level is chosen (see Fig. 4–3B). Clearly, many of the diabetics will not be identified as positive; on the other hand, most of the non-diabetics will be correctly identified as negative. If these results are distributed on a 2 $\times$ 2 table, the sensitivity of the test using this cut-off level will be 25% (5/20) and the specificity will be 90% (18/20).

What if a low cut-off level is chosen (see Fig. 4–3C)? Very few diabetics would be misdiagnosed. What then is the problem? A large proportion of the non-diabetics are now identified as positive by the test. As seen in the 2 $\times$ 2 table, the sensitivity is now 85% (17/20), but the specificity is only 30% (6/20).

The difficulty is that in the real world, no vertical line separates the diabetics and non-diabetics, and they are even mixed together (see Fig. 4–3D); in fact, they are not even distinguishable by black or cross-hatched circles (see Fig. 4–3E). So if a high cut-off level is used (see Fig. 4–3F), all those with results below the line will be assured they do not have the disease and will not be followed further; if the low cut-off is used (see Fig. 4–3G), all those with results above the line will be brought back for further testing.

Figure 4–4 shows actual data regarding the distribution of blood sugar levels in diabetics and non-diabetics. Suppose we were to go out and screen this population. If we decide to set the cut-off level so that we identify all of the diabetics (100% sensitivity), we could set the level at 80 mg/100 cc. The problem is, however, that in so doing we will also call many of the non-diabetics positive (very low specificity). On the other hand, if we set the level at 200 mg/100 cc so that we call all the non-diabetics negative (100% specificity), we now miss many of the true diabetics (very low sensitivity). Thus, there is a trade-off between sensitivity and specificity: if we increase the sensitivity by lowering the cut-off level, we decrease the specificity; if we increase the specificity by raising the cut-off level, we decrease the sensitivity. To quote an unknown sage: ''There is no such thing as a free lunch.''

The dilemma involved in deciding whether to set a high cut-off or a low cut-off rests in the problem of the false positives and the false negatives that result from the testing. It is important to remember

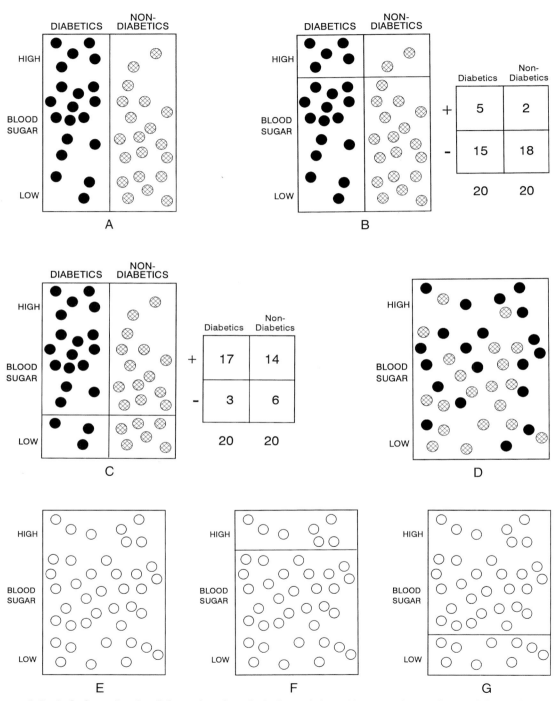

Figure 4–3. *A–G*, Screening for diabetes in a hypothetical population with a prevalence of 50%: Effects of choosing different cut-off levels for a positive test. (See text.)

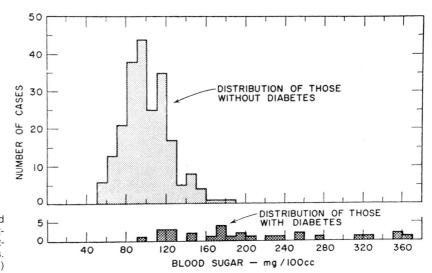

Figure 4–4. Distribution of blood sugar in diabetics and non-diabetics. (From Blumberg M: Evaluating health screening procedures. Operations Res 5:351–360, 1957.)

that in screening we end up with groups classified only on the basis of their test results, such as positives and negatives. We have no information regarding their true disease status, which, of course, is the reason for the screening. In effect we end up not with four groups, as seen in Figure 4–5, but rather with two groups: one group of people who tested positive and who will be brought back for additional examinations and one group who tested negative who will not be brought back for further testing (Fig. 4–6).

The choice of a high or a low cut-off level for screening therefore depends on the importance we attach to false positives and false negatives. False positives are associated with costs—emotional and financial—as well as with the difficulty of "delabeling" a person who tests positive and is later found not to have the disease. In addition, false

positives pose a major burden to the health care system in that a large group of people need to be brought back for a retest, when only a few of them may turn out to have the disease. False negatives, on the other hand, will be told they do not have the disease and will not be followed, so serious disease might possibly be missed at an early treatable stage. Thus, the choice of cut-off level relates to the relative importance of false positivity and false negativity for the disease in question.

TWO-STAGE SCREENING

Screening is often carried out in stages: a less expensive, less invasive, or less uncomfortable test is carried out first, and those who screen positive on this test are recalled for further testing with a

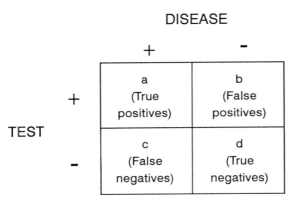

Figure 4–5. Box diagram indicating four possible groups resulting from screening using a dichotomous test.

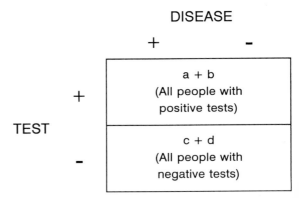

Figure 4–6. Box diagram indicating grouping of all people with positive test results and all people with negative test results on screening.

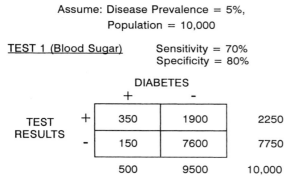

Figure 4–7. Hypothetical example of a two-stage screening program: I.

more expensive or more invasive test, which may have greater sensitivity and specificity. It is hoped that bringing back for further testing those who screen positive will reduce the problem of false positives.

Consider the hypothetical example in Figure 4–7, in which a population is screened for diabetes using a test with a sensitivity of 70% and a specificity of 80%. How are the data shown in this table obtained? The disease prevalence in this population is given as 5%, so that in the population of 10,000, 500 persons have the disease. With a sensitivity of 70%, the test will correctly identify 350 of the 500 people who have the disease. With a specificity of 80%, the test will correctly identify as non-diabetic 7,600 of the 9,500 people who are free of diabetes; however, 1,900 of these 9,500 will have positive results. Thus a total of 2,250 people will test posi-

tive and will be brought back for a second test. (Remember that in real life we do not have the vertical line separating diabetics and non-diabetics, and we do not know that 350 of the 2,250 have diabetes.)

Now those 2,250 people are brought back and screened using a second test (such as a glucose tolerance test), which for purposes of this example we assume to have a sensitivity of 90% and a specificity of 90%. Figure 4–8 again shows test 1 together with test 2, which deals only with the 2,250 people who tested positive in the first screening test and have been brought back for second-stage screening.

Since 350 people (of the 2,250) have the disease and the test has a sensitivity of 90%, 315 of those 350 will be correctly identified as positive. Because 1,900 (of the 2,250) do not have diabetes and the test specificity is 90%, 1,710 of the 1,900 will be correctly identified as negative and 190 will be false positives.

We are now able to calculate the *net sensitivity* and the *net specificity* of using both tests in sequence. After finishing both tests, 315 people of the total 500 in this population of 10,000 will have been correctly called positive: 315/500 = 63% *net sensitivity*. Thus there is a loss in net sensitivity by using both tests. To calculate *net specificity*, note that 7,600 people of the 9,500 in this population who do not have diabetes were correctly called negative in the first-stage screening and were not tested further; an additional 1,710 of those 9,500 non-diabetics were correctly called negative in the

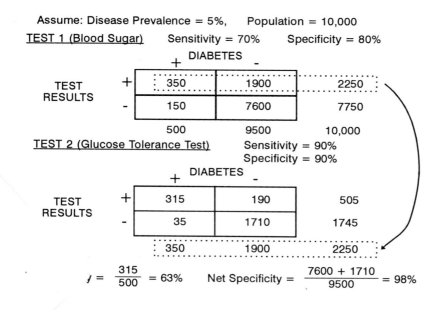

$$\not = \frac{315}{500} = 63\% \qquad \text{Net Specificity} = \frac{7600 + 1710}{9500} = 98\%$$

Figure 4–8. Hypothetical example of a two-stage screening program: II.

second-stage screening. Thus a total of 7,600 + 1,710 of the 9,500 non-diabetics were correctly called negative: 9,310/9,500 = 98% *net specificity*. Thus, use of both tests has resulted in a gain in net specificity.

PREDICTIVE VALUE OF A TEST

So far, we have asked, How good is the test at identifying people with the disease and people without the disease? This is an important issue, particularly in screening free-living populations. We are in effect asking, If we screen a population, what proportion of people who have the disease will be correctly identified? This is clearly an important public health consideration. In the clinical setting, however, a different question may be important for the physician: If the test results are positive in this patient, what is the probability that this patient has the disease? This is called the *positive predictive value* of the test. In other words, what proportion of patients who test positive actually have the disease in question? To calculate the predictive value we divide the number of true positives by the total number who tested positive (true positives + false positives).

Let us return to the example presented in Table 4–1, in which a population of 1,000 persons is screened. As seen in Table 4–3, a 2 × 2 table shows the results of a dichotomous screening test in a population. Of the 1,000 subjects, 180 have a positive test; of these 180, 80 have the disease. The *positive predictive value* is therefore 80/180 or 44%.

A parallel question can be asked relating to negative tests: If the test result is negative, what is the probability that this patient does not have the disease? This is called the *negative predictive value* of the test. It is calculated by dividing the number of true negatives by all those who tested negative (true negatives + false negatives). Looking again at the

example in Table 4–3, 820 people have a negative test result, and of these, 800 do not have the disease. Thus, the *negative predictive value* is 800/820 or 98%. In the discussion of predictive value that follows, the term *predictive value* is used to denote the positive predictive value of the test.

Every test that a physician carries out—history, physical examination, laboratory tests, x-rays, electrocardiograms, and other procedures—is used to enhance the physician's ability to make a correct diagnosis. What he or she wants to know after administering a test to a patient is: Given this positive test result, what is the likelihood that the patient has the disease?

Unlike the sensitivity and specificity of the test, which can be considered characteristic of the test being used, the predictive value is affected by two factors: the prevalence of the disease in the population tested and, when the disease is infrequent, the specificity of the test being used. Both of these relationships are discussed in the following sections.

Relation of Predictive Value to Disease Prevalence

The relation between predictive value and disease prevalence can be seen in the example given in Table 4–4.

First, let us direct our attention to the upper part of the table. Assume we are using a test with a sensitivity of 99% and a specificity of 95% in a population of 10,000 people in which the disease prevalence is 1%. Because the prevalence is 1%, 100 of the 10,000 persons have the disease and 9,900 do not. With a sensitivity of 99%, the test correctly identifies 99 of the 100 people who have the disease. With a specificity of 95%, the test correctly identifies as negative 9,405 of the 9,900 people who do not have the disease.

Thus, in this population with a 1% prevalence, 594 people are called positive by the test (99 + 495). However, of these 594, 495 (83%) are false positives and the positive predictive value is therefore 99/594 or only 17%.

Let us now apply the same test—with the same sensitivity and specificity—to a population with a higher disease prevalence, 5%, as seen in the lower part of Table 4–4. Using calculations similar to those that we used in the upper part of the table, the positive predictive value is now 51%. Thus, the higher prevalence in the screened population has led to a marked increase in the positive predictive value using the same test.

Table 4–3. Predictive Value of a Test

Test Results	Disease	No Disease	Total
Positive	80	100	180
Negative	20	800	820
Total	100	900	1,000

Positive predictive value = $\frac{80}{180}$ = 44%   Negative predictive value = $\frac{800}{820}$ = 98%

Table 4–4. Relationship of Disease Prevalence to Predictive Value

| Disease Prevalence | Test Results | Example: Sensitivity = 99%, specificity = 95% | | | Predictive Value |
		Sick	Not Sick	Totals	
1%	+	99	495	594	$\frac{99}{594} = 17\%$
	−	1	9,405	9,406	
	Totals	100	9,900	10,000	
5%	+	495	475	970	$\frac{495}{970} = 51\%$
	−	5	9,025	9,303	
	Totals	500	9,500	10,000	

Figure 4–9 shows the relation between disease prevalence and predictive value: Clearly, most of the gain in predictive value occurs with increases in prevalence at the lowest rates of disease prevalence.

Why should we be concerned about the relation of predictive value and disease prevalence? We have seen that the higher the prevalence, the higher the predictive value. Therefore, a screening program is most productive and efficient if it is directed to a high-risk target population. Screening a total population for a relatively infrequent disease can be very wasteful of resources and may yield few previously undetected cases for the amount of effort involved. However, if a high-risk subset can be identified and the screening can be directed to them, the program is likely to be far more productive. In addition, a high-risk population may be more motivated to participate in such a screening program and be more likely to take recommended action if their screening results are positive.

The relationship between predictive value and disease prevalence also demonstrates that the results of any test must be interpreted in the context of the prevalence of the disease in the population from which the subject originates. An interesting example is seen with the use of α-fetoprotein (AFP) determinations in amniotic fluid for the prenatal diagnosis of spina bifida. Figure 4–10 shows the distribution of AFP levels in amniotic fluid in normal pregnancies and in pregnancies in which the fetus has spina bifida, a neural tube defect. Although the distribution is bimodal, a range exists in which the curves overlap, and within that range, it may not always be clear to which curve the mother and baby belong. Sheffield and co-workers[1] reviewed the literature and constructed artificial populations of 10,000 women screened for amniotic fluid AFP to identify fetuses with spina bifida. They created two populations: one at high risk for spina bifida and the other at normal risk.

Table 4–5 shows the calculations for both high-risk and low-risk women. Which women are at high risk for having a child with spina bifida? It is known that women who have previously had a child with

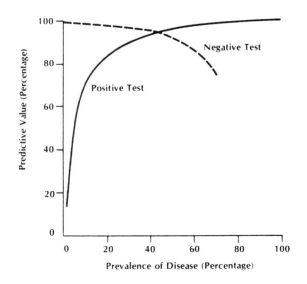

Figure 4–9. Relationship between disease prevalence and predictive value in a test with 95% sensitivity and 95% specificity. (From Mausner JS, Kramer S: Mausner and Bahn Epidemiology: An Introductory Text. Philadelphia, WB Saunders, 1985, p 221.)

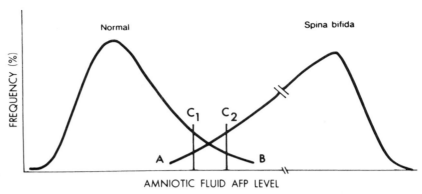

Figure 4–10. Amniotic fluid α-fetoprotein (AFP) levels in normal subjects and in subjects with spina bifida. (From Sheffield LJ, Sackett DL, Goldsmith CH, et al: A clinical approach to the use of predictive values in the prenatal diagnosis of neural tube defects. Am J Obstet Gynecol 145:319–324, 1983.)

a neural tube defect are at increased risk because the defect is known to repeat in siblings. In these calculations, the positive predictive value is found to be 82.9%. Which women are at low risk but would still have an amniocentesis? These are older women who are having amniocentesis because of concern over possible Down's syndrome or some other defect associated with advanced-maternal-age pregnancies. The risk of spina bifida, however, is not related to maternal age, so that these women are not at any increased risk. The calculation shows that, using the same test for AFP as was used for the high-risk women, the positive predictive value of the test is only 41.7%, considerably less than it was in a high-risk group.

Thus, we see that the same test can have a very different predictive value when it is administered to a high-risk (high prevalence) population or to a low-risk (low prevalence) population. This has clear clinical implications: A woman may make a decision to terminate a pregnancy and a physician may formulate advice to such a woman on the basis of

the test results. But the same test result must be interpreted differently depending on whether the woman comes from a pool of high-risk or low-risk women, which will be reflected in the positive predictive value of the test. Consequently, the test result by itself may not be sufficient to serve as a guide without taking into account the other considerations just described.

The following true examples highlight the importance of this issue:

The head of a firemen's union consulted a university cardiologist because the fire department physician had read an article in a leading medical journal reporting that a certain electrocardiographic finding was highly predictive of serious, generally unrecognized, coronary heart disease. On the basis of this paper, the fire department physician was disqualifying many young able-bodied firemen from active duty. The cardiologist read the paper and found that the study had been carried out in hospitalized patients.

What was the problem? Because hospitalized patients have a much higher prevalence of heart dis-

Table 4–5. Calculations of Predictive Values for Neural Tube Defects (NTD)* for α-Fetoprotein (AFP) Test in High- and Low-Risk Women

AFP Test	Pregnancy Outcome			Predictive Values (%)
	NTD	Normal	Total	
High-Risk Women				
Abnormal	87	18	105	82.9
Normal	13	9,882	9,895	99.9
Total	100	9,900	10,000	
Low-Risk Women				
Abnormal	128	179	307	41.7
Normal	19	99,674	99,693	99.98
Total	147	99,853	100,000	

*Spina bifida or encephalocele.
From Sheffield LJ, Sackett DL, Goldsmith CH, et al: A clinical approach to the use of predictive values in the prenatal diagnosis of neural tube defects. Am J Obstet Gynecol 145:319–324, 1983.

ease than does a group of young firemen, the fire department physician had erroneously taken the high predictive value obtained in studying a high-prevalence population and inappropriately applied it to a low-prevalence population of healthy fire-fighters, in whom the same test would actually have a much lower predictive value.

Another example:

A physician visited his general internist for a regular annual medical examination, which included a stool examination for occult blood. One of the three stool specimens examined in the test was positive. The internist told his physician-patient that the result was of no significance because he regularly encountered many false-positive test results in his busy practice. The test was repeated, and all three stool specimens were now negative. Nevertheless, sensing his patient's lingering concerns, the internist referred his physician-patient to a gastroenterologist. The gastroenterologist said, "In my experience the positive stool finding is serious. Such a finding is almost always associated with gastrointestinal pathological disorders. The subsequent negative tests mean nothing, because you could have a tumor that only bleeds intermittently."

Who was correct in this episode? The answer is that both the general internist and the gastroenterologist were correct. The internist gave his assessment of predictive value based on his experience in his general medical practice—a population with a low prevalence of serious gastrointestinal disease. The gastroenterologist, on the other hand, gave his assessment of the predictive value of the test based on his experience in his referral practice—a practice in which most patients are referred because of a likelihood of serious gastrointestinal illness—a high-prevalence population.

Relation of Predictive Value to the Specificity of the Test

A second factor that affects the predictive value of a test is the *specificity* of the test. Examples of this are shown first in graphic form and then in tabular form.

Figures 4–11A through D diagrams the results of screening a population; however, the 2 × 2 tables in these figures differ from those in earlier figures: The size of each cell is proportional to the population it represents. In each figure the cells that represent persons who tested positive are shaded gray; these are the cells that will be used in calculating the positive predictive value.

Figure 4–11A presents the baseline screened population that is used in our discussion: A population of 1,000 people in whom the prevalence is 50%; thus, 500 people have the disease and 500 do not. In analyzing this figure we also assume that the screening test employed has a sensitivity of 50% and a specificity of 50%. Because 500 people tested positive, and 250 of these have the disease, the predictive value is 250/500 or 50%.

Fortunately, the prevalence of most diseases is much lower than 50%; we are generally dealing with relatively infrequent diseases. Figure 4–11B therefore assumes a lower prevalence, 20% (although even this would be an unusually high prevalence for most diseases); both the sensitivity and specificity remain at 50%. Now only 200 of the 1,000 people have the disease, and the vertical line separating diseased from non-diseased persons is shifted to the left. The predictive value is now calculated as 100/500 or 20%.

Given that we are screening a population with the lower prevalence rate, can we improve the predictive value? What would be the effect on predictive value if we increased the sensitivity of the test? Figure 4–11C shows the results when we leave the prevalence at 20% and the specificity at 50% but increase the sensitivity to 90%. The predictive value is now 180/580 or 31%, a modest increase.

What if, instead of increasing the sensitivity of the test, we increase the specificity? Figure 4–11D shows the results when prevalence remains 20% and sensitivity remains 50% but specificity is increased to 90%. The predictive value is now 100/180 or 56%. Thus, an increase in specificity resulted in a much greater increase in predictive value than did the same increase in sensitivity.

Why does specificity have a greater effect than sensitivity on predictive value? The answer becomes clear by examining these figures. Because we are dealing with infrequent diseases, most of the population falls to the right of the vertical line. Consequently, any change to the right of the vertical affects a greater number of people than would a comparable change to the left. Thus a change in specificity has a greater effect on predictive value than does a change in sensitivity. If we were dealing with a high-prevalence disease, the situation would be different.

The effect of changes in specificity on predictive value is also seen in Table 4–6 in a form similar to that used in Table 4–4.

As seen in this example, even with 100% sensitivity, a change in specificity from 70% to 95% has a dramatic effect on the positive predictive value.

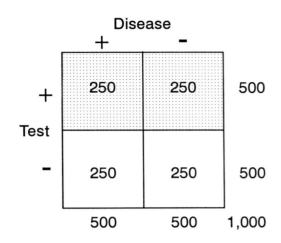

Prevalence = 50%
Sensitivity = 50%
Specificity = 50%

$$PV = \frac{250}{500} = 50\%$$

A

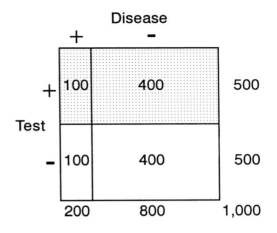

Prevalence = 20%
Sensitivity = 50%
Specificity = 50%

$$PV = \frac{100}{500} = 20\%$$

B

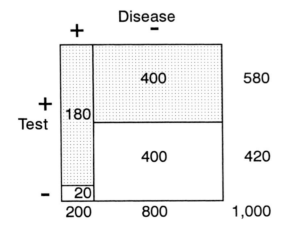

Prevalence = 20%
Sensitivity = 90%
Specificity = 50%

$$PV = \frac{180}{580} = 31\%$$

C

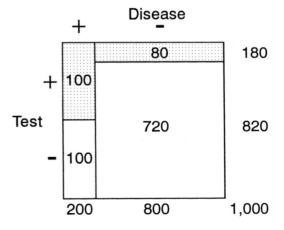

Prevalence = 20%
Sensitivity = 50%
Specificity = 90%

$$PV = \frac{100}{180} = 56\%$$

D

Figure 4–11. *A–D,* Relationship of specificity to predictive value.

Table 4–6. Relationship of Specificity to Predictive Value

Specificity	Test Results	Sick	Not Sick	Totals	Predictive Value
	Example: Prevalence = 10%, sensitivity = 100%				
70%	+	1,000	2,700	3,700	$\frac{1,000}{3,700} = 27\%$
	−	0	6,300	6,300	
	Totals	1,000	9,000	10,000	
95%	+	1,000	450	1,450	$\frac{1,000}{1,450} = 69\%$
	−	0	8,550	8,550	
	Totals	1,000	9,000	10,000	

RELIABILITY (REPEATABILITY) OF TESTS

Let us consider another aspect of assessing diagnostic and screening tests—the question of whether a test is reliable or repeatable. Can the results obtained be replicated if the test is repeated? Clearly, regardless of the sensitivity and specificity of a test, if the test results cannot be reproduced, the value and usefulness of the test are minimal. This chapter focuses on the reliability or repeatability of diagnostic and screening tests. The factors that contribute to the variation between test results are discussed first: intrasubject variation (variation within individual subjects) and interobserver variation (variation between those reading the test results).

Intrasubject Variation

The values obtained in measuring many human characteristics often vary over time, even during a short period. Table 4–7 shows changes in blood pressure readings over a 24-hour period in three individuals. Variability over time is considerable. This, as well as the conditions under which certain tests are conducted (e.g., postprandially or postexercise, at home or in a physician's office), can clearly lead to different results in the same individual. Therefore, in evaluating any test result, it is important to take into consideration the conditions under which the test was carried out, including the time of day.

Interobserver Variation

Another important consideration is variation between observers. Two examiners often do not derive the same result. The extent to which observers agree or disagree is an important issue, whether we are considering physical examinations, laboratory tests, or other means of assessing human characteristics. We therefore need to be able to express the extent of agreement in quantitative terms.

Overall Percent Agreement

Table 4–8 presents a schema for examining variation between observers. Two observers were instructed to categorize each test result into one of four categories: abnormal, suspect, doubtful, or normal. This diagram might refer, for example, to readings performed by two radiologists. In this diagram the readings of observer 1 are cross-tabulated against those of observer 2. The number of readings in each cell is denoted by a letter of the alphabet. Thus, A x-rays were read as abnormal by both radiologists. C x-rays were read as abnormal by radiologist 2 and as doubtful by radiologist 1. M x-rays were read as abnormal by radiologist 1 and as normal by radiologist 2.

To calculate the overall percent agreement we add up all the cells in which readings by both radiologists agreed (A + F + K + P), divide that sum by the total number of x-rays read, and multiply the result by 100 to yield a percentage.

Table 4–7. Examples Showing Variation in Blood Pressure Readings During a 24-Hour Period

Blood Pressure (mm Hg)	Female Aged 27 yr	Female Aged 62 yr	Male Aged 33 yr
Basal	110/70	132/82	152/109
Lowest hour	86/47	102/61	123/78
Highest hour	126/79	172/94	153/107
Casual	108/64	155/93	157/109

From Richardson DW, Honour AJ, Fenton GW, et al: Variation in arterial pressure throughout the day and night. Clin Sci 26:445, 1964.

Table 4–8. Observer or Instrument Variation: Percent Agreement

Reading No. 2	Reading No. 1			
	Abnormal	*Suspect*	*Doubtful*	*Normal*
Abnormal	A	B	C	D
Suspect	E	F	G	H
Doubtful	I	J	K	L
Normal	M	N	O	P

$$\text{Percent Agreement} = \frac{A + F + K + P}{\text{Total Readings}} \times 100$$

In general, most persons who are tested have negative results. There is likely to be considerable agreement between the two observers regarding these negative, or normal, subjects. Therefore, when percent agreement is calculated for all study subjects, its value may be high only because of the large number of negative findings on which the observers agree. The high value may thus conceal significant disagreement between the observers in regard to identification of subjects as positive.

One approach to this problem is to disregard the subjects who were labeled negative by both observers (cell d), and to calculate percent agreement using as a denominator only subjects who were labeled abnormal by at least one observer (cells a, b, and c) (Fig. 4–12).

Thus, in the *paired observations* in which at least one of the findings in each pair was positive, the following equation is applicable:

$$\text{percent agreement} = \frac{a}{a + b + c} \times 100$$

Kappa Statistic

Percent agreement is also significantly affected by the fact that even if two observers use completely different criteria for calling subjects positive or negative, we would expect agreement about certain subjects solely as a function of chance.

This can be shown intuitively in the following example: You are director of a radiology department that is short of staff one day, and a large number of chest x-rays remain to be read. To solve your problem, you go out in the street and collar a few neighborhood residents, who have no background in biology or medicine, and ask them to read x-rays as either positive or negative. The first person goes through the pile of x-rays, reading them haphazardly as positive, negative, negative, positive, etc. The second person does the same, in

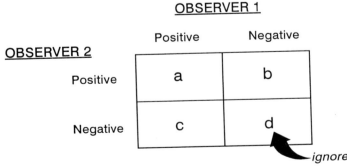

Figure 4–12. Percent agreement when examining paired observations between observer 1 and observer 2.

In the <u>paired observations</u> in which at least one of the observations in each pair was positive, the percent

$$\text{agreement} = \frac{a}{a + b + c} \times 100$$

$$\text{Kappa} = \frac{(\text{Percent Observed Agreement}) - (\text{Percent Agreement Expected by Chance Alone})}{100\% - (\text{Percent Agreement Expected by Chance Alone})}$$

(4.1)

the same way. Given that both readers have no knowledge, criteria, or standards for reading x-rays, would any of their readings on a specific x-ray agree? The answer is clearly yes; they would agree in some cases, *purely by chance.*

If we want to know how well two observers read x-rays, we might ask: To what extent do their readings agree *beyond what we would expect by chance alone?* Or, stated differently: To what extent does the agreement between the two observers exceed the level of agreement that would result just from chance?

One approach to answering these questions is to calculate the *kappa statistic*, proposed by Cohen in 1960.[2] The kappa statistic can be defined by equation 4.1, shown at the top of the page.

What does the numerator of kappa represent? We want to know how much better is the agreement between the observers' readings than would be expected by chance alone, or the *percent observed agreement* minus the *percent agreement expected by chance alone.* Now look at the denominator. The 100% in the denominator represents full agreement—the two observers agree completely. The most the observers could improve their results over the results expected by chance alone is the difference between *full agreement* and the *percent agreement expected by chance alone,* as denoted by the denominator. Thus, kappa quantifies the extent to which the observed agreement exceeds that which would be expected by chance alone, and expresses it as the proportion of the maximum improvement that could occur beyond the agreement expected by chance alone, that the observers achieved.

To calculate kappa, we must first calculate the amount of agreement that might be expected on the basis of chance alone. Consider data reported on the histologic classification of lung cancer that focused on the reproducibility of subtyping of non–small cell lung carcinoma.[3]

Figure 4–13 shows data comparing the findings of two pathologists in subtyping such cases.

The first question is: What is the observed agreement between the two pathologists? Figure 4–14 shows the readings by pathologist A of the entire group of slides along the bottom of the table, and those of pathologist B along the righthand margin of the table. Thus, pathologist A identified 45 or 60% of all of the 75 slides as grade II, and pathologist B identified 44 or 58.6% of all of the slides as grade II. As discussed earlier in the chapter, the percent agreement is determined by the following equation:

$$\frac{41 + 27}{75} \times 100 = 90.7\%$$

That is, the pathologists agreed in 90.7% of the readings.

The next question is: If the two pathologists had used entirely different sets of criteria, how much agreement would have been expected solely on the basis of chance? Pathologist A read 60% of all 75 slides (45 slides) as being grade II. If his readings had used criteria independent of those used by pathologist B (i.e., if pathologist A were to read 60% of any group of slides as being grade II), we would expect that pathologist A would read as grade II both 60% of the slides that pathologist B had called grade II and 60% of the slides that pathologist B had called grade III. We would therefore expect that 60% (26.4) of the 44 slides called grade II by pathologist B would be called grade II by pathologist A, and that 60% (18.6) of the 31 slides called grade III by pathologist B would also be called grade II by pathologist A (Fig. 4–15).

Thus, the agreement expected by chance alone would be (26.4 + 12.4 = 38.8)/75 or 51.7% of all slides read. Kappa can therefore be calculated using the same formula (equation 4.2), shown below.

(4.2)

$$\text{Kappa} = \frac{(\text{Percent Observed Agreement}) - (\text{Percent Agreement Expected by Chance Alone})}{100\% - (\text{Percent Agreement Expected by Chance Alone})}$$

$$= \frac{90.7\% - 51.7\%}{100\% - 51.7\%} = \frac{39\%}{48.3\%} = .81$$

Figure 4–13. Histologic classification by subtype of 75 slides of non–small cell carcinoma, by two pathologists (A and B). (Data from Ghandur-Mnaymneh L, Raub WA, Sridhar KS, et al: The accuracy of the histological classification of lung carcinoma and its reproducibility: A study of 75 archival cases of adenosquamous carcinoma. Cancer Invest 11:641, 1993.)

		Grading by Pathologist A		
		Grade II	Grade III	Totals by B
Grading by Pathologist B	Grade II	41	3	44 (58.6%)
	Grade III	4	27	31 (41.4%)
	Totals by A	45 (60%)	30 (40%)	75 (100%)

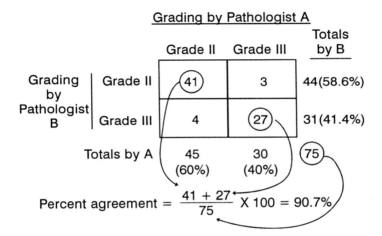

		Grading by Pathologist A		
		Grade II	Grade III	Totals by B
Grading by Pathologist B	Grade II	41	3	44(58.6%)
	Grade III	4	27	31(41.4%)
	Totals by A	45 (60%)	30 (40%)	75

$$\text{Percent agreement} = \frac{41 + 27}{75} \times 100 = 90.7\%$$

Figure 4–14. Percent agreement by pathologist A and pathologist B. (Data from Ghandur-Mnaymneh L, Raub WA, Sridar KS, et al: The accuracy of the histological classification of lung carcinoma and its reproducibility: A study of 75 archival cases of adenosquamous carcinoma. Cancer Invest 11:641, 1993.)

		Grading by Pathologist A		
		Grade II	Grade III	Totals by B
Grading by Pathologist B	Grade II	26.4	17.6	44(58.6%)
	Grade III	18.6	12.4	31(41.4%)
	Totals by A	45 (60%)	30 (40%)	75

$$\text{Percent agreement} = \frac{26.4 + 12.4}{75} \times 100 = 51.7\%$$

Figure 4–15. Percent agreement by pathologist A and pathologist B expected by chance alone. (Data from Ghandur-Mnaymneh L, Raub WA, Sridar KS, et al: The accuracy of the histological classification of lung carcinoma and its reproducibility: A study of 75 archival cases of adenosquamous carcinoma. Cancer Invest 11:641, 1993.)

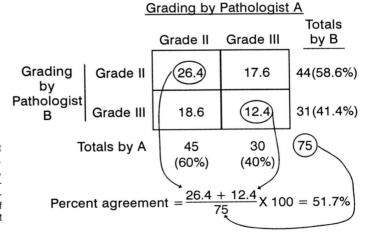

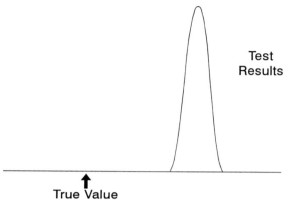

Test
Results

True Value

Figure 4–16. Graph of hypothetical test results that are reliable but invalid.

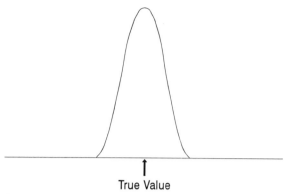

True Value

Figure 4–18 Graph of hypothetical test results that are both valid and reliable.

Landis and Koch[4] suggested that a kappa greater than .75 represents excellent agreement beyond chance, that a kappa below .40 represents poor agreement, and that a kappa of .40 to .75 represents intermediate to good agreement. Testing for the statistical significance of kappa is described by Fleiss.[5] Considerable discussion has arisen regarding appropriate use of kappa, a subject addressed by MacLure and Willett.[6]

RELATION BETWEEN VALIDITY AND RELIABILITY

To conclude this chapter, let us compare validity and reliability using a graphic presentation.

The horizontal line in Figure 4–16 is a scale of values for a given variable, such as blood glucose level, with the true value indicated. The test results obtained are shown by the curve. The curve is a narrow one, indicating that the results are quite reliable (repeatable); unfortunately, however, they cluster far from the true value, so they are not valid. Figure 4–17 shows a curve that is broad, and therefore has low reliability. But the values obtained cluster around the true value, and are thus valid. Clearly, what we would like to achieve are results that are both valid and reliable (Fig. 4–18).

It is important to point out that in Figure 4–17, in which the distribution of the test results is a broad curve centered on the true value and we say the results are valid, the results are only valid for a group (i.e., they tend to cluster around the true value). However, what may be valid for a group or for a population may not be so for an individual in a clinical setting. When the reliability or repeatability of the test is poor, the validity of the test for a given individual may also be poor. The distinction between group validity and individual validity is therefore an important one to keep in mind when assessing the quality of diagnostic and screening tests.

CONCLUSION

This chapter has discussed the validity of diagnostic and screening tests as measured by their sensitivity and specificity, their predictive value, and the reliability or repeatability of these tests. Clearly, regardless of how sensitive and specific a test may be, if its results cannot be replicated, the test is of little use. All these characteristics must, therefore, be borne in mind when evaluating such tests, together with the purpose for which the test will be used.

References

1. Sheffield LJ, Sackett DL, Goldsmith CH, et al: A clinical approach to the use of predictive values in the prenatal diagnosis of neural tube defects. Am J Obstet Gynecol 1465:319–324, 1983.
2. Cohen J: A coefficient of agreement for nominal scales. Educ Psychol Meas 20:37, 1960.
3. Ghandur-Mnaymneh L, Raub WA, Sridhar KS, et al: The accuracy of the histological classification of lung carcinoma

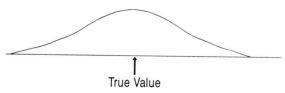

True Value

Figure 4–17. Graph of hypothetical test results that are valid but not reliable.

and its reproducibility: a study of 75 archival cases of adeno-squamous carcinoma. Cancer Invest 11:641, 1993.
4. Landis JR, Koch GG: The measurement of observer agreement for categorical data. Biometrics 33:159, 1977.

5. Fleiss JL: Statistical Methods for Rates and Proportions, ed 2. New York, John Wiley & Sons, 1981.
6. MacLure M, Willett WC: Misinterpretation and misuse of the kappa statistic. Am J Epidemiol 126:161, 1987.

Review Questions

Questions 1, 2, and 3 are based on the information given below:

A physical examination was used to screen for breast cancer in 2,500 women with biopsy-proven adenocarcinoma of the breast and in 5,000 age- and race-matched control women. The results of the physical examination were positive (i.e., a mass was palpated) in 1,800 cases and in 800 control women, all of whom showed no evidence of cancer at biopsy.

1. The sensitivity of the physical examination was: _____

2. The specificity of the physical examination was: _____

3. The positive predictive value of the physical examination was: _____

4. A screening test is used in the same way in two similar populations, but the proportion of false-positive results among those who test positive in population A is lower than that among those who test positive in population B. What is the likely explanation for this finding?
 a. It is impossible to determine what caused the difference
 b. The specificity of the test is lower in population A
 c. The prevalence of disease is lower in population A
 d. The prevalence of disease is higher in population A
 e. The specificity of the test is higher in population A

Question 5 is based on the following information:

A physical examination and an audiometric test were given to 500 persons with suspected hearing problems, of whom 300 were actually found to have them. The results of the examinations were as follows:

Physical Examination

| | Hearing Problems | |
Result	Present	Absent
Positive	240	40
Negative	60	160

Audiometric Test

| | Hearing Problems | |
Result	Present	Absent
Positive	270	60
Negative	30	140

5. Compared to the physical examination, the audiometric test is:
 a. Equally sensitive and specific
 b. Less sensitive and less specific
 c. Less sensitive and more specific
 d. More sensitive and less specific
 e. More sensitive and more specific

Question 6 is based on the following information:

Two pediatricians want to investigate a new laboratory test that identifies streptococcal infections. Dr. Kidd uses the standard culture test, which has a sensitivity of 90% and a specificity of 96%. Dr. Childs uses the new test, which is 96% sensitive and 96% specific.

6. If 200 patients undergo culture with both tests, which of the following is correct?
 a. Dr. Kidd will correctly identify more people *with* streptococcal infection than Dr. Childs
 b. Dr. Kidd will correctly identify fewer people *with* streptococcal infection than Dr. Childs
 c. Dr. Kidd will correctly identify more people *without* streptococcal infection than Dr. Childs
 d. The prevalence of streptococcal infection *is* needed to determine which pediatrician will correctly identify the larger number of people with the disease

Questions 7 and 8 are based on the following information:

A colon cancer screening study is being conducted in Nottingham, England. Individuals aged 50 to 75 years will be screened with the Hemoccult test. In this test, a stool sample is tested for the presence of blood.

7. The Hemoccult test has a sensitivity of 70% and a specificity of 75%. If Nottingham has a prevalence of 12/1,000 for colon cancer, what is the *positive predictive value* of the test? _____

8. If the Hemoccult test is negative, no further testing is done. If the Hemoccult test is positive, the individual will have a second stool sample tested with the Hemoccult II test. If this second sample also tests positive for blood, the individual will be referred for more extensive evaluation. The effect on net sensitivity and net specificity of this method of screening is:
   a. Net sensitivity and net specificity are both increased
   b. Net sensitivity is decreased, net specificity is increased
   c. Net sensitivity remains the same and net specificity is increased
   d. Net sensitivity is increased and net specificity is decreased
   e. The effect on net sensitivity and net specificity cannot be determined from the data

Questions 9 to 12 are based on the information given below:

Two physicians were asked to classify 100 chest x-rays as "abnormal" or "normal" independently. The comparison of their classification is shown in the following table:

Classification of Chest X-Rays by Physician 1 Compared to Physician 2

		Physician 2		
		Abnormal	*Normal*	**Total**
Physician 1	Abnormal	40	20	60
	Normal	10	30	40
	Total	50	50	100

9. The simple, overall percent agreement between the two physicians out of the total is: _____

10. The overall percent agreement between the two physicians, removing the x-rays that both physicians classified as normal, is: _____

11. The value of kappa is: _____

12. This kappa represents which kind of agreement?
    a. Excellent
    b. Intermediate to good
    c. Poor

CHAPTER 5

The Natural History of Disease: Ways of Expressing Prognosis

At this point we have learned how diagnostic and screening tests permit the categorization of sick and healthy individuals. Once a person is identified as having a disease, the question arises, How can we characterize the natural history of the disease in quantitative terms? Such quantification is important for several reasons: First, it is necessary to describe the severity of a disease to establish priorities for clinical services and public health programs. Second, patients often ask questions relating to prognosis. Third, such quantification is important to establish a baseline for natural history, so that as new treatments become available, the effects of such treatments can be compared with the expected outcome that existed without them. Furthermore, if different types of therapy are available for a given disease, such as surgical or medical treatments or two different types of surgical procedures, we want to be able to compare the effectiveness of the various types of therapy. We therefore need a quantitative means of expressing the prognosis in each group, to enable comparison of different therapies.

This chapter presents some of the ways in which prognosis can be described in quantitative terms for a group of patients. Thus, the natural history of disease (prognosis) is discussed in this chapter; in later chapters the issue of how to intervene in the natural history of disease to improve prognosis is addressed: How is the most appropriate drug or other treatment selected (Chapters 6 and 7), and how can disease be detected at an earlier point than usual in its natural history to maximize the effectiveness of treatment (Chapter 17)?

To discuss prognosis, let us begin with a schematic representation of the natural history of disease in a patient as shown in Figure 5–1.

Point A marks the biologic onset of disease.

Often this point cannot be identified: It occurs sub-clinically, perhaps as a subcellular change such as an alteration in DNA. At some point in the progression of the disease process (point P), pathologic evidence of disease could be obtained if it were sought. Subsequently, signs and symptoms of the disease develop in the patient (point S), and at some time after that the patient may seek medical care (point M). The patient may then receive a diagnosis (point D), after which treatment may be given (point T). The subsequent course of the disease might result in cure, control of the disease (with or without disability), or even death.

At what point do we begin to quantify survival time? Ideally, we might prefer to do so from the onset of the disease. Generally this is not possible, because the time of biologic onset is not known in an individual. If we were to count from the time at which symptoms begin, we would introduce a major variable in the subjective recognition of symptoms. In general, duration of survival is counted from the time of diagnosis in order to standardize the calculations. Even with the use of this starting point, however, variability occurs, because patients differ in the point at which they seek medical care. In addition, when survival is counted from time of diagnosis, any patients who may have died before a diagnosis was made are excluded from the count.

An important related question is: How is the diagnosis made? Is there a clear-cut pathognomonic test for the disease in question? Such a test is often not available. Sometimes a disease may be diagnosed by the isolation of an infectious agent, but because people can be carriers of organisms without actually being infected, we do not always know that the isolated organism is the cause of disease. In some diseases we might prefer to make

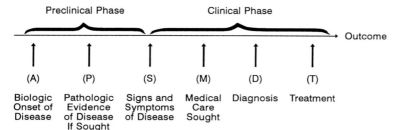

Figure 5–1. The natural history of disease in a patient.

a diagnosis by tissue confirmation, but there is often variability in interpretation of tissue slides by different pathologists. Consequently, when we say that survivorship is measured from the time of diagnosis, the situation is not always precise and clear. These issues should be kept in mind as we proceed to discuss different approaches to estimating prognosis.

Prognosis can be expressed either in terms of deaths from the disease or in terms of survivors with the disease. Both approaches are utilized in the following discussion. Finally, the endpoint used for the purposes of discussion is death. Because death is universal, we are not talking about dying or not dying, but rather about extending the time period until death occurs. It should be clear that other endpoints might be used, including the interval from diagnosis to recurrence of disease or from diagnosis to the time of functional impairment, disability, or changes in the patient's quality of life, which may be affected by the invasiveness of the available treatment or the extent to which some of the symptoms can be relieved even if the life span cannot be extended. These are all important measures, but they are not discussed in this chapter.

CASE-FATALITY RATE

The first way of expressing prognosis is the *case-fatality rate*, which was discussed in Chapter 3. This is defined as the number of people who die of a disease divided by the number of people who have the disease. Given that a person has the disease, what is the likelihood that he or she will die of the disease? Note that the denominator for case-fatality is the number of people who have the disease. This differs from a mortality rate, in which the denominator includes anyone at risk of dying of the disease—both persons who have the disease and persons who do not (yet) have the disease, but in whom it could develop.

The case-fatality rate does not include any explicit statement of time. However, time is expressed implicitly, because case-fatality is generally used for acute diseases in which death, if it occurs, occurs relatively soon after diagnosis. Thus, if the usual natural history of the disease is known, the use of *case-fatality* refers to the period after diagnosis during which death might be expected to occur.

The case-fatality rate is ideally suited to diseases that are short-term, acute conditions. However, in chronic diseases, in which death may occur many years after diagnosis and the possibility of death from other causes becomes more likely, the case-fatality rate becomes a less useful measure. We therefore use different approaches for expressing prognosis in such diseases.

FIVE-YEAR SURVIVAL

The next term for expressing prognosis is *5-year survival*. This term is frequently employed in clinical medicine, particularly in evaluating treatments for cancer.

Five-year survival is the percent of patients who are alive 5 years after treatment begins or 5 years after diagnosis. Despite the use of the 5-year interval, it should be pointed out that there is nothing magical about 5 years. Certainly, no significant biologic change occurs abruptly at 5 years in the natural history of a disease that would justify its use as an endpoint. However, most deaths from cancer occur during this period after diagnosis, so 5-year survival has been used as an index of success in cancer treatment.

One problem in using the 5-year survival has become more prominent in recent years, with the advent of screening programs. Let us examine a hypothetical example: Figure 5–2 shows a timeline for a woman who in 1987 had biologic onset of breast cancer. Because the disease was subclinical at that time, she had no symptoms; not until 1991 did she feel a lump in her breast that precipitated a visit to the doctor who made the diagnosis, after

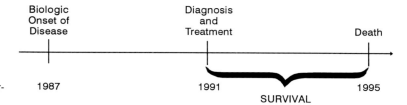

Figure 5–2. The problem of 5-year survival in a screened population: I.

which the patient underwent a mastectomy. In 1995 she died of metastatic cancer. As measured by the 5-year survival, which is often used as a measure of successful therapy in oncology, this patient is not a "success," as she survived for only 4 years.

Let us now imagine that this woman lived in a community in which there was an aggressive breast cancer screening campaign (Fig. 5–3). As before, biologic onset was in 1987, but in 1989 she was identified through screening as having a very small mass in her breast. She was operated on in 1989 and died in 1995. Having survived 6 years after the therapy, she would now be identified as a therapeutic success in terms of 5-year survival. But this apparently longer survival is an artifact. Death still occurred in 1995; the patient's life was not lengthened by early detection and therapy. What has happened is that the interval between diagnosis (and treatment) and death was increased by earlier diagnosis, but there was no delay in time of death. (The interval by which the diagnosis has been made earlier is called the *lead time*, and is discussed in detail in Chapter 17 in the context of evaluating screening.) So it is misleading to conclude that, given the patient's increased 5-year survival, the outcome of the second scenario is any better than the first, because no change in the natural history of the disease has occurred as reflected by the year

of death. Indeed, the only change that has taken place is that when the diagnosis was made 2 years earlier (1989 vs. 1991), the patient received medical care for breast cancer, with all its attendant difficulties, for an additional 2 years. Thus, when screening is carried out, a higher 5-year survival may be observed, not because people live longer but only because an earlier diagnosis has been made. This type of potential bias must be taken into account in the evaluation of any screening program before it can be concluded that the screening is beneficial.

Another problem with 5-year survival is that if we want to look at the survival experience of a group of patients who were diagnosed less than 5 years ago, we clearly cannot use this criterion, because 5 years of observation are necessary in these patients to calculate 5-year survival. Therefore, if we want to assess a therapy that was introduced less than 5 years ago, 5-year survival is not an appropriate measure.

OBSERVED SURVIVAL

Another approach is to use the actual observed survival over time. For this purpose we use a *life-table* approach. Let us examine the conceptual

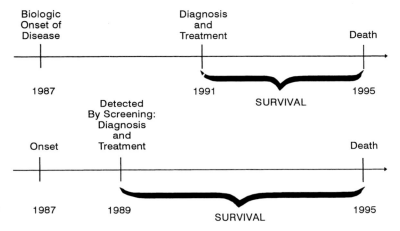

Figure 5–3. The problem of 5-year survival in a screened population: II.

Table 5–1. Hypothetical Study of Treatment Results in Patients Treated From 1990 to 1994 and Followed to 1995 (None Lost to Follow-up)

Year of Treatment	No. of Patients Treated	No. Alive on Anniversary of Treatment				
		1991	*1992*	*1993*	*1994*	*1995*
1990	84	44	21	13	10	8
1991	62		31	14	10	6
1992	93			50	20	13
1993	60				29	16
1994	76					43

framework underlying the calculation of survival rates using a life table.

Table 5–1 shows a hypothetical study of treatment results in patients who were treated from 1990 to 1994 and followed to 1995. (By just glancing at this table you can tell that the example is a hypothetical one, because the title indicates "none lost to follow-up.")

For each calendar year of treatment the table shows the number of patients enrolled in treatment and the number alive at each calendar year following initiation of that treatment. For example, of 84 patients enrolled in treatment in 1990, 44 were alive in 1991; a year after beginning treatment, 21 were alive in 1992; and so on.

The results in Table 5–1 are all the data that are available for assessing the treatment. If we want to describe the prognosis in these treated patients using all the data in the table, obviously we cannot use 5-year survival, because the entire group of 375 patients has not been observed for 5 years. We could calculate 5-year survival using only the 84 patients who were enrolled in 1990 and who were observed until 1995, because they were the only ones observed for 5 years. However, this would require us to discard the rest of the data, which would be unfortunate given the effort and expense involved in obtaining the data, and also given the

additional light that the survival experience of those patients would cast on the effectiveness of the treatment. So the question is how to use *all* the information in Table 5–1 to describe the survival experience of the patients in this study?

In order to use all the data, we rearrange the data from Table 5–1 as shown in Table 5–2. In this table the data are shown as the number of patients started on treatment each calendar year, and the number of these who are alive on each anniversary of the beginning of treatment. Note that the patients who came in 1994 were observed for only 1 year, since the study ended in 1995.

With the data in this format, how do we use the table? First we ask, What is the probability of surviving 1 year after the beginning of treatment (Table 5–3)? To answer this, we total the number of patients started on treatment (375), and add up the number of patients who were alive 1 year after treatment (197). The probability of surviving the first year is as follows:

$$\frac{197}{375} = .52$$

Next, we ask, What is the probability that, having survived the first year after beginning treatment, the patient will survive the second year? We see in Table 5–4 that 197 people survived the first year,

Table 5–2. Rearrangement of Data in Table 5–1, Showing Survival Tabulated by Years Since Enrollment in Treatment (None Lost to Follow-up)

Year of Treatment	No. of Patients Treated	No. Alive at End of Year				
		1st Year	*2nd Year*	*3rd Year*	*4th Year*	*5th Year*
1990	84	44	21	13	10	8
1991	62	31	14	10	6	
1992	93	50	20	13		
1993	60	29	16			
1994	76	43				

Table 5–3. Analysis of Survival in Patients Treated From 1990 to 1994 and Followed to 1995 (None Lost to Follow-up): I

Year of Treatment	No. of Patients Treated	No. Alive at End of Year				
		1st Year	2nd Year	3rd Year	4th Year	5th Year
1990	84	44	21	13	10	8
1991	62	31	14	10	6	
1992	93	50	20	13		
1993	60	29	16			
1994	76	43				
Total	375	197				

$$\text{Probability of surviving the 1st year} = \frac{197}{375} = 0.52$$

but for 43 of them (the ones who were enrolled in 1994) we have no further information, because they were only observed for 1 year. Because 71 survived the second year, we calculate the probability of surviving the second year, if the patient has survived the first year, as follows:

$$P = \frac{71}{197 - 43} = .46$$

We subtract the 43 for whom we have no data.

Following this pattern, we ask, Given that a person has survived to the end of the second year, what is the probability that he or she will survive to the end of the third year?

In Table 5–5, we see that 36 survived the third year. Although 71 had survived the second year, we have no further information on survival for 16 of them because they were enrolled late in the study. We therefore subtract 16 from 71, and calculate the probability of surviving the third year, given survival to the end of the second year, as follows:

$$\frac{36}{71 - 16} = .65$$

We then ask, if a person survives to the end of the third year, what is the probability that he or she will survive to the end of the fourth year?

As seen in Table 5–6, 36 people survived the third year, but we have no further information for 13 of them. Since 16 survived the fourth year, the probability of surviving the fourth year, if the person has survived the third year, is as follows:

$$\frac{16}{36 - 13} = .70$$

Finally, we do the same calculation for the fifth year (Table 5–7). We see that 16 people survived the fourth year, but that no further information is available for 6.

Since eight people were alive at the end of the fifth year, the probability of surviving the fifth year, if the person has survived the fourth year, is as follows:

Table 5–4. Analysis of Survival in Patients Treated From 1990 to 1994 and Followed to 1995 (None Lost to Follow-up): II

Year of Treatment	No. of Patients Treated	No. Alive at End of Year				
		1st Year	2nd Year	3rd Year	4th Year	5th Year
1990	84	44	21	13	10	8
1991	62	31	14	10	6	
1992	93	50	20	13		
1993	60	29	16			
1994	76	43				
Total	375	197	71			

$$\text{Probability of surviving the 2nd year} = \frac{71}{197 - 43} = 0.46$$

Table 5–5. Analysis of Survival in Patients Treated From 1990 to 1994 and Followed to 1995 (None Lost to Follow-up): III

Year of Treatment	No. of Patients Treated	No. Alive at End of Year				
		1st Year	2nd Year	3rd Year	4th Year	5th Year
1990	84	44	21	13	10	8
1991	62	31	14	10	6	
1992	93	50	20	13		
1993	60	29	16			
1994	76	43				
Total			71	36		

$$\text{Probability of surviving the 3rd year} = \frac{36}{71 - 16} = 0.65$$

Table 5–6. Analysis of Survival in Patients Treated From 1990 to 1994 and Followed to 1995 (None Lost to Follow-up): IV

Year of Treatment	No. of Patients Treated	No. Alive at End of Year				
		1st Year	2nd Year	3rd Year	4th Year	5th Year
1990	84	44	21	13	10	8
1991	62	31	14	10	6	
1992	93	50	20	13		
1993	60	29	16			
1994	76	43				
Total				36	16	

$$\text{Probability of surviving the 4th year} = \frac{16}{36 - 13} = 0.70$$

Table 5–7. Analysis of Survival in Patients Treated From 1990 to 1994 and Followed to 1995 (None Lost to Follow-up): V

Year of Treatment	No. of Patients Treated	No. Alive at End of Year				
		1st Year	2nd Year	3rd Year	4th Year	5th Year
1990	84	44	21	13	10	8
1991	62	31	14	10	6	
1992	93	50	20	13		
1993	60	29	16			
1994	76	43				
Total					16	8

$$\text{Probability of surviving the 5th year} = \frac{8}{16 - 6} = 0.80$$

Table 5–8. Probability of Survival for Each Year of the Study

P_1 = Probability of surviving the first year $= \dfrac{197}{375} = 0.52 = 52\%$

P_2 = Probability of surviving the second year given survival to the end of the first year $= \dfrac{71}{197 - 43} = 0.46 = 46\%$

P_3 = Probability of surviving the third year given survival to the end of the second year $= \dfrac{36}{71 - 16} = 0.65 = 65\%$

P_4 = Probability of surviving the fourth year given survival to the end of the third year $= \dfrac{16}{36 - 13} = 0.70 = 70\%$

P_5 = Probability of surviving the fifth year given survival to the end of the fourth year $= \dfrac{8}{16 - 6} = 0.80 = 80\%$

$$\frac{8}{16 - 6} = .80$$

Using all data that we have calculated, we ask, What is the probability of surviving for all 5 years? Table 5–8 shows all the probabilities of surviving for each individual year that we have calculated.

Returning to our original question: If a person is enrolled in the study, what is the probability that he or she will survive 5 years after beginning treatment? The probability of surviving for 5 years is the product of each of the probabilities of surviving each year, shown in Table 5–8. So the probability of surviving for 5 years

$$= P_1 \times P_2 \times P_3 \times P_4 \times P_5$$
$$= .52 \times .46 \times .65 \times .70 \times .80$$
$$= .088, \text{ or } 8.8\%$$

The probabilities for surviving different lengths of time are shown in Table 5–9. These calculations can be presented graphically in a survival curve as seen in Figure 5–4. Note that these calculations use all of the data we have obtained, including the data for patients who were not observed for the full 5 years of the study. As a result, the use of data is very economical and efficient.

Two important assumptions are made in using life tables. The first is that there has been no secular (temporal) change in the effectiveness of treatment or in survivorship over calendar time. That is, we assume that over the period of the study there has been no improvement in treatment and that survivorship in one calendar year of the study is the same as in another calendar year of the study. Clearly, if a study is conducted over many years, this assumption may not be valid as–fortunately– therapies improve over time.

The second assumption relates to follow-up of persons enrolled in the study. In every study, persons are lost to follow-up. (As mentioned previously, this problem does not appear in the hypothetical example just presented.) People can be lost to follow-up for many reasons: Some may die and not be traced. Some may move or seek care elsewhere. Some may be lost because their disease disappears and they feel well. In most studies, we do not know the actual reasons for loss to follow-up. How can we handle people lost to follow-up for whom we therefore have no further information on survival? Because we have baseline data on these people, we could compare their characteristics with those of persons who remained in the study, but it nevertheless remains a problem. If a large proportion of the study population is lost to follow-up, the

Table 5–9. Cumulative Probabilities of Surviving Different Lengths of Time

Probability of surviving 1 year $= P_1$
$= .52 = 52\%$

Probability of surviving 2 years $= P_1 \times P_2$
$= .52 \times .46 = .239 = 23.9\%$

Probability of surviving 3 years $= P_1 \times P_2 \times P_3$
$= .52 \times .46 \times .65 = .156 = 15.6\%$

Probability of surviving 4 years $= P_1 \times P_2 \times P_3 \times P_4$
$= .52 \times .46 \times .65 \times .70 = .109 = 10.9\%$

Probability of surviving 5 years $= P_1 \times P_2 \times P_3 \times P_4 \times P_5$
$= .52 \times .46 \times .65 \times .70 \times .80 = .088 = 8.8\%$

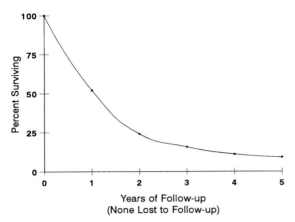

Figure 5–4. Survival curve for hypothetical example of patients treated from 1990–1994 and followed to 1995.

findings will be less valid. The challenge is to minimize loss to follow-up. In any case, the second assumption made in life tables is that the survival experience of people who are lost to follow-up is the same as the experience of those who are followed up. Although this assumption is made for purposes of calculation, in actual fact its validity may often be questionable.

Life tables are used in virtually every clinical area. They are the standard means by which survival is expressed and compared. Let us examine a few examples. One of the great triumphs of pediatrics in recent decades has been the treatment of leukemia in children. However, the improvement

has been much greater for whites than for blacks, and the reasons for this are not clear. At a time when survival rates from childhood acute leukemia were increasing rapidly, a study was carried out to explore the racial differences in survivorship. Figures 5–5 through 5–7 show data from this study.[1] The curves are based on life tables that were constructed using the approach just discussed.

Figure 5–5 shows survival for white and black children with leukemia in Baltimore over a 15-year period. No black children survived more than 4 years, while there were white children who survived up to 11 years in this 15-year period of observation.

What changes took place in survivorship during the 15 years of the study? Figure 5–6 and Figure 5–7 show changes in leukemia mortality over time in whites and blacks, respectively. The 15-year period was divided into three 5-year periods: 1960–1964 (dotted line), 1965–1969 (dashed line), and 1970–1975 (solid line).

In whites (see Fig. 5–6), survivorship increased in each successive time period. For example, if we examine 3-year survival by looking at the 3-year point on each successive curve, we see that survival has improved from 8% to 25% to 58%. In contrast, in blacks (see Fig. 5–7), there was much less improvement in survival over time; the curves for two later 5-year periods almost overlap.

What accounts for this racial difference? First, we must take account of the small numbers involved and the possibility that the observations

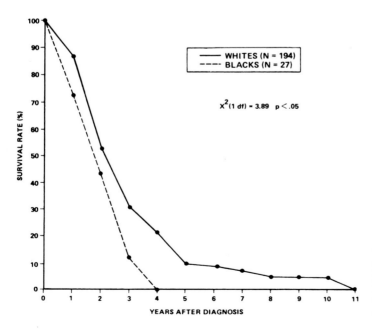

Figure 5–5. Survival of children aged 0 to 19 years with acute lymphocytic leukemia by race, metropolitan Baltimore, 1960–1975. (From Szklo M, Gordis L, Tonascia J, Kaplan E: The changing survivorship of white and black children with leukemia. Cancer 42:59–66, 1978.)

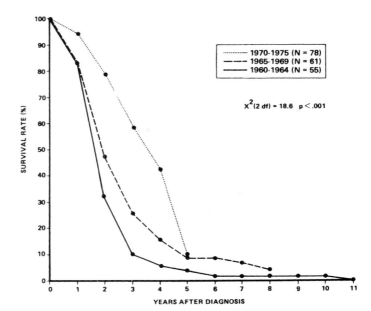

Figure 5–6. Temporal changes in survival of white children aged 0 to 19 years with acute lymphocytic leukemia, metropolitan Baltimore, 1960–1975. (From Szklo M, Gordis L, Tonascia J, Kaplan E: The changing survivorship of white and black children with leukemia. Cancer 42:59–66, 1978.)

could have been due to chance. Let us assume, however, that the differences are real. During the past several decades tremendous strides have occurred in the treatment of leukemia through combined therapy, including central nervous system radiation added to chemotherapy. Why then does a racial difference exist in survivorship? Why is it that the improvement in therapy that has been so effective in whites has not had a comparable benefit in black children? Further analyses of the interval from the time the mother noticed symptoms to the time of diagnosis and treatment indicated that the

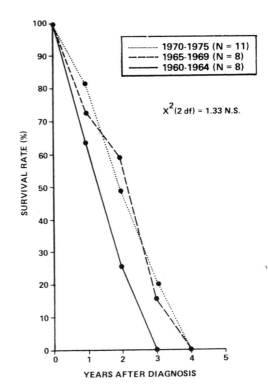

Figure 5–7. Temporal changes in survival of black children aged 0 to 19 years with acute lymphocytic leukemia, metropolitan Baltimore, 1960–1975. (From Szklo M, Gordis L, Tonascia J, Kaplan E: The changing survivorship of white and black children with leukemia. Cancer 42:59–66, 1978.)

differences in survival did not appear to be due to a delay in blacks seeking or obtaining medical care. Because acute leukemia is more severe in blacks and more advanced at the time of diagnosis, the racial difference could also reflect biologic differences in the disease, such as a more aggressive and rapidly progressive form of the illness. The definitive explanation is not yet clear.

MEDIAN SURVIVAL TIME

Another approach to expressing prognosis is the *median survival time,* which is defined as the length of time that half of the study population survives. Why should we use median survival time rather than mean survival time, which is an average of the survival times? Median survival offers two advantages over mean survival: First, it is less affected by extremes, whereas the mean is significantly affected by even a single outlier. One or two persons with a very long survival time could significantly affect the mean, even if all the other survival times were much shorter. Second, if we used mean survival, we would have to observe all the deaths in the study population before the mean could be calculated. However, to calculate median survival, we would only have to observe the deaths of half the group.

RELATIVE SURVIVAL RATE

Let us consider 5-year survival for a group of 30-year-old men with colon cancer. What would we expect their survival to be if they did not have colon cancer? Clearly, it would be near 100%. So we are comparing the survival rate observed in young men with colon cancer to an expected survival of almost 100% in the absence of colon cancer. What if we consider a group of 80-year-old men with colon cancer? We would not expect anything near 100% survival in a population of this age, even without colon cancer. Again, we would want to compare the observed survival in 80-year-old men with colon cancer to the survival expected in the absence of colon cancer. So for any group of people with a disease, we want to compare their survival to the survival we would expect in this age group if they did *not* have the disease. This is known as the *relative survival rate.*

The relative survival rate is defined as the ratio of the observed survival to the expected survival rate:

$$\text{Relative survival rate} = \frac{\text{Observed survival in people with the disease}}{\text{Expected survival if disease were absent}}$$

Does relative survival really make any difference?

Table 5–10 shows data for cancer of the rectum, both relative survival and the observed survival. When we look at the older age groups, whose numbers have high mortality from other causes, there is a large difference between the observed and the relative survival rates. But in young persons, who generally do not die of other causes, the observed survival and the relative survival rates for cancer of the rectum do not differ significantly.

GENERALIZABILITY OF SURVIVAL DATA

A final point in connection with the natural history and prognosis of disease is the question of which patients are selected for study. Let us look at one example.

Febrile seizures are common in infants: Children who are otherwise normal often experience a seizure in association with high fever. The question arises whether these children should be put on a regimen of phenobarbital or another long-term anticonvulsant medication. That is, is a febrile seizure a sign of subsequent epilepsy, or is it just a phenomenon associated with fever in infants, in which case children are unlikely to have subsequent nonfebrile seizures?

To make a rational decision regarding treatment, the question is: What is the risk that a child who has had a febrile seizure will have a subsequent nonfebrile seizure? Figure 5–8 shows the results of an analysis by Ellenberg and Nelson of published studies.[2]

Table 5–10. Five-Year Observed and Relative Survival Rates (%) by Age for Colon Cancer in White Males and Females: SEER* Program, 1981–1987

Age (yr)	Observed Rate (%)	Relative Rate (%)
<45	55.6	56.3
45–54	57.1	59.2
55–64	53.6	58.5
65–74	47.8	57.8
≥75	31.7	54.1

*Surveillance, Epidemiology, and End Results Study.
From Ries LAG, Hankey BF, Miller BA, et al: Cancer Statistics Review, 1973–88. Bethesda, Md, National Cancer Institute, NIH Publication No. 91–2789, 1991.

Each dot shows the percent of children with febrile seizures who later developed nonfebrile seizures in a different study. The authors divided the studies into two groups: Studies that were population-based and studies that were based on individual clinics, such as epilepsy or pediatric clinics. Examining the results from different clinic-based studies, we see a considerable range of risks of development of later nonfebrile seizures. But when the results of population-based studies are examined, very little variation in the risks is seen, and the results of all of the studies tend to cluster at a very low level.

Why should the two types of studies differ? Which results would you believe? Each of the clinics probably had different selection criteria, and different referral patterns. Consequently, the different risks observed in the different clinic-based studies are probably the result of selection of different populations to each of the clinics. In the population-based studies, on the other hand, this type of varia-

Table 5–11. Five Approaches to Expressing Prognosis

1. Case-fatality rate
2. 5-year survival
3. Observed survival rate
4. Median survival time
5. Relative survival rate

tion due to selection is reduced or eliminated, which accounts for the clustering of the data and the resultant finding that the risk of nonfebrile seizures is very low. The important point is that it may be very tempting to go to a single hospital, look at patient records, and generalize to all patients in the general population. But it is not legitimate to do so, because patients who come to a specific clinic or hospital, for example, are often not representative of all patients in the community. This does not mean that studies conducted at single hospitals cannot be of value. Indeed, there is much to be learned from doing studies at single hospitals. But such studies are particularly prone to selection bias, and this possibility must always be kept in mind when findings and their potential generalizability are being interpreted.

SUMMARY

This chapter has discussed five ways of expressing prognosis (Table 5–11). Which approach is best depends on the kind of data that are available and on the purpose of the analysis for which the data will be used. Chapters 6 and 7 address the use of randomized trials for selecting the optimal means of intervention.

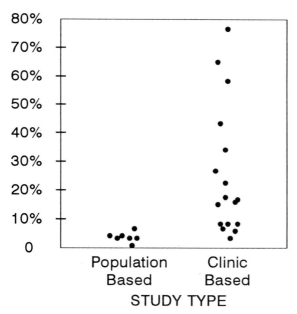

Figure 5–8. Percentage of children who experienced non-febrile seizures after one or more febrile seizures, by study design. (Adapted from Ellenberg JH, Nelson KB: Sample selection and the natural history of disease: Studies on febrile seizures. JAMA 243:1337–1340, 1980.)

References

1. Szklo M, Gordis L, Tonascia J, Kaplan E: The changing survivorship of white and black children with leukemia. Cancer 42:59–66, 1978.
2. Ellenberg JH, Nelson KB: Sample selection and the natural history of disease: Studies on febrile seizures. JAMA 243:1337–1340, 1980.

Review Questions

1. Which of the following is/are a good index of the severity of a short-term, acute disease:
   a. Cause-specific death rate
   b. 5-year survival
   c. Case-fatality rate
   d. Standardized mortality ratio
   e. None of the above

Question 2 is based on the information given below:

One hundred eighty patients were treated for disease X from 1991 to 1993, and their progress was followed to 1994. The treatment results are given in the following table. No patients were lost to follow-up.

Year of Treatment	No. of Patients Treated	No. of Patients Alive on Each Anniversary		
		1st	2nd	3rd
1991	75	60	56	48
1992	63	55	31	
1993	42	37		
	180	152	87	48

2. The probability of surviving 3 years is _____.
3. An important assumption in this type of analysis is that:
   a. Treatment has improved during the period of the study
   b. Quality of record-keeping has improved during the period of the study
   c. No change has occurred in the effectiveness of the treatment during the period of the study
   d. An equal number of men and women were enrolled each year
   e. None of the above

4. A diagnostic test has been introduced that will detect a certain disease 1 year earlier than it is usually detected. Which of the following is *most likely* to happen to the disease within the 10 years after the test is introduced? (Assume that early detection has no effect on the natural history of the disease. Also assume that no changes in death certification practices occur during the 10 years.)
   a. The period prevalence rate will decrease
   b. The apparent 5-year survival rate will increase
   c. The age-adjusted mortality rate will decrease
   d. The age-adjusted mortality rate will increase
   e. The incidence rate will decrease

5. Which of the following statement(s) pertains to relative survival?
   a. Refers to survival of first-degree relatives
   b. Is generally closer to observed survival in elderly populations
   c. Is generally closer to observed survival in young populations
   d. Generally differs from observed survival by a constant amount, regardless of age
   e. None of the above

CHAPTER 6

Assessing the Efficacy of Preventive and Therapeutic Measures: Randomized Trials

Some ways of quantifying the natural history of disease and of expressing disease prognosis were discussed in Chapter 5. Our objective, both in public health and in clinical practice, is to modify the natural history of a disease so as to prevent or delay death or disability and to improve the health of the patient or the population. The challenge is to select the best available preventive or therapeutic measures to achieve this goal. To do so, we need to carry out studies that determine the value of these measures. The randomized trial is considered the ideal design for evaluating both the effectiveness and the side effects of new forms of intervention.

The notion of using a rigorous methodology to assess the efficacy of new drugs, or of any new modalities of care, is not new. In 1883, Sir Francis Galton, the British anthropologist, explorer, and eugenicist, who had a strong interest in human intelligence, wrote as follows:

It was asserted by some that men possess the faculty of obtaining results over which they have little or no direct personal control, by means of devout and earnest prayer, while others doubt the truth of this assertion. The question regards a matter of fact, that has to be determined by observation and not by authority; and it is one that appears to be a very suitable topic for statistical inquiry . . . Are prayers answered or are they not? . . . Do sick persons, who pray or are prayed for, recover on the average more rapidly than others?[1]

As with many pioneering ideas in science and medicine, many years were to pass before this suggestion was actually implemented. In 1965, Joyce and Welldon reported the results of a double-blind clinical trial of the efficacy of prayer.[2] The findings of this study did not indicate that patients who were prayed for derived any benefits from that prayer. However a more recent study by Byrd[3] evaluated the effectiveness of intercessory prayer in a coronary care unit population using a randomized double-blind protocol. The findings from this study suggested that prayer had a beneficial therapeutic effect.

In this chapter and the one following, we discuss the possible study designs that can be used for evaluating new approaches to treatment and prevention, and focus on the randomized trial. Although the term *randomized clinical trial* is often used, the randomized trial design also has major applicability to studies outside of the clinical setting, such as community-based trials. For this reason, we use the term *randomized trial*. To facilitate our discussion, reference is generally made to treatments and drugs; the reader should bear in mind that the principles described apply equally to evaluations of preventive and other measures.

Suggestions of many of the elements that are important to randomized trials can be seen in many anecdotal descriptions of early trials. In a review of the history of clinical trials, Bull describes an unintentional trial conducted by Ambroise Paré (1510–1590), a leading figure in surgery during the Renaissance.[4] Paré lived at a time when the standard treatment for war wounds was the application of boiling oil. In 1537, Paré was responsible for the treatment of the wounded after the capture of the castle of Villaine. The wounded were so numerous that, he says:

At length my oil lacked and I was constrained to apply in its place a digestive made of yolks of eggs, oil of roses and turpentine. That night I could not sleep at my ease, fearing that by lack of cauterization I would find the wounded upon which I had not used the said oil, dead from the poison. I raised myself early to visit them, when beyond my hope I found those to whom I had applied the digestive medicament feeling but little pain, their wounds neither swollen nor inflamed, and having slept through the night. The others to whom I had applied the boiling oil were feverish with much pain and swelling about their wounds. Then I determined never again to burn thus so cruelly the poor wounded.

Although this was not a randomized trial, it was a form of unplanned trial, which has been carried out many times when a therapy thought to be the best available has been in short supply and has not been available for all of the patients who needed it.

A planned trial was described by James Lind in 1747. He wrote on scurvy as follows:

I took 12 patients in the scurvy on board the Salisbury at sea. The cases were as similar as I could have them . . . they lay together in one place and had one diet common to them all. Two of these were ordered a quart of cider per day. . . . Two others took 25 gutts of elixir vitriol. . . . Two others took two spoonfuls of vinegar. . . . Two were put under a course of sea water. . . . Two others had two oranges and one lemon given them each day. . . . Two others took the bigness of nutmeg. The most sudden and visible good effects were perceived from the use of oranges and lemons, one of those who had taken them being at the end of 6 days fit for duty. . . . The other . . . was appointed nurse to the rest of the sick.[5]

Randomized trials can be used for many purposes. They can be used for evaluating new drugs and other treatments of disease, including tests of new health and medical care technology. Such trials can be used to assess new programs for screening and early detection, or new ways of organizing and delivering health services.

The basic design of a randomized trial is shown in Figure 6–1.

We begin with a defined population that is randomized to new treatment or current treatment and we follow the subjects in each group to see how many are improved in the new treatment group compared with the current treatment group. If the new treatment is associated with a better outcome, we would expect to find better outcome in more of

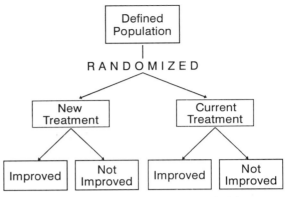

Figure 6–1. Design of a randomized trial.

the new treatment group than the current treatment group.

We may choose to compare two different therapies, or we may compare more than two groups. Although at times a treatment may be compared with no treatment, a decision may be made not to use an untreated group. For example, if we wanted to evaluate a newly developed therapy for acquired immunodeficiency syndrome (AIDS), would we be willing to have a group of AIDS patients in our study who were untreated? The answer is clearly no; we would compare the newly developed therapy with the best therapy currently available and in use, which although not ideal is presumably better than no therapy at all.

Let us now turn to some of the issues that must be considered in the design of randomized trials.

SELECTION OF SUBJECTS

The criteria for determining who will or will not be included in the study must be spelled out with great precision, and *in writing*. An excellent test of the adequacy of these written criteria is to ask: If we have spelled out our criteria in writing, and someone walks in off the street and applies our criteria to the same population, will they select the same subjects whom we would have selected? There should be no element of subjective decision-making on the part of the investigator in deciding who is included or not in the study. Any study must in principle be replicable by others, just as is the case with laboratory experiments. Clearly, this is easier said than done, because in randomized trials we are often dealing with relatively large populations. The principle is nevertheless important, and the criteria must therefore be precisely stated.

ALLOCATION OF SUBJECTS TO TREATMENT GROUPS

Before discussing the process of randomization, let us ask whether there might not be some alternatives to randomization that could be employed.

Studies Without Comparison

The first possible alternative is the *case study* or *case series:* that is, no comparison is made with an untreated group or with a group receiving some other treatment. The following story was told by Dr. Earl Peacock when he was chairman of the Department of Surgery at the University of Arizona:

> One day when I was a junior medical student, a very important Boston surgeon visited the school and delivered a great treatise on a large number of patients who had undergone successful operations for vascular reconstruction. At the end of the lecture, a young student at the back of the room timidly asked, "Do you have any controls?" Well, the great surgeon drew himself up to his full height, hit the desk, and said, "Do you mean did I not operate on half of the patients?" The hall grew very quiet then. The voice at the back of the room very hesitantly replied, "Yes, that's what I had in mind." Then the visitor's fist really came down as he thundered, "Of course not. That would have doomed half of them to their death." God, it was quiet then, and one could scarcely hear the small voice ask, "Which half?"[6]

The issue of comparison is important because we want to be able to derive a causal inference regarding the relationship of a treatment and subsequent outcome. The problem of inferring a causal relationship from a sequence of events without any comparison is demonstrated in a story cited by Ederer.[7]

> During World War II, rescue workers digging in the ruins of an apartment house blown up in the London blitz, found an old man lying naked in a bathtub, fully conscious. He said to his rescuers: "You know, that was the most amazing experience I ever had. When I pulled the plug and the water started down the drain, the whole house blew up."

The problem exemplified by this story is: If we administer a drug and the patient improves, can we attribute the improvement to the administration of that drug? Professor Hugo Muensch of Harvard articulated his Second Law: "Results can always be improved by omitting controls."[8]

Studies With Comparison

If we therefore recognize the need for our study to include some type of comparison, what are the possible designs?

Historical Controls

We could use a comparison group from the past, called *historical controls.* We have a therapy today that we believe will be quite effective, and we would like to test it in a group of patients; we realize we need a comparison group. So for comparison, we will go back to the records of patients with the same disease who were treated before the new therapy became available. This type of design seems inherently simple and attractive.

What are the problems in using historical controls? First, if today we decide to carry out the study just described, we may set up a very meticulous system for data collection from the patients currently being treated. But of course we cannot do that for the patients who were treated in the past, for whom we must abstract data from medical records. Those records were generated for clinical purposes at the time and not for research purposes. Consequently, if at the end of the study we find a difference in outcome between patients treated in the early period (historical controls) and patients treated in the later (current) period, we will not know whether there was a true difference in outcome or whether the observed difference was due only to a difference in the quality of the data collection. The data obtained from the study groups must be comparable in kind and quality; in studies using historical controls, this is often not the case.

The second problem is that if we observe a difference in outcome between the early group and the later group, we will not be sure that the difference is due to the therapy, because many things other than the therapy change over calendar time (e.g., ancillary supportive therapy, living conditions, nutrition, and lifestyles). Hence, if we observe a difference and if we have ruled out differences in data quality as the reason for the observed difference, we will not know whether the difference is a result of the drug we are studying or of changes that take place in many other factors over calendar time.

At times, however, this type of design may be

desirable. For example, when a disease is uniformly fatal initially and a new drug becomes available, a significant decline in case-fatality would strongly support the conclusion that the new drug is having an effect, although the possibility that the decline could have resulted from other changes in the environment would have to be ruled out.

Simultaneous Non-randomized Controls

Because of the importance of the problems posed by historical controls and the difficulties of dealing with changes over calendar time, an alternative approach is to use simultaneous controls that are not selected in a randomized manner. The problem with selecting simultaneous controls in a non-randomized manner is illustrated by the following story:

A sea captain was given samples of anti-nausea pills to test during a voyage. The need for controls was carefully explained to him. Upon return of the ship, the captain reported the results enthusiastically. "Practically every one of the controls was ill, and not one of the subjects had any trouble. Really wonderful stuff." A skeptic asked how he had chosen the controls and the subjects. "Oh, I gave the stuff to my seamen and used the passengers as controls."[9]

There are a number of possible approaches for selecting controls in such a non-randomized fashion. One is to assign patients by the day of the month on which the patient is admitted to the hospital: for example, if admission is on an odd-numbered day of the month the patient is in group A, and if admission is on an even-numbered day of the month the patient is in group B. In a trial of anticoagulant therapy after World War II, in which this day-of-the-month method was used, it was discovered that more patients than expected were admitted on odd-numbered days. The investigators reported that "as physicians observed the benefits of anticoagulant therapy, they speeded up, where feasible, the hospitalization of those patients . . . who would routinely have been hospitalized on an even day in order to bring as many as possible under the odd-day deadline."[10]

The problem here is that the assignment system was predictable: it was possible for the physicians to know what the assignment of the next patient would be. What randomization accomplishes is to eliminate the possibility of knowing what the as-

signment of the next patient will be, as such knowledge introduces the possibility of a selection bias.

Many years ago a study was carried out of the effects of bacille Calmette-Guérin (BCG) vaccination against tuberculosis in children from tuberculous families in New York City.[11] The physicians were told to divide the group of eligible children into a group to be immunized and a control group.

As seen in Table 6–1, tuberculosis mortality was almost five times higher in the controls than in the vaccinated children. However, as the investigators wrote: "Subsequent experience has shown that by this method of selection, the tendency was to inoculate the children of the more intelligent and cooperative parents and to keep the children of the noncooperative parents as controls. This was probably of considerable error since the cooperative parent will not only keep more careful precautions, but will usually bring the child more regularly to the clinic for instruction as to child care and feeding."

Recognizing that the vaccinations were selectively performed in children from families more likely to be conscious of health and related issues, it was possible that the mortality rate from tuberculosis was lower in the vaccinated group not because of the vaccination itself, but because these children were selected from more health-conscious families that had a lower risk of mortality from tuberculosis, with or without a vaccination. To address this problem, a change was made in the study design: Alternate children were vaccinated and the remainder served as controls: this does not constitute randomization, but it was a marked improvement over the initial design. As seen in Table 6–2, there was now no difference between the groups.

Randomization

In view of the problems discussed, randomization is the best approach in design of a trial. Randomization means, in effect, tossing a coin to decide assignment of a patient to a study group. The critical

Table 6–1. Results of a Trial of BCG Vaccination—I

	No. of Children	TB Deaths	
		No.	%
Vaccinated	445	3	0.67
Controls	545	18	3.30

Data from Levine MI, Sackett MF: Results of BCG immunization in New York City. Am Rev Tuberculosis 53:517–532, 1946.

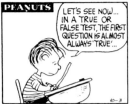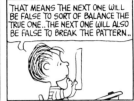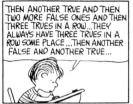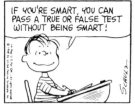

Figure 6–2. How to predict the next patient's treatment assignment in a randomized study. (From Schulz C: Peanuts cartoon of October 3, 1968. Reproduced by permission of United Features Syndicate.)

element of randomization is the unpredictability of the next assignment. Ederer cited Figure 6–2 to demonstrate the problem of predictability of the next assignment.[12]

How is randomization accomplished? This example uses a selection from a table of random numbers (Table 6–3). (Such random-number tables are available in most statistics textbooks.) Today, particularly for large trials, randomization is carried out using a computer.

First, how do we look at this table? Note that the table is divided into groups of five rows and five columns. This division is only made to enhance readability. The columns are numbered along the top, 00, 01, 02, and so on. Similarly, the rows are numbered along the left, 00, 01, 02, and so on. Thus, it is possible to refer to any digit in the table by giving its column and row numbers. This is important if the quality of the randomization process is to be checked by an outsider.

How do we use this table? Let us say we are doing a study in which there will be two groups: therapy A and therapy B. In this example, we will consider every odd number an assignment to A and every even number an assignment to B. We close our eyes and put a finger anywhere on the table, and write down which column and row number was our starting point. We also write down the direction in which we will move in the table from that starting point (horizontally to the right, horizontally to the left, up, or down). Let us assume we point to

the "5" at the intersection of column 7 and row 7, and move horizontally to the right. The first patient is then designated by an odd number, and will receive therapy A. The second patient is also designated by an odd number and will receive therapy A. The third is designated by an even number and will receive therapy B, and so on. Note that the next patient assignment is not predictable; it is *not* a strict alternation, which would be predictable.

There are other ways of using a table of random numbers. For example, we could say that digits 0 to 4 would be treatment A, and digits 5 to 9 treatment B. If we are studying three groups, we could say that digits 1 to 3 are treatment A, digits 4 to 6 treatment B, digits 7 to 9 treatment C, and digit 0 would be ignored. Any of these approaches is valid; the important point is to spell out in writing whatever approach is selected, before the randomization is actually started.

One way of using the table is to prepare a series of opaque envelopes that are numbered sequentially on the outside: 1, 2, 3, 4, 5, and so on. Inside each envelope a card is placed: a card for therapy A in the first one, for therapy B in the second one, and so on, as determined by the random numbers. The envelopes are then sealed. When the first patient is enrolled, envelope 1 is opened and the assignment is read: this is repeated for each of the remaining patients in the study.

Table 6–2. Results of a Trial of BCG Vaccination—II

| | No. of Children | TB Deaths | |
		No.	%
Vaccinated	556	8	1.44
Controls	528	8	1.52

Data from Levine MI, Sackett MF: Results of BCG immunization in New York City. Am Rev Tuberculosis 53:517–532, 1946.

Table 6–3. A Table of Random Numbers

	00–04	05–09	10–14	15–19
00	56348	01458	36236	07253
01	09372	27651	30103	37004
02	44782	54023	61355	71692
03	04383	90952	57204	57810
04	98190	89997	98839	76129
05	16263	35632	88105	59090
06	62032	90741	13468	02647
07	48457	78538	22759	12188
08	36782	06157	73084	48094
09	63302	55103	19703	74741

In a randomized study comparing radical and simple mastectomy for breast cancer, one of the surgeons participating was convinced that radical mastectomy was the treatment of choice and could not reconcile himself to performing simple mastectomy on any of his patients who were included in the study. When randomization was carried out for his patients and an envelope was opened which indicated simple mastectomy for the next assignment, he would set the envelope aside and keep opening envelopes until he reached one with an assignment to radical mastectomy.

What is reflected here is the conflict felt by many clinicians who enroll their patients in randomized trials. On the one hand, the clinician has the obligation to do the best he or she can for the patients; on the other hand when he or she participates in a clinical trial he or she is, in effect, asked to step aside from a decision-making role and to "flip a coin" to decide on the therapy that the patient will receive. Thus, there is often an underlying conflict between the clinician's role and the role of the physician participating in a clinical trial; and as a result, unintentional biases may occur.

This is such a common problem, particularly in large multi-centered trials, that randomization is not carried out in each clinical center but is rather done in a separate coordinating and statistical center. When a new patient is registered at a clinical center, the coordinating center is called and the patient's name is given. A randomized assignment is then made for that patient by the center and the assignment is noted in both locations.

What do we hope to accomplish by randomization? If we randomize properly, we achieve non-predictability of the next assignment; we do not have to worry that any subjective biases of the investigators, either overt or covert, may be introduced into the process of selecting patients for one treatment group or the other. Also, in the long run, we hope that randomization will increase the likelihood that the groups will be comparable in regard to characteristics about which we may be concerned such as sex, age, race, and severity of disease, which may affect prognosis. However, randomization is not a guarantee of comparability, because chance may play a role in the process. But over the long term, the groups will tend to be similar.

Figure 6–3 presents a hypothetical example of the effect of lack of comparability on a comparison of mortality rates of the groups being studied. Let us assume a study population of 2,000 subjects with

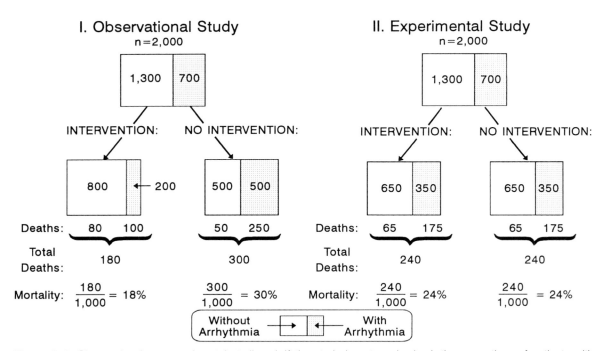

Figure 6–3. Observational vs. experimental studies. *I,* If the study is not randomized, the proportions of patients with arrhythmia in the two groups may differ. *II,* If the study is randomized, the proportions of patients with arrhythmia in the two groups are more likely to be similar.

myocardial infarctions, of whom half receive an intervention and the other half do not. Let us further assume that of the 2,000 patients, 700 have an arrhythmia X and 1,300 do not. Case-fatality in patients with the arrhythmia is 50% and in patients without the arrhythmia it is 10%.

Looking at the left side of Figure 6–3, if the groups are not comparable in the proportion of patients with the arrhythmia, by chance perhaps 200 in the intervention group will have the arrhythmia (and a case-fatality of 50%) and 500 in the no-intervention group will have the arrhythmia (and its 50% case-fatality). The result will be a case-fatality rate of 18% in the intervention group and 30% in the no-intervention group, and we might be tempted to conclude that the intervention is effective.

Let us now look at the right side of this figure, in which the groups are comparable, as we are more likely to find when we randomize—350 of the 1,000 intervention group patients and 350 of the 1,000 no-intervention group patients have the arrhythmia. When case-fatality is calculated for this example, we find it to be 24% in both groups. Thus the difference observed between intervention and no-intervention when the groups were not comparable in terms of the arrhythmia was entirely due to the non-comparability and not to any effects of the intervention itself.

One might ask, if we are so concerned about the comparability of the groups, why not just match the groups on the specific variables about which we are concerned, rather than randomizing? The answer is that we can only match on variables that we know about and that we can measure. Thus, we cannot match on many variables that may affect prognosis, such as an individual's genetic constitution, elements of an individual's immune status, or other variables of which we may not even be aware. Randomization increases the likelihood that the groups will be comparable not only in terms of variables that we recognize and can measure, but also in terms of variables that we may not recognize and may not be able to measure, but that may nevertheless affect prognosis.

Stratified Randomization

Let us say that we are particularly concerned about age as a prognostic variable: prognosis is much worse in older patients. We are therefore concerned that the two treatment groups be comparable in terms of age. Although randomization may increase the likelihood of such comparability, it

does not guarantee it. It is still possible that after we randomize we may, by chance, find that most of the older patients are in one group and most of the younger patients are in the other. Our results would then be impossible to interpret because the high-risk patients would be clustered in one group and the low-risk patients in the other, and the difference in outcome may be attributable to this difference in distribution rather than to the effects of the intervention.

One approach for dealing with this problem is called *stratified randomization*. In this approach, we first stratify (stratum = layer) our study population by each variable that we consider important, and then randomize to treatment groups within each stratum.

Let us consider the example shown in Figure 6–4. We are studying 1,000 patients and are concerned that age and sex are important determinants of prognosis. If we randomize, we do not know what the composition of the groups may be in terms of age and sex; therefore we decide to use stratified randomization.

We first stratify the 1,000 patients by sex into 600 males and 400 females. We then stratify the males by age and the females by age. We now have four groups (strata): young males, old males, young females, and old females. We now randomize *within each group,* and the result is a therapy A group and a therapy B group for each of the four groups. We end up with two randomized groups, but having initially stratified the groups, we increase the likelihood that the two groups will be comparable in terms of age and sex.

DATA COLLECTION ON SUBJECTS

As mentioned earlier, it is essential that the data collected for each of the study groups be of the same quality. Let us consider some of the variables about which data need to be obtained on the subjects.

Treatment (Assigned and Received)

What data are needed? First, we must know to which treatment group the patient was assigned. In addition, we must know which therapy the patient actually received. It is important to know, for example, if the patient was assigned to receive treatment A and did not comply. A patient may agree to be randomized, but may later change his or her mind

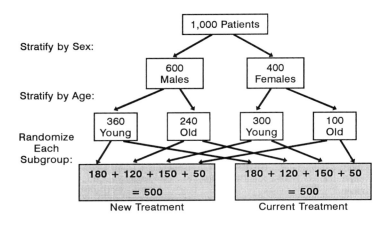

Stratify by Sex:

Stratify by Age:

Randomize Each Subgroup:

New Treatment

Current Treatment

Figure 6–4. Stratified randomization.

and refuse to comply. Conversely, it is also clearly important to know whether a patient was not assigned to treatment A but took treatment A on his own.

Outcome

The need for comparable measurements in all study groups is particularly true for measurements of outcome. Such measurements include both improvement (the desired effect) and any side effects that may appear. There is, therefore, a need for explicitly stated criteria for all outcomes to be measured in a study. Once the criteria are explicitly stated, we must be certain that they are measured comparably in all study groups. In particular, the potential pitfall of outcomes being measured more carefully in those receiving a new drug than in those receiving currently available therapy must be avoided. Blinding can prevent much of this problem, but because blinding is not always possible, attention must be given to ensuring comparability of measurements and of data quality in all of the study groups.

Prognostic Profile at Entry

If we know the risk factors for a bad outcome, we want to check that the randomization has provided a reasonable similarity between the two groups in terms of these risk factors. For example, if age is a significant risk factor, we would want to know that randomization has resulted in groups that are comparable for age. Data for prognostic factors should be obtained at the time of subject entry into the study.

Masking (Blinding)

Masking involves several components: First, we would like the subjects not to know which group they are in. This is of particular importance when the outcome is a subjective measure, such as headache or low back pain. If the patient knows that he or she is getting a new therapy, enthusiasm and certain psychological factors may operate to elicit an improved response.

How can subjects be masked? One way is by using a *placebo,* an inert substance that looks, tastes, and smells like the active agent. However, use of a placebo does not automatically guarantee that the patients are blinded. Some participants may try to determine whether they are taking the placebo or active drug. For example, in a randomized trial of vitamin C for the common cold, patients were blinded by use of a placebo and were then asked whether they knew or suspected which drug they were taking.

As seen in Table 6–4, of the 52 people who were receiving vitamin C and were willing to make a

Table 6–4. A Randomized Trial of Vitamin C and Placebo for the Common Cold: Results of a Questionnaire Study to Determine Whether Subjects Suspected Which Agent They Had Been Given

	Suspected Drug		
Actual Drug	*Vitamin C*	*Placebo*	**Total**
Vitamin C	40	12	52
Placebo	11	39	50
Total	51	51	102

$P<0.001$.
From Karlowski TR, Chalmers TC, Frenkel LD, et al: Ascorbic acid for the common cold. JAMA 231(10):1038, 1975.

Table 6–5. Physicians' Health Study: Side Effects According to Treatment Group

Side Effect	Aspirin Group (%)	Placebo Group (%)	P Value
GI symptoms (except ulcer)	34.8	34.2	0.48
Upper GI ulcers	1.5	1.3	0.08
Bleeding problems	27.0	20.4	<0.00001

Data from Steering Committee of the Physicians' Health Study Research Group: Final report on the aspirin component of the Ongoing Physicians' Health Study. N Engl J Med 321:129–135, 1989.

guess, 40 stated they had been receiving vitamin C. Of the 50 who were receiving placebo, 39 said they were receiving placebo. How did they know? They had bitten into the capsule and could tell by the bitter taste. Does it make any difference that they knew? The data suggest that the rate of colds was higher in subjects who received vitamin C but thought they were receiving placebo than in subjects who received placebo but thought they were receiving vitamin C. Thus, we must be very concerned about lack of blinding of the subjects and its potential effects on the results of the study, particularly when we are dealing with subjective endpoints.

A placebo is also important for studying the rates of side effects and reactions. The Physicians' Health Study was a randomized trial of use of aspirin as a preventive for myocardial infarctions. Table 6–5 shows side effects in groups receiving aspirin and those receiving placebo in this study.

Note the high rates of reported reactions in people receiving placebos. Thus it is not sufficient to say that 34% of the people receiving aspirin had gastrointestinal symptoms; what we really want to know is the extent to which the risk of side effects is increased in people taking aspirin compared to those not taking aspirin (i.e., those taking placebo). Thus the placebo plays a major role in identifying both the real benefits of an agent and its side effects.

In addition to blinding the subjects, we also want to mask or blind the data collectors and the data analysts in regard to which group a patient is in. This is called "double blinding." Some years ago, a study was being conducted to evaluate coronary care units in the treatment of myocardial infarction. It was planned in the following manner:

Patients who met strict criteria for categories of myocardial infarction [were to] be randomly assigned either to the group that was admitted immediately to the coronary care unit or to the group that was returned to their homes for domiciliary care. When the preliminary data were presented, it was apparent in the early phases of the experiment that the group of patients labeled as having been admitted to the coronary care unit did somewhat better than the patients sent home. An enthusiast for coronary care units was uncompromising in his insistence that the experiment was unethical and should be terminated and that the data showed that all such patients should be admitted to the coronary care unit. The statistician then revealed the headings of the data columns had been interchanged and that really the home care group seemed to have a slight advantage. The enthusiast then changed his mind and could not be persuaded to declare coronary care units unethical.[13]

The message of this example is that each of us comes to whatever study we are doing with a certain number of subconscious or conscious biases and preconceptions. The methods discussed in this chapter and the next are designed to shield the study from the biases of the investigators.

References

1. Galton F: Inquiries into Human Faculty and Its Development. London, Macmillan Co, 1883.
2. Joyce CRB, Welldon RMC: The efficacy of prayer: A double blind clinical trial. J Chron Dis 18:367, 1965.
3. Byrd RC: Positive therapeutic effects of intercessory prayer in a coronary care unit population. South Med J 81:826, 1988.
4. Bull JP: The historical development of clinical therapeutic trials. J Chron Dis 10:218, 1959.
5. Lind J: A treatise of the scurvy. Edinburgh, Sands, Murray & Cochran, 1753.
6. Peacock E. Cited in Tufte ER: Data Analyses for Politics and Policy. Englewood, NJ, Prentice Hall, 1974.
7. Ederer F: Why do we need controls? Why do we need to randomize? Am J Ophthalmol 79:758, 1975.
8. Bearman JE, Loewenson RB, Gullen WH: Muensch's Postulates, Laws and Corollaries. Biometrics note No. 4. Bethesda, Md, Office of Biometry and Epidemiology, National Eye Institute, April 1974.
9. Wilson EB. Cited in Ederer F: Why do we need controls? Why do we need to randomize? Am J Ophthalmol 79:761, 1975.
10. Wright IS, Marple CD, Beck DF. Cited in Ederer F: Why do we need controls? Why do we need to randomize? Am J Ophthalmol 79:761, 1975.
11. Levine MI, Sackett MF: Results of BCG immunization in New York City. Am Rev Tuberculosis 53:517–532, 1946.
12. Ederer F: Practical problems in collaborative clinical trials. Am J Epidemiol 102:111–118, 1975.
13. Ballintine EJ: Objective measurements and the double-masked procedure. Am J Ophthalmol 79:763–766, 1975.
14. Cochrane AL. Cited in Ballintine EJ: Objective measurements and the double-masked procedure. Am J Ophthalmol 79:764, 1975.

(Review questions for material in this chapter can be found at the end of Chapter 7, pp. 112–113.)

CHAPTER 7

Randomized Trials: Some Further Issues

SAMPLE SIZE

At a scientific meeting some years ago, an investigator presented the results of a study he had conducted to evaluate a new drug in sheep. "After taking the drug," he reported, "one third of the sheep were markedly improved, one third of the sheep showed no change, and the other one ran away."

This story introduces one of the most frequent questions asked by physicians conducting trials of new agents, or for that matter by anyone conducting evaluative studies: "How many subjects do we have to study?" The time to answer this question is *before* the study is done. All too often studies are conducted, large amounts of money and other resources are invested, and only after the study has been completed do the investigators find that from the beginning they had too few subjects to obtain meaningful results.

The question of how many subjects are needed for study is not based on mystique. This section presents the logic of how to approach the question of sample size. Let us begin this discussion of sample size with Figure 7–1.

We have two jars of beads, each containing 100 beads, some white and some black. The jars are opaque, so (despite their appearance in the figure) we cannot see the colors of the beads in the jars just by looking at the jars. We want to know whether the distribution of the beads by color differs in jars A and B: that is, is there a larger (or smaller) proportion of black beads in jar A than in jar B?

To answer this question, let us take a sample of 10 beads from jar A in one hand and a sample of 10 beads from jar B in the other. On the basis of the color distribution of the 10 beads in each hand, we will try and make a conclusion about the color distribution of the 100 beads in each of the jars.

Let us assume that (as shown in Fig. 7–2) in one hand we have 9 black beads and 1 white bead from jar A, and in the other hand we have 2 black beads and 8 white beads from jar B. Can we conclude that 90% of the beads in jar A are black and that 10% are white? Clearly, we cannot. It is possible, for example, that of the 100 beads in jar A, 90 are

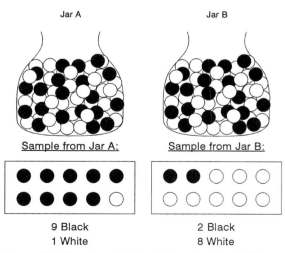

Figure 7–2. Samples of 10 beads from jar A and 10 from jar B.

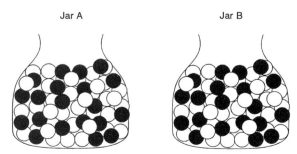

Figure 7–1. Two opaque jars, each holding 100 beads, some black and some white.

white and 10 are black, but that *by chance* our 10-bead sample includes 9 black and 1 white. This is possible, but highly unlikely. Similarly, in regard to jar B we cannot conclude that 20% of the beads are black and 80% are white. It is conceivable that 90 of the 100 beads are black and 10 are white, but that *by chance* the 10-bead sample includes 2 black beads and 8 white beads. This is conceivable, but, again, highly unlikely.

On the basis of the distributions of the 10-bead samples in each hand, could we say that the distributions of the 100 beads in the two jars are different? Given the samples in each hand, could it be, for example, that the distribution of beads in each jar is 50 black and 50 white? Again, it is possible, but it is not likely. We cannot exclude this possibility on the basis of our samples. We are looking at samples and trying to draw a conclusion regarding a whole universe—the jars from which we have drawn the samples.

Let us consider a second example, shown in Figure 7–3. Again we draw two samples. This time the 10-bead sample from jar A consists of 7 black and 3 white beads, and the 10-bead sample from jar B also consists of 7 black and 3 white beads. Could the color distribution of the beads in the two jars be the same? Clearly it could. Could I have drawn these two samples of 7 black and 3 white beads from both jars if the distribution is actually 90 white beads and 10 black in jar A and 90 black beads and 10 white in jar B? Yes, possibly, but highly unlikely.

When we carry out a study we are only looking at the sample of subjects in our study, such as a sample of patients with a certain illness who are being treated with treatment A or with treatment B. From the study results we want to draw a conclusion that goes beyond the study population—is treatment A more effective than treatment B in the total universe of all patients with this disease who might be treated with drug A or drug B? The same issue that arose with the 10-bead samples arises when we want to derive a conclusion regarding all patients from the sample of patients included in our study. Rarely, if ever, is a study conducted in all patients with a disease or in all patients who might be treated with the drugs in question.

Given this background, let us now consider a trial in which groups receiving one of two therapies, therapy A and therapy B, are being compared. (Keep in mind the sampling of beads just discussed.) Before beginning our study, we can list the four possible study outcomes (Table 7–1):

1. It is possible that in reality there is no difference in effectiveness between therapy A and B (i.e., therapy A is no better and no worse than therapy B), and when we do our study we correctly conclude on the basis of our samples that the two groups do not differ.

2. It is possible that in reality there is no difference between therapies A and B (i.e., therapy A is no better and no worse than therapy B), but in our study we found a difference between the groups and therefore concluded, on the basis of our samples, that there is a difference between the therapies. This conclusion, based on our samples, is in error.

3. It is possibile that in reality there is a difference between therapy A and B, but when we examine the groups in our study we find no difference between them. We therefore conclude, on the basis of our samples, that there is no difference between therapy A and B. This conclusion is in error.

4. It is possible that in reality there is a differ-

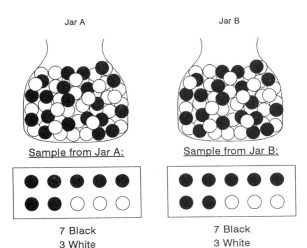

Jar A   Jar B

Sample from Jar A: Sample from Jar B:

7 Black   7 Black
3 White   3 White

Figure 7–3. Samples of 10 beads from jar A and 10 from jar B.

Table 7–1. Four Possibilities in Testing Whether the Treatments Differ

1. The treatments do not differ and we correctly conclude that they do not differ.
2. The treatments do not differ but we conclude that they do differ.
3. The treatments differ but we conclude that they do not differ.
4. The treatments do differ and we correctly conclude that they do differ.

ence between therapy A and B, and when we examine the groups in our study we find that they differ. On the basis of these samples, we correctly conclude that therapy A differs from therapy B.

These four possibilities constitute the universe of outcomes after we complete our study. Let us look at these four possibilities presented in a 2×2 table (Fig. 7–4): Two columns represent reality—either therapy A differs from therapy B or therapy A does not differ from therapy B. The two rows represent our decision: We conclude either that they differ or that they do not differ. In this figure, the four possibilities that were just listed are represented as four cells in the table. If there is no difference, and on the basis of the samples included in our study we conclude there is no difference, this is a correct decision (*cell a*). If there is a difference, and on the basis of our study we conclude that there is a difference (*cell d*), this too is a correct decision. In the best of all worlds, all of the possibilities would fall into one of these two cells. Unfortunately, this is rarely if ever the case. There are times when there is no difference between the therapies, but on the basis of the samples of subjects included in our study we erroneously conclude that they differ (*cell c*). This is called a *type I error*. It is also possible that there really is a difference between the therapies, but on the basis of the samples included in our study we erroneously conclude that there is no difference (*cell b*); this is called a *type II error*. (In this situation, the therapies differ, but we fail to detect the difference in our study samples.)

The *probability* that we will make a type I error is designated α, and the *probability* that we will make a type II error is designated β (as shown in Fig. 7–5).

α is the so-called *P value*, which is seen in many

published papers and has been sanctified by many years of use. When you see "$P < 0.05$," the reference is to α. What does $P < 0.05$ mean? It tells us that we have concluded that therapy A differs from therapy B on the basis of the sample of subjects included in our study, which we found to differ. The probability that such a difference could have arisen by chance alone, and that this difference between our groups does not reflect any true difference between therapies A and B, is only 0.05 (or 1 in 20).

Let us now direct our attention to the right half of this 2 × 2 table, which shows the two possibilities when there is a true difference between therapies A and B, as shown in Figure 7–6.

If, as seen here, the reality is that there is a

REALITY

DECISION	Treatments are not different	Treatments are different
Conclude treatments are not different	Correct decision	Type II error (Probability = β)
Conclude treatments are different	Type I error (Probability = α)	Correct decision

Figure 7–5. Possible outcomes of a randomized trial: types I and II errors.

REALITY

DECISION	Treatments are not different	Treatments are different
Conclude treatments are not different	Correct decision (Cell a)	Type II error (Cell b)
Conclude treatments are different	Type I error (Cell c)	Correct decision (Cell d)

Figure 7–4. Possible outcomes of a randomized trial.

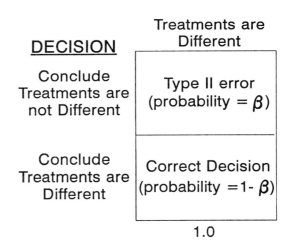

REALITY

DECISION	Treatments are Different
Conclude Treatments are not Different	Type II error (probability = β)
Conclude Treatments are Different	Correct Decision (probability =1- β)

1.0

Figure 7–6. Possible outcomes of a randomized trial when the treatments differ.

REALITY

DECISION	Treatments are not different	Treatments are different
Conclude treatments are not different	Correct decision	Type II error (probability = β)
Conclude treatments are different	Type I error (Probability = α)	Correct decision (Probability = 1- β) (power)

Figure 7–7. Possible outcomes of a randomized trial: summary.

difference between the therapies, there are only two possibilities: We might conclude, in error, that the therapies do not differ (type II error). The probability of making a type II error is designated β. Or we might conclude, correctly, that the therapies differ. Because the total of all probabilities must equal 1, and the probability of a type II error = β, the probability that we shall correctly decide on the basis of our study that the therapies differ if there is a difference will equal $1 - \beta$. This probability, $1 - \beta$, is called the *power* of the study. It tells us how good our study is at correctly identifying a difference between the therapies if in reality they are different. How likely is our study not to miss a difference if one exists?

The full 2 × 2 table in Figure 7–7 includes all of the terms that have been discussed. Table 7–2 provides multiple definitions of these terms.

How do these concepts help us to arrive at an estimate of the sample size that we need? If we ask the question, How many people do we have to study in a clinical trial? We must be able to specify a number of items as listed in Table 7–3.

First, we must specify the expected difference in

Table 7–2. Summary of Terms

Term	Definitions
α	= Probability of making a type I error
	= Probability of concluding the treatments differ when in reality they do not differ
β	= Probability of making a type II error
	= Probability of concluding that the treatments do not differ when in reality they do differ
Power	= 1 − Probability of making a type II error
	= 1 − β
	= Probability of correctly concluding that the treatments differ
	= Probability of detecting a difference between the treatments if the treatments do in fact differ

Table 7–3. What Must Be Specified in Order to Estimate the Sample Size Needed in a Randomized Trial?

1. The difference in response rates to be detected
2. An estimate of the response rate in one of the groups
3. Level of statistical significance (α)
4. The value of the power desired ($1 - \beta$)
5. Whether the test should be one-sided or two-sided

response rate. Let us say that the existing therapy cures 40% of patients, and we are going to test a new therapy. We must be able to say whether we expect the new therapy to cure 50%, 60%, or some other proportion of treated patients. That is, will the new therapy be 10% better than the current therapy and cure 50% of people, 20% better than current therapy and cure 60%, or some other difference? What is the size of the difference between current therapy and new therapy that we want to be able to detect with our study?

How do we generally arrive at such a figure? What if we do not have information on which to base an estimate of the improvement in effectiveness that might be anticipated? Perhaps we are studying a new therapy for which we have no prior experience. One approach is to search for data in human populations for similar diseases and therapies. We can also search for relevant data from animal studies. At times, we simply have no way of producing such an estimate. In this situation, we can make a guess—say, 30% improvement—but *bracket* the estimate: that is, calculate the sample size needed based on a 40% improvement in response rate and also calculate the sample size needed based on a 20% improvement in response rate.

Second, we must have an estimate of the response rate (rate of cure, rate of improvement) in one of the groups. In the example just used, we said the current cure rate (or response rate) is 40%. This is the estimate of the response rate for one of the groups based on current clinical experience.

Third, we must specify the level of α with which we will be satisfied. The choice is up to the investigator; there is nothing sacred about any specific value, but values of 0.05 or 0.01 are commonly used.

Fourth, we must specify the power of the study. Again, no specific value is sacred, but powers of 80% or 90% are commonly used.

Finally, we must specify whether the test should be one-sided or two-sided. What does this mean? Our present cure rate is 40% and we are trying a

Table 7–4. Number of Patients Needed in Each Group to Detect Various Differences in Cure Rates; $\alpha = .05$; Power $(1 - \beta) = .80$ (Two-Sided Test)

Lower of the Two Cure Rates	Differences in Cure Rates Between the Two Treatment Groups													
	0.05	*0.10*	*0.15*	*0.20*	*0.25*	*0.30*	*0.35*	*0.40*	*0.45*	*0.50*	*0.55*	*0.60*	*0.65*	*0.70*
0.05	420	130	69	44	36	31	23	20	17	14	13	11	10	8
0.10	680	195	96	59	41	35	29	23	19	17	13	12	11	8
0.15	910	250	120	71	48	39	31	25	20	17	15	12	11	9
0.20	1,090	290	135	80	53	42	33	26	22	18	16	12	11	9
0.25	1,250	330	150	88	57	44	35	28	22	18	16	12	11	—
0.30	1,380	360	160	93	60	44	36	29	22	18	15	12	—	—
0.35	1,470	370	170	96	61	44	36	28	22	17	13	—	—	—
0.40	1,530	390	175	97	61	44	35	26	20	17	—	—	—	—
0.45	1,560	390	175	96	60	42	33	25	19	—	—	—	—	—
0.50	1,560	390	170	93	57	40	31	23	—	—	—	—	—	—

Modified from Gehan E: Clinical trials in cancer research. Environ Health Perspect 32:31, 1979.

new therapy that we believe will have a higher cure rate—perhaps 50% or 60%. We want to detect a difference that is in the direction of improvement with the new therapy—an increase in cure rate. So we might say we will only test for a difference in that direction because that is the direction in which we are interested—that is, a one-sided test.

The problem is that in the history of medicine and of public health we have at times been surprised, and have found that new therapies that we thought would be beneficial have actually been harmful. If such a possibility is a problem, we would want to find a difference in cure rate *in either direction* from the current rate in our study—that is, we would use a two-sided test, testing not only for a difference that is better than the current cure rate, but also for one that is worse than the current rate. Clinicians and other investigators often prefer to use a one-sided test in their studies because such

tests require smaller sample sizes than do two-sided tests. Because the number of patients available for study is often limited, a one-sided test is attractive. At times investigators may make a practical decision to use a one-sided test, even if there is no conceptual justification for this decision.

Opinions differ on this subject. Some believe that if the investigator is only interested in one direction—that is, improvement—a one-sided test is justified. Others believe that as long as the difference could go in either direction, a two-sided test is required. In a situation in which a particular disease is currently 100% fatal, any difference with a new therapy could only be in the direction of improvement, and a one-sided test would be appropriate.

Let us now turn to the application of these five factors to estimating the needed sample size from a sample size table. Tables 7–4 and 7–5 are selections

Table 7–5. Number of Patients Needed in Each Group to Detect Various Differences in Cure Rates; $\alpha = .05$; Power $(1 - \beta) = .80$ (One-Sided Test)

Lower of the Two Cure Rates	Differences in Cure Rates Between the Two Treatment Groups													
	0.05	*0.10*	*0.15*	*0.20*	*0.25*	*0.30*	*0.35*	*0.40*	*0.45*	*0.50*	*0.55*	*0.60*	*0.65*	*0.70*
0.05	330	105	55	40	33	24	20	17	13	12	10	9	9	8
0.10	540	155	76	47	37	30	23	19	16	13	11	11	9	8
0.15	710	200	94	56	43	32	26	22	17	15	11	10	9	8
0.20	860	230	110	63	42	36	27	23	17	15	12	10	9	8
0.25	980	260	120	69	45	37	31	23	17	15	12	10	9	—
0.30	1,080	280	130	73	47	37	31	23	17	15	11	10	—	—
0.35	1,160	300	135	75	48	37	31	23	17	15	11	—	—	—
0.40	1,210	310	135	76	48	37	30	23	17	13	—	—	—	—
0.45	1,230	310	135	75	47	36	26	22	16	—	—	—	—	—
0.50	1,230	310	135	73	45	36	26	19	—	—	—	—	—	—

Modified from Gehan E: Clinical trials in cancer research. Environ Health Perspect 32:31, 1979.

from sample size tables published by Gehan in 1979.[1] (Similar tables are available in many standard statistics texts.) Both tables give the number of patients needed *in each group* to detect various differences in cure rates with an α of 0.05 and a power $(1 - \beta)$ of .80. Table 7–4 is intended to be used for a two-sided test and Table 7–5 for a one-sided test.

Let us say that we are conducting a clinical trial of two therapies: one that is a currently in use and one that is new. The current therapy has a cure rate of 40%, and we believe that the new therapy may have a cure rate of 60%—that is, we wish to detect an improvement in cure rate of 20%. How many subjects do we have to study? Let us say we will use an α of .05, a power of 80%, and a two-sided test. We therefore will use Table 7–4. The first column of this table is designated the lower of the two cure rates. As the current cure rate is 40%, and we expect a cure rate of 60% with our new therapy, the lower of the two cure rates is 40%, and we move to that row of the table. We expect the new therapy to have a cure rate of 60%, so the difference in cure rates will be 20%. We therefore move down the 20% column (the difference in cure rates) to the point at which it intersects the row of 40% (the lower of the cure rates), where we find the value 97. We need 97 subjects *in each of our study groups.*

Another approach is to use the table in a reverse direction: For example, a clinic for a rare disease, which each year treats 30 patients with the disease, wishes to test a new therapy. Given this maximum number of 30 patients, we could ask, What size difference in cure rates could we hope to detect? We may find a difference of a certain size that may be acceptable, or we may find that the number of subjects available for study is simply too small. If the number of patients is too small we have several options: We can decide not to do the study, and such a decision should be made early on, before most of the effort has been invested. Or we could decide to extend the study in time to accumulate more subjects. Finally, we could decide to collaborate with investigators at other institutions to increase the total number of subjects available for the study. An advantage of the last approach is that in such a multi-center study, a major selection bias at one of the centers would be manifest in the results in subjects recruited at that center and would differ from the results in the other subjects in the study. The presence of such a bias would be readily recognizable.

This section has demonstrated the use of a sample size table. Formulas are also available for calculating these figures directly, and computer programs are also available for this purpose. Sample sizes can be calculated not only for randomized trials but also for cohort and case-control studies.

CROSSOVER

Another important issue in clinical trials is *crossover*. Crossover may be of two types: planned or unplanned.

A *planned crossover* is shown in Figure 7–8. Subjects are randomized to therapy A or therapy B, and after being observed for a certain period of time on one therapy, they are switched to the other therapy. In effect, each patient can serve as his or her own control, thus holding constant the variation between individuals in many characteristics that

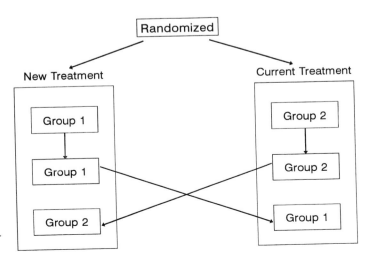

Figure 7–8. Design of a planned crossover trial.

could potentially affect a comparison of the effectiveness of two agents.

This type of design is very attractive and useful provided that certain cautions are taken into account. First is that of *carryover*: If a subject is changed from therapy A to therapy B and observed under each therapy, the observations under therapy B will be valid only if there is no residual carryover from therapy A. There must be enough of a washout period to be sure none of therapy A or its effect remains. Second, the order in which the therapies are given may elicit psychological responses. Patients may react differently to the first therapy given in a study as a result of the enthusiasm that is often accorded a new study; this enthusiasm may diminish over time. We therefore want to be sure that any differences observed are indeed due to the agents being evaluated, and not to any effect of order.

A more important consideration is that of an *unplanned crossover*. Figure 7–9 shows the design of a randomized trial of coronary bypass surgery, comparing it with medical care for coronary heart disease. Randomization is carried out after informed consent has been obtained.

Although the initial design is straightforward, in reality, unplanned crossovers may occur. Some subjects assigned by the randomization to bypass surgery may begin to have second thoughts and decide not to go through with the surgery. They are therefore crossovers into the medical care group. In addition, the condition of some subjects assigned to medical care may begin to deteriorate and urgent bypass surgery may be required—these subjects are crossovers from the medical to the surgical care group.

This problem, seen schematically in Figure 7–10, poses a serious problem in analysis of the data. If we analyze according to the original assignment, we will include in the surgical group some patients

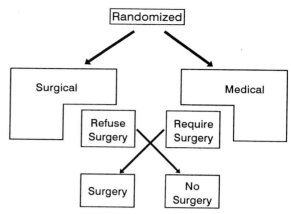

Figure 7–10. Unplanned crossover in a study of cardiac bypass surgery: II. Reality: unplanned crossovers.

who received only medical care, and in the medical group we will include some patients who had surgery. If, however, we analyze according to the treatment that the patients actually receive, we will have broken the randomization.

No perfect solution is available for this dilemma. Current practice is to perform the primary analysis by intention to treat—according to the original randomized assignment. We would hope that the results of other comparisons would be consistent with this primary approach. The bottom line is that because there are no perfect solutions, the number of crossovers must be kept to a minimum. Obviously, if we analyze according to original randomization and there have been many crossovers, the meaning of the study results will be questionable. If the number of crossovers becomes large, the problem may be insurmountable.

FACTORIAL DESIGN

An attractive variant on the study designs discussed in these chapters is *factorial design*. Assuming that two drugs are to be tested, the anticipated outcomes for the two drugs are different, and their modes of action are independent, one can economically use the same study population for testing both drugs. This factorial type of design is shown in Figure 7–11.

If the effects of the two treatments are indeed completely independent, we could evaluate the effects of treatment A by comparing the results in $a + b$ to the results in $c + d$. Similarly, the results for treatment B could be evaluated by comparing the effects in $a + c$ to those in $b + d$. In the event

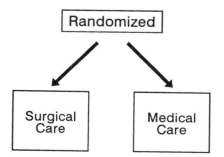

Figure 7–9. Unplanned crossover in a study of cardiac bypass surgery: I. Original study design.

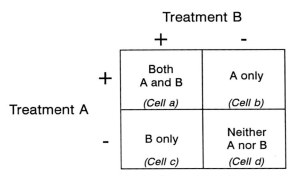

Figure 7–11. Factorial design for studying effects of two treatments.

that it is decided to terminate the study of treatment A, this design permits the continuation of the study for the effects of treatment B.

NON-COMPLIANCE

Patients may agree to be randomized, but following randomization they may not comply with the assigned treatment. Non-compliance may be overt or covert: On the one hand, people may overtly articulate their refusal to comply or may stop participating in the study. These non-compliers are also called *dropouts* from the study. On the other hand, people may just stop taking the agent assigned without admitting this to the investigator or the study staff. Whenever possible, checks on potential non-compliance are built into the study. These may include, for example, urine tests for the agent being tested or for one of its metabolites.

Another problem in randomized trials has been called *drop-ins*. Patients in one group may inadvertently take the agent assigned to the other group. For example, in a trial of the effect of aspirin for prevention of myocardial infarction, patients were randomized to aspirin or to no aspirin. However, a problem arose in that because of the large number of over-the-counter preparations that contain aspirin, many of the control patients might well be taking aspirin without knowing it. Two steps were taken to address this problem: (1) controls were provided with lists of aspirin-containing over-the-counter preparations that they should avoid, and (2) urine tests for salicylates were carried out both in the aspirin group and the controls.

The net effect of non-compliance on the study results will be to reduce any observed differences, because the treatment group will include some who did not receive the therapy and the no-treatment group may include some who received the treatment. Thus the groups will be less different in terms of therapy than they would have been had there been no non-compliance, so that even if there is a difference in the effects of the treatments, it will appear much smaller.

One approach that was used in the Veterans Administration Study of the Treatment of Hypertension was to carry out a pilot study in which compliers and non-compliers were identified. When the actual full study was later carried out, the study population was limited to those who had been compliers during the pilot study. The problem with this approach is that when we want to generalize from the results of such a study, we can only do so to other populations of compliers, which may be very different from the population in any free-living community, which would consist of both compliers and non-compliers.

Table 7–6 shows data from the Coronary Drug Project reported by Canner and co-workers.[2] This study was a comparison of clofibrate and placebo for lowering cholesterol. The table presents the mortality in the two groups.

No large difference in 5-year mortality was seen between the two groups. The investigators speculated that perhaps this was the result of the patients not having taken their medication. Table 7–7 shows the results of separating the clofibrate subjects into good compliers and poor compliers.

Here we see the 5-year mortality was 24.6% in the poor-complier group compared to 15% in the good-complier group. We might thus be tempted to conclude that compliance was indeed the factor that produced the results seen in Table 7–7: no significant difference between the clofibrate and placebo groups.

Table 7–8 separates both groups, clofibrate and placebo, into compliers and non-compliers. Even in the placebo group, 5-year mortality in the poor

Table 7–6. Coronary Drug Project: Five-Year Mortality in Patients Given Clofibrate or Placebo

	No. of Patients	Mortality (%)
Clofibrate	1,065	18.2
Placebo	2,695	19.4

Adapted from Canner PL, Forman SA, Prud'homme GJ, for the Coronary Drug Project Research Group: Influence of adherence to treatment and response to cholesterol on mortality in the coronary drug project. N Engl J Med 303:1038–1041, 1980.

Table 7–7. Coronary Drug Project: Five-Year Mortality in Patients Given Clofibrate or Placebo According to Level of Compliance

	No. of Patients	Mortality (%)
Clofibrate		
Poor complier (<80%)	357	24.6
Good complier (≥80%)	708	15.0
Placebo	2,695	19.4

Adapted from Canner PL, Forman SA, Prud'homme GJ, for the Coronary Drug Project Research Group: Influence of adherence to treatment and response to cholesterol on mortality in the coronary drug project. N Engl J Med 303:1038–1041, 1980.

compliers was higher than in the good compliers: 28% compared to 15%.

What can we learn from these tables? People who do not comply or who do not participate in studies differ from those who do comply and who do participate. Therefore, in conducting a study to evaluate a therapy or other intervention, we cannot offer the agent to a population and compare the effects in those who take the agent to the effects in those who refuse or do not, because the two groups are basically different in terms of many demographic, social, psychological, and cultural variables that may have important roles in determining outcome. That is why randomization, or other approaches that reduce selection bias, is essential.

GENERALIZABILITY OF RESULTS

Whenever we carry out a trial, the ultimate objective is to generalize the results beyond the study population itself. In this context, it is useful

to introduce two concepts: internal validity and external validity, as shown in Figure 7–12.

This diagram represents a randomized trial in which the study population is our sample, identified as a subset of some reference population. For example, the reference population might be all patients with lupus erythematosus, and the study population will be patients with the disease attending several clinics in our city. We then randomize the study population to one of two therapies, A or B. If the study is properly done without major methodologic problems, and it takes into account all the issues discussed thus far, the study is said to have *internal validity*.

Another issue relates to the *generalizability* or *external validity* of the study. If, for example, we carry out a study in one city and find a new therapy to be better than a current therapy, we would like to be able to say that the new therapy is better for the disease regardless of where the patients are treated, and not just for patients in that city. We want to be able to generalize from the study findings to all patients with the disease. To do so, we must know to what extent the patients we have studied are representative of all patients with the disease in question. To do so, we must characterize those who did not participate in the study, and identify characteristics of study patients that might preclude our generalizing the results to other patients who were not in the study. Thus, the issues of internal validity—whether the study was well done and whether the findings are valid—and of external validity or generalizability are basic concerns in the conduct of any randomized trial.

Table 7–8. Coronary Drug Project: Five-Year Mortality in Patients Given Clofibrate or Placebo According to Level of Compliance

	Clofibrate		Placebo	
Compliance	No. of Patients	Mortality (%)	No. of Patients	Mortality (%)
Poor (<80%)	357	24.6	882	28.2
Good (≥80%)	708	15.0	1,813	15.1
Total group	1,065	18.2	2,695	19.4

Adapted from Canner PL, Forman SA, Prud'homme GJ, for the Coronary Drug Project Research Group: Influence of adherence to treatment and response of cholesterol on mortality in the coronary drug project. N Engl J Med 303:1038–1041, 1980.

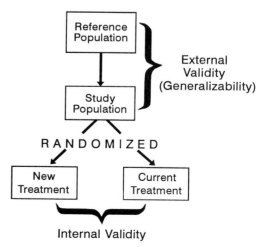

Figure 7–12. Internal and external validity in a randomized trial.

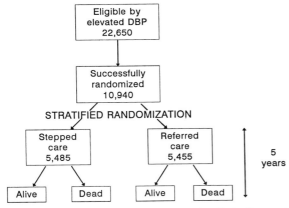

Figure 7–13. Schema of the Hypertension Detection and Follow-up Program (HDFP).

TWO MAJOR U.S. RANDOMIZED TRIALS

The Hypertension Detection and Follow-up Program

Many years ago a Veterans Administration study demonstrated that treating people with large increases in blood pressure can significantly reduce their mortality.[3] The question of the value of antihypertensive therapy for people who have only a slight increase in blood pressure (diastolic blood pressure of 90 to 104 mm Hg) was left unanswered. Although we might be able to reduce blood pressure in such persons, the problem exists of the side effects of antihypertensive agents. Unless some health benefit to the patients can be demonstrated, use of these agents would not be justified in people whose blood pressure is only elevated minimally.

The multi-center Hypertension Detection and Follow-up Program (HDFP) study was designed to investigate the benefits of treating mild to moderate hypertension. In this study, of 22,994 subjects who were eligible because they had elevated diastolic blood pressure, almost 11,000 were randomized either to the stepped care or to the referred care group (Fig. 7–13).

Stepped care meant treatment according to a precisely defined protocol, under which treatment was changed when a specified decrease in blood pressure had not been obtained during a certain period. The comparison group posed a problem: from the standpoint of study design, a group receiving no care for hypertension might have been desirable. However, the investigators felt it would be ethically unjustifiable to withhold antihypertensive care from known hypertensive subjects. So the subjects in the comparison group were referred back to their own physicians, and this group was therefore called the *referred care group*. Mortality in both groups over a 5-year period was then studied.[4]

Figure 7–14 shows that at every interval following entry into the study, the patients in the stepped care group had lower mortality than did those in the referred care group. In Figure 7–14 we see that the same pattern held in those with mild increases in blood pressure.

The results are shown in greater detail in Table 7–9, in which the data are presented according to diastolic blood pressure at entry into the study. The righthand column shows the percent reduction in mortality for the stepped care group: the greatest reduction is seen to have occurred in those subjects with a minimal increase in diastolic pressure.

This study has had considerable impact in en-

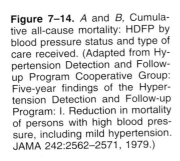

Figure 7–14. *A* and *B*, Cumulative all-cause mortality: HDFP by blood pressure status and type of care received. (Adapted from Hypertension Detection and Follow-up Program Cooperative Group: Five-year findings of the Hypertension Detection and Follow-up Program: I. Reduction in mortality of persons with high blood pressure, including mild hypertension. JAMA 242:2562–2571, 1979.)

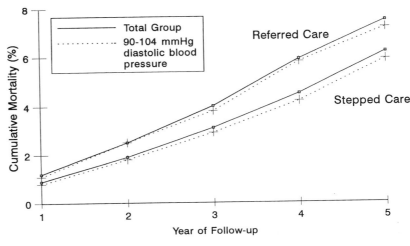

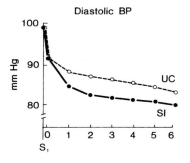

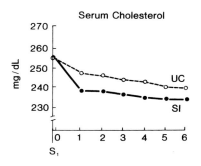

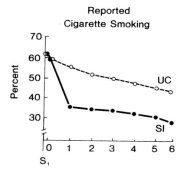

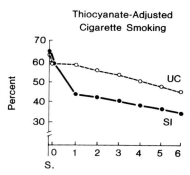

Figure 7–15. Mean risk factor levels by year of follow-up for Multiple Risk Factor Intervention Trial Research Group participants. Abbreviations: SI, special intervention; UC, usual care; S_1, first screening visit. (From Multiple Risk Factor Intervention Trial Research Group: Multiple Risk Factor Intervention Trial: Risk factor changes and mortality results. JAMA 248:1465–1477, 1982.)

couraging physicians to treat even mild to moderate elevations in blood pressure. It has been criticized, however, because of the absence of an untreated group for comparison. Not only were these patients referred back to their own physicians, but there was no monitoring of the care that was provided to them by their physicians. There is therefore some problem in interpreting these data. Even today, people differ on whether there was indeed a legitimate ethical objection to including an untreated placebo group in this study or whether there was an ethical problem in designing an expensive study that was difficult to mount and left so much uncertainty and difficulty in interpretation.

The Multiple Risk Factor Intervention Trial

A serious problem in large-scale trials that require the investment of tremendous resources, financial and otherwise, and take years to complete is that their interpretation is often clouded by a problem in design or methodology that may not have been appreciated at an early stage of the study. The Multiple Risk Factor Intervention Trial (MRFIT) was a randomized study designed to determine whether mortality from myocardial infarction could be reduced by changes in lifestyle and other measures. In this study, one group re-

Table 7–9. Mortality From All Causes During the Hypertension Detection and Follow-up Program

Diastolic Blood Pressure at Entry (mm Hg)	Stepped Care (SC)	Referred Care (RC)	5-yr Death Rate		% Mortality Reduction in SC Group
			SC	*RC*	
90–104	3,903	3,922	5.9	7.4	20.3
105–114	1,048	1,004	6.7	7.7	13.0
≥115	534	529	9.0	9.7	7.2
Total	5,485	5,455	6.4	7.7	16.9

From Hypertension Detection and Follow-up Program Cooperative Group: Five-year findings of the Hypertension Detection and Follow-up Program: I. Reduction in mortality of persons with high blood pressure, including mild hypertension. JAMA 242:2562–2571, 1979.

ceived special intervention (SI), consisting of stepped care for hypertension and intensive education and counseling about lifestyle changes. The comparison group received its usual care (UC) in the community. Over an average follow-up period of 7 years, levels of coronary heart disease (CHD) risk factors declined more in SI men than in UC men (Fig. 7–15).

However, by the end of the study, no statistically significant differences were evident between the groups in either CHD mortality or all-cause mortality (Fig. 7–16).

Serious problems occurred in the interpretation of these results. First of all, the study was unfortunately conducted at a time when mortality from coronary disease was declining in the United States. In addition, it was not clear whether the lack of difference found in this study was because lifestyle change made no difference or because the control group, on its own, had made the same lifestyle changes as those made by many other people in the United States during this period. Widespread dietary changes, increases in exercise, and quitting smoking have taken place in much of the population, so the control group may have been ''contaminated'' with some of the behavior changes that had been encouraged in the study group in a formal and structured manner.

This study also points up the problem of using intermediate measures as endpoints of effectiveness in randomized trials. Because any effect on mortality may take years to be manifested, it is tempting to utilize measures that might be affected sooner by the intervention. However, as seen here, although the intervention succeeded in reducing smoking, cholesterol levels, and diastolic blood pressure, one could not conclude on the basis of these changes that the intervention was effective, because the objective of the study was to determine whether the intervention could reduce CHD mortality, which it did not.

Because of these problems, which often lead to problems in interpretation of the findings in very large and expensive studies, some have advocated that the same funds invested in a number of smaller studies by different investigators in different populations might be a wiser choice: if the results were consistent they might be more credible, despite the problems of smaller sample size that would be introduced in the individual studies.

PHASES IN TESTING OF NEW DRUGS IN THE UNITED STATES

As new drugs are developed, the U.S. Food and Drug Administration follows a standard sequence

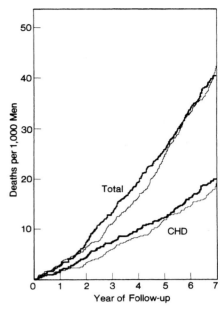

Figure 7–16. Cumulative coronary heart disease (CHD) and total mortality rates for Multiple Risk Factor Intervention Trial Research Group participants. *Heavy line* indicates men receiving usual care; *thin line,* men receiving special intervention. (From Multiple Risk Factor Intervention Trial Research Group: Multiple Risk Factor Intervention Trial: Risk factor changes and mortality results. JAMA 248:1465–1477, 1982.)

in testing these new agents: *phase I* studies are clinical pharmacologic studies—small studies of 20 to 80 patients that look at toxic and pharmacologic effects. If the drug passes these studies, it then undergoes *phase II* studies, clinical investigations of 100 to 200 patients for effectiveness and relative safety. If the drug passes phase II studies, it is then tested in *phase III* studies—large-scale randomized controlled trials for effectiveness and relative safety, which are often multi-centered. If the drug passes phase III testing, it will be licensed for marketing. It has been increasingly recognized, however, that certain adverse effects of drugs, such as carcinogenesis and teratogenesis, may not become manifest for many years, or that these effects may be so infrequent that they may not be detectable even in relatively large clinical trials but may become evident only when the drug is in use by large populations. For this reason, *phase IV* studies, postmarketing surveillance, are important for monitoring new agents as they come into general use by the public.

This rigorous sequence has protected the American public against many hazardous agents. In recent years, however, the pressure to speed up the processing of new agents for the treatment of AIDS has led to a re-examination of this approval process. It seems likely that whatever modifications are made in the approval process will not remain limited to drugs used against AIDS, but will in fact have extensive ramifications for the general process of approving new drugs and will therefore have major implications for the health of the public both in the United States and throughout the world.

ETHICAL CONSIDERATIONS

Many ethical issues arise in the context of clinical trials, and the reader is referred to the excellent monographs listed at the end of this chapter for a full discussion.

One frequently raised question is whether randomization is ethical. How can we knowingly withhold a drug from patients, particularly those with serious and life-threatening diseases? Randomization is ethical only when we do not know that drug A is better than drug B. We may have some suggestion that this is so (and often this is the rationale for doing a trial in the first place) but we are not certain. Often, however, it is not precisely clear at what point we "know" that drug A is better than drug B. The question may be better stated as: When do we have adequate evidence to support the conclusion that drug A is better than drug B?

The question can also be posed in the reverse: Is it ethical not to randomize? When we are considering drugs, preventive measures, or systems of health care delivery that apply to large numbers of people both in the United States and in other countries, the mandate may be to carry out a randomized trial and resolve the questions of benefit and harm, and not to continue to subject people to unnecessary toxic effects and raise false hopes, often at tremendous expense. Hence, the question regarding ethics of randomization should be asked in both directions: randomizing and not randomizing.

Another important question is whether truly informed consent can be obtained. Many protocols for multi-centered clinical trials require that patients be entered into the study immediately after diagnosis. The patient may be incapable of giving consent, and the family may be so shocked by the diagnosis and its implications that they have great difficulty in dealing with the notion of randomization. For example, much of the progress of recent decades in the treatment of childhood leukemia has been a result of the rigorous multi-centered protocols that have required enrollment of the child immediately after the diagnosis of leukemia has been made. Clearly, at such a time the parents are so distressed that one may question whether they are capable of giving truly informed consent. Nevertheless, only through such rigorous trials has the progress been made that has saved so many lives of children with acute leukemia.

Finally, under what circumstances should a trial be stopped earlier than originally planned? This is also a difficult issue and could arise because either harmful effects or beneficial effects of the agent become apparent early, before the full sample has been enrolled, or before subjects have been studied for the full follow-up period. In many studies, an outside data monitoring board monitors the data as they are received, and the board makes that decision. For example, in the Physicians' Health Study, the factorial design employed permitted the effects both of aspirin and of β-carotene to be examined. As the study was being conducted, the data monitoring committee decided that the findings for aspirin were sufficiently clear that the aspirin part of the study should be terminated; however, the β-carotene portion of the study continued.

CONCLUSION

The randomized trial is the gold standard for evaluating effectiveness of therapeutic, preventive, and other measures, both in clinical medicine and public health. Chapters 6 and 7 have provided an overview of approaches to study design in randomized trials and the measures used for minimizing or avoiding selection and other types of bias. From the societal viewpoint, issues of generalizability and ethical considerations are major concerns and have been discussed. For those who wish to explore further this important type of study, a list of selected monographs on this topic is provided at the end of this chapter.

EPILOGUE

We shall conclude this discussion of randomized trials by citing an article by Caroline and Schwartz published in the journal *Chest* in 1975. The article was entitled "Chicken Soup Rebound and Relapse of Pneumonia: Report of a Case."[5]

The authors introduced their topic by saying:

Chicken soup has long been recognized to possess unusual therapeutic potency against a wide variety of viral and bacterial agents. Indeed, as early as the 12th century, the theologian, philosopher and physician, Moses Maimonides wrote, "Chicken soup . . . is recommended as an excellent food as well as medication." Previous anecdotal reports regarding the therapeutic efficacy of this agent, however, have failed to provide details regarding the appropriate length of therapy. What follows is a case report in which abrupt withdrawal of chicken soup led to a severe relapse of pneumonia.

The authors then present a case report of a 47-year-old physician who was treated with chicken soup for pneumonia. Chicken soup administration was terminated prematurely, and the patient suffered a relapse. Chicken soup being unavailable, the relapse was treated with intravenous penicillin.

The authors' discussion is of particular interest. It reads in part:

The therapeutic efficacy of chicken soup was first discovered several thousand years ago when an epidemic highly fatal to young Egyptian males seemed not to affect an ethnic minority residing in the same area. Contemporary epidemiologic inquiry revealed that the diet of the group not afflicted by the epidemic contained large amounts of a preparation made by boiling chicken with various vegetables and herbs. It is notable in this regard that the dietary injunctions given to Moses on Mount Sinai, while restricting consumption of no less than 19 types of fowl, exempted chicken from the prohibition. Some scholars believe that the recipe for chicken soup was transmitted to Moses on the same occasion, but was relegated to the oral tradition when the scriptures were canonized. . . . While chicken soup is now widely employed against a variety of organic and functional disorders, its manufacture remains largely in the hands of private individuals and standardization has proved nearly impossible. Preliminary investigation into the pharmacology of chicken soup (Bohbymycetin®) has shown that it is readily absorbed after oral administration. . . . Parenteral administration is not recommended.

This report stimulated several letters to the editor. In one, Dr. Laurence F. Greene, Professor of Urology at the Mayo Clinic, wrote:

You may be interested to know that we have successfully treated male impotence with another chicken-derived compound, sodium cytarabine hexamethyl-acetyl lututria tetrazolamine (Schmaltz [Upjohn]). This compound, when applied in ointment form to the penis, not only cures impotence, but also increases libido and prevents premature ejaculation. . . . Preliminary studies indicate that its effects are dose related inasmuch as intercourse continues for 5 minutes when 5% ointment is applied, 15 minutes when 15% ointment is applied, and so forth.

We have received a grant in the sum of $650,000 from the National Scientific Foundation to carry out a prospective randomized, controlled double-blind study. Unfortunately, we are unable to obtain a suitable number of subjects inasmuch as each volunteer refuses to participate unless we assure him that he will be a subject rather than a control.[6]

References

1. Gehan E: Clinical trials in cancer research. Environ Health Perspect 32:31, 1979.
2. Canner PL, Forman SA, Prud'homme GJ: Influence of adherence to treatment and response of cholesterol on mortality in the coronary drug project. N Engl J Med 303:1038–1041, 1980.
3. Veterans Administration Cooperative Study Group on Hypertensive Agents: Effects of treatment on morbidity in hypertension: Results in patients with diastolic blood pressure averaging 115 through 129 mm Hg. JAMA 213:1028–1034, 1967.
4. Hypertension Detection and Follow-up Program Cooperative Group: Five year findings of the Hypertension Detection and Follow-up Program: I. Reduction of mortality of persons with high blood pressure, including mild hypertension. JAMA 242:2562, 1979.
5. Caroline NL, Schwartz H: Chicken soup rebound and relapse of pneumonia: Report of a case. Chest 67:215–216, 1975.
6. Greene LF: The chicken soup controversy [letter]. Chest 68:605, 1975.

Monographs on Randomized Trials

Friedman LM, Furberg CD, DeMets DL: Fundamentals of Clinical Trials. Boston, PSG, 1982.
Johnson FN, Johnson S: Clinical Trials. Oxford, Blackwell Scientific Publications, 1977.
Meinert CL: Clinical Trials: Design, Conduct, and Analysis: Monographs in Epidemiology, vol 8. New York, Oxford University Press, 1986.

Pocock SJ: Clinical Trials: A Practical Approach. New York, John Wiley & Sons, 1983.

Silverman WA: Human Experimentation: A Guided Step into the Unknown. New York, Oxford University Press, 1985.

Review Questions

These questions pertain to both Chapters 6 and 7.

1. The major purpose of random assignment in a clinical trial is to:
   a. Help ensure that study subjects are representative of the general population
   b. Facilitate double blinding
   c. Facilitate measurement of outcome variables
   d. Try to have the study groups comparable on baseline characteristics
   e. Reduce selection bias in allocation of treatment

2. An advertisement in a medical journal stated that "2,000 subjects with sore throats were treated with our new medicine. Within four days, 94% were asymptomatic." The advertisement claims that the medicine was effective. Based on the evidence given above, the claim:
   a. Is correct
   b. May be incorrect because the conclusion is not based on a rate
   c. May be incorrect because of failure to recognize a long-term cohort phenomenon
   d. May be incorrect because no test of statistical significance was used
   e. May be incorrect because no control or comparison group was involved

3. The purpose of a *double-blind* or *double-masked* study is to:
   a. Achieve comparability of treated and untreated subjects
   b. Reduce the effects of sampling variation
   c. Avoid observer and subject bias
   d. Avoid observer bias and sampling variation
   e. Avoid subject bias and sampling variation

4. In many studies examining the association between estrogens and endometrial cancer of the uterus, a one-sided significance test was used. The underlying assumption justifying a one-sided rather than a two-sided test is:
   a. The distribution of the proportion exposed followed a "normal" pattern
   b. The expectation prior to doing the study was that estrogens cause endometrial cancer of the uterus

   c. The pattern of association could be expressed by a straight line function
   d. The type II error was the most important potential error to avoid
   e. Only one control group was being used

5. A study is performed in which one group of patients is given a new drug and the other group is not. Assignment to treatment groups is made on the basis of hospital admission number. All individuals with an even hospital admission number are assigned to the first group, and all individuals with an odd hospital admission number are assigned to the second group. The main purpose(s) of this procedure is(are) to:
   a. Prevent investigator bias with respect to the assignment of treatment
   b. Prevent investigator bias with respect to the outcome
   c. Improve the likelihood that the two groups will be comparable with regard to other relevant factors
   d. Ensure a double-masked study
   e. Both *a* and *c* are correct

6. In a randomized trial, a planned crossover design
   a. Eliminates the problem of a possible order effect
   b. Must take into account the problem of possible residual effects of the first therapy
   c. Requires a stratified randomization
   d. Eliminates the need for monitoring compliance and non-compliance
   e. Enhances the generalizability of the results of the study

7. A randomized trial comparing the efficacy of two drugs showed a difference between the two (with a *P* value of <0.05). Assume that in reality, however, the two drugs do not differ. This is therefore an example of:
   a. Type I error (α error)
   b. Type II error (β error)
   c. $1 - \alpha$
   d. $1 - \beta$
   e. None of the above

Question 8 is based on the following table:

Number of Patients Needed in an Experimental and a Control Group for a Given Probability of Obtaining a Significant Result (Two-Sided Test)

Lower of the Two Cure Rates	Differences in the Cure Rates Between the Two Treatment Groups					
	0.05	*0.10*	*0.15*	*0.20*	*0.25*	*0.30*
0.05	420	130	69	44	36	31
0.10	680	195	96	59	41	35
0.15	910	250	120	71	48	39
0.20	1,090	290	135	80	53	42
0.25	1,250	330	150	88	57	44
0.30	1,380	360	160	93	60	44
0.35	1,470	370	170	96	61	44
0.40	1,530	390	175	97	61	44

$\alpha = 0.05$; power $(1 - \beta) = .80$.
Modified from Gehan E: Clinical trials in cancer research. Environ Health Perspect 32:31, 1979.

8. A drug company maintains that a new drug G for a certain disease has a 50% cure rate as compared with drug H, which only has a 25% cure rate. You are asked to design a clinical trial, comparing drugs G and H. Using the preceding table, estimate the number of patients needed in each therapy group to detect such a difference with $\alpha = 0.05$, two-sided, and $\beta = 0.20$.

   The number of patients needed in each therapy group is: _____

9. All of the following are potential benefits of a randomized clinical trial, *except*:
   a. The likelihood that the study groups will be comparable is increased
   b. Self-selection for a particular treatment is eliminated
   c. External validity of the study is increased
   d. Assignment of the next subject cannot be predicted
   e. The therapy a subject receives is not influenced by either conscious or subconscious bias of the investigator

Using Epidemiology to Identify the Cause of Disease

In Section I we addressed issues of defining and diagnosing disease, and of describing its transmission, acquisition, and natural history. We then discussed the use of randomized trials for evaluating and selecting pharmacologic agents or other interventions to modify the natural history, both through disease prevention and through effective treatment. In Section II we turn to a different issue: How do we design and conduct studies to elucidate the etiology of and risk factors for human disease? Such studies are critically important both in clinical medicine and in public health practice.

Why should a clinician be concerned with disease etiology? Has not the clinician's traditional role been to treat disease once it has become apparent? To answer this question, several points should be made. First, *prevention* is a major responsibility of the physician; both prevention and treatment should be viewed by the physician as essential elements in his or her professional role. Indeed, many patients take the initiative and ask their physicians questions about what measures to take for maintaining health and preventing certain diseases. Most opportunities for preventing disease require an understanding of the *etiology* or *cause* of disease, so that exposure to a causative environmental factor can be reduced or the pathogenic chain leading from the causal factor to the development of clinical illness can be interrupted.

Second, patients and their families often ask the physician questions about the *risk* of disease. What is the risk that the disease will recur? What is the risk that other family members may develop the disease? For example:

A man who suffers a myocardial infarction at a young age may ask, ''Why did it happen to me? Can I prevent my having a second infarction? Are my children also at high risk for having an infarction at a young age? If so, can anything be done to lower their risk?''

A woman who delivers a baby with a congenital malformation may ask, ''Why did it happen? Is it because of something I did during the pregnancy? If I get pregnant again, is that child also likely to have a malformation?''

Third, in the course of doing clinical work and making bedside observations, a physician often ''gets a hunch'' regarding a possible relationship between a factor and the risk of a disease that is as yet not understood. For example, Alton Ochsner, the famous surgeon, noted that virtually all the patients on whom he operated for lung cancer were cigarette smokers; this observation led him to suggest that smoking was causally related to the development of lung cancer and indicated the need to clarify the nature of this relationship by means of rigorously conducted studies in defined human populations.

Whereas clinical practice focuses on individuals, public health practice focuses on populations. In view of the tremendous potential impact of public health actions, which often affect entire communities, public health practitioners must understand how conclusions regarding health risks to a community are arrived at, and how a foundation for preventive measures and actions is developed on the basis of population-centered data that are properly interpreted in their biologic context. Only in this way can rational policies be adopted for preventing disease and for enhancing the health of populations at the lowest possible cost.

Alert and astute physicians and other public health practitioners in academic, clinical, and health department settings have many opportunities to conduct studies of disease etiology or disease risk to confirm or refute preliminary clinical or other impressions regarding the origins of diseases. The findings may be of critical importance in providing the rationale for preventing these diseases, for enhancing our understanding of their pathogenesis, and for suggesting directions for future laboratory and epidemiologic research. Consequently, an understanding of the types of study design that are employed for investigating etiology and identifying risk factors, together with an appreciation of the methodologic problems involved in such studies, is fundamental to both clinical medicine and public health practice.

This section discusses the basic study designs that are used in etiologic studies (Chapters 8 and 9) and how the findings from such studies may be used to estimate risks of disease associated with specific exposures (Chapters 10 and 11). Because we ultimately wish to answer questions of disease etiology or cause, the chapters that follow discuss how observed associations can be interpreted and how causal inferences are derived from them (Chapters 13 and 14). Finally, this section closes with a discussion of how epidemiology can be used to assess the relative contributions of genetic and environmental factors to the causation of human disease, an assessment that has major clinical and public health policy implications (Chapter 15).

CHAPTER 8

Cohort Studies

In this chapter and in the following chapters in Section II, we turn to the uses of epidemiology in elucidating etiologic or causal relationships. The two steps that underlie the study designs that are discussed in Chapters 8 and 9 are shown schematically in Figure 8–1.

1. First, we determine whether there is an association between a factor or a characteristic and the development of a disease. This can be accomplished by studying the characteristics of groups, by studying the characteristics of individuals, or both (Chapters 8 through 11).

2. Second, we derive appropriate inferences regarding a possible causal relationship from the patterns of association that have been found (Chapters 13 and 14).

Chapters 8 and 9 describe the study designs used for step 1. In this chapter, cohort studies are discussed; case-control and cross-sectional studies are discussed in Chapter 9.

DESIGN OF A COHORT STUDY

In a cohort study (also called a *prospective study*), the investigator selects a group of exposed individuals and a group of non-exposed individuals and follows up both groups to compare the incidence of disease (or rate of death from disease) in the two groups (Fig. 8–2). The design may include more than two groups, although only two groups are shown for diagrammatic purposes.

If a positive association exists between the exposure and the disease, we would expect that the proportion of the exposed group in whom the disease develops (incidence in the exposed group) would be greater than the proportion of the non-exposed group in whom the disease develops (incidence in the non-exposed group).

The calculations involved are seen in Table 8–1. We begin with an exposed group and a non-exposed group. Of the $a + b$ exposed persons, the disease develops in a but not in b. Thus, the incidence of the disease among the exposed is: $\frac{a}{a + b}$. Similarly, in the c and d non-exposed persons in the study, the disease develops in c but not in d. Thus, the incidence of the disease among the non-exposed is $\frac{c}{c + d}$.

The use of these calculations is seen in a hypothetical example of a cohort study shown in Table 8–2. In this cohort study, the association of smoking with coronary heart disease (CHD) is investigated by selecting for study a group of 3,000 smokers (exposed) and a group of 5,000 non-smokers (non-exposed) who are free of heart disease at baseline.

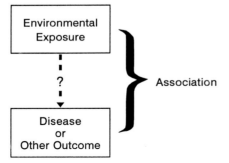

Figure 8–1. If we observe an association between an exposure and a disease or other outcome, the question is: Is it causal?

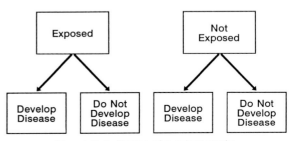

Figure 8–2. Design of a cohort study.

Table 8–1. Design of a Cohort Study

		Then Follow to See Whether			Incidence Rates of Disease
		Disease Develops	Disease Does Not Develop	Totals	
First select	Exposed	a	b	a + b	$\dfrac{a}{a + b}$
	Not exposed	c	d	c + d	$\dfrac{c}{c + d}$

Both groups are followed for the development of CHD, and the *incidence* of CHD in both groups is compared. CHD develops in 84 of the smokers and in 87 of the non-smokers. The result is a CHD incidence of 28.0/1,000 in the smokers and of 17.4/1,000 in the non-smokers.

Note that because we are identifying *new* (incident) cases of disease as they occur, we can determine whether a temporal relationship exists between the exposure and the disease—that is, whether the exposure preceded the onset of the disease. Clearly, such a temporal relationship must be established if we are to consider the exposure a possible cause of the disease in question.

COMPARING COHORT STUDIES WITH RANDOMIZED TRIALS

At this point, it is useful to compare the observational cohort study just described with the randomized trial (experimental cohort) design described previously, in Chapters 6 and 7 (Fig. 8–3).

Both types of studies compare exposed with non-exposed groups (or a group with a certain exposure to a group with another exposure). Because for ethical and other reasons we cannot randomize people to receive a putatively harmful substance, such as a suspected carcinogen, the "exposure" in most randomized trials is a treatment or preventive measure. In cohort studies that propose to investigate

etiology, however, the "exposure" is often to a possibly toxic or carcinogenic agent. In both types of design the comparison is of an exposed group with a non-exposed group or of an exposed group with another.

The difference between these two designs—the presence or absence of randomization—is critical in regard to interpreting the study findings. The advantages of randomization have been discussed in the previous Chapters 6 and 7. In a non-randomized study, when we observe an association of an exposure with a disease, we are left with uncertainty as to whether the association may be a result of the fact that people were not randomized to the exposure; perhaps it is not the exposure, but rather the factors that led people to be exposed, that are associated with the disease. For example, if an increased risk of a disease is found in workers at a certain factory, and if workers at this factory tend to live in a certain area, the increased risk of disease could result from an exposure associated with their place of residence rather than with their occupation or place of work. This issue is discussed in Chapters 13 and 14.

SELECTION OF STUDY POPULATIONS

The essential characteristic in the design of cohort studies is the comparison of outcome(s) in an exposed group and a non-exposed group (or a group

Table 8–2. Results of a Hypothetical Cohort Study of Smoking and Coronary Heart Disease (CHD)

		Then Follow to See Whether			Incidence per 1,000 per Year
		Develop CHD	Do Not Develop CHD	Totals	
First select	Smoke cigarettes	84	2,916	3,000	28.0
	Do not smoke cigarettes	87	4,913	5,000	17.4

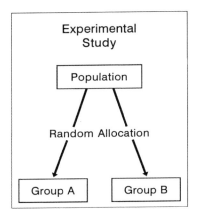
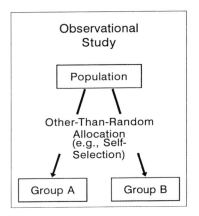

Figure 8–3. Selection of study groups in experimental and observational epidemiologic studies.

with a certain characteristic and a group without that characteristic). There are two basic ways to generate such groups:

1. We can create a study population by selecting groups for inclusion in the study on the basis of whether or not they were exposed (e.g., occupationally exposed cohorts) (Fig. 8–4).
2. Or we can select a defined population before any of its members become exposed or before their exposures are identified. We could select a population on the basis of some factor not related to exposure (such as community of residence) (Fig. 8–5) and take histories of, or perform blood tests or other assays on, the entire population. Using the results of the histories and/or the tests, the individuals can then be separated into *exposed* and *non-exposed* groups (or those who have and those who do not have certain biologic characteristics), such as was done in the Framingham Study, described later in this chapter.

Cohort studies, in which we wait for an outcome to develop in a population, often require a long follow-up period until enough events (outcomes) have occurred. When the second approach is used—in which a population is identified for study

based on some characteristic unrelated to the exposure in question—the exposure of interest may not take place for some time, even for many years, after the population has been defined. Consequently, the length of follow-up required is even greater with the second approach than it is with the first.

Note that with either approach the study design is fundamentally the same: we *compare exposed and non-exposed* persons. This comparison is the hallmark of the cohort design.

TYPES OF COHORT STUDIES

A major problem with the cohort design just described is that the study population must often be followed up for a long period to determine whether the outcome of interest has developed. Consider as an example a hypothetical study of the relationship of smoking to lung cancer. We identify a population of elementary school students and follow them up; 10 years later, when they are teenagers, we identify those who smoke and those who do not. We then

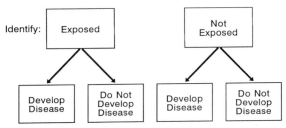

Figure 8–4. Design of a cohort study beginning with exposed and non-exposed groups.

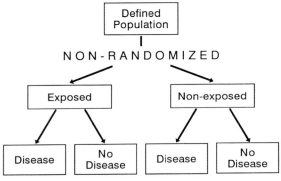

Figure 8–5. Design of a cohort study beginning with a defined population.

follow up both groups—smokers and nonsmokers—to see who develops lung cancer and who does not. For purposes of this example, let us assume that the latent period from beginning smoking to development of lung cancer is 10 years. Let us say that we begin our study in 1995 (Fig. 8–6). Because the interval from the time of identification of the elementary school children to the time of identification of their smoking status as teenagers or college students is 10 years, exposure status (smoker or nonsmoker) will not be ascertained until the year 2005. Development of lung cancer will not be ascertained until 10 years later, in 2015.

This type of study design is called a *concurrent cohort study* (also a *concurrent prospective* or *longitudinal study*). It is *concurrent* because the investigator identifies the original population at the beginning of the study and, in effect, accompanies the subjects concurrently through calendar time until the point at which the disease develops or not.

What is the problem with this approach? The difficulty is that, as just described, the study will take at least 20 years to complete. Several problems can result. If one is fortunate enough to obtain a research grant, such funding is generally limited to a maximum of only 3 to 5 years. In addition, with a study of this length, there is the risk that the study subjects will outlive the investigator, or at least that the investigator may not survive to the end of the study. Given these issues, the concurrent cohort study often proves unattractive to investigators who are contemplating new research.

Do these problems mean that the cohort design is not practical? Is there any way to shorten the time period needed to conduct a cohort study? Let us consider an alternate approach using the cohort design (Fig. 8–7). Suppose that we again begin our study in 1995, but now we find that an old roster of elementary schoolchildren from 1975 is available in our community, and that they had been surveyed

regarding their smoking habits in 1985. Using these data resources in 1995, we can begin to determine who in this population has developed lung cancer and who has not. This is called a *retrospective cohort study* (also called a *historical cohort* or *nonconcurrent prospective study*). Note, however, that the study design does not differ from that of the concurrent cohort design—we are still comparing exposed and non-exposed groups; what we have done in the retrospective cohort design is to use historical data from the past so that we can telescope the frame of calendar time for the study and obtain our results sooner. It is no longer a concurrent design, because we are beginning the study with a pre-existing population to reduce the duration of the study. But, as shown in Figure 8–8, *the designs for both the concurrent cohort study and the retrospective cohort study are identical: we are comparing exposed and non-exposed populations.* The only difference between them is calendar time. In a *concurrent cohort design*, exposure and non-exposure are ascertained as they occur during the study; the groups are then followed up for several years into the future and incidence is measured. In a *retrospective cohort design*, exposure is ascertained from past records and outcome (development or no development of disease) is ascertained at the time the study is begun.

It is also possible to conduct a study that is a *combination* of concurrent cohort and retrospective cohort designs. With this approach, exposure is ascertained from objective records in the past (as in a historical cohort study), and follow-up and measurement of outcome continue into the future.

EXAMPLES OF COHORT STUDIES

Example 1: The Framingham Study
One of the most important and best-known

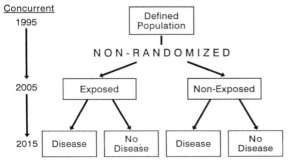

Figure 8–6. Time frame for a hypothetical concurrent cohort study begun in 1995.

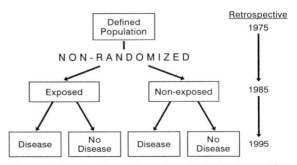

Figure 8–7. Time frame for a hypothetical retrospective cohort study begun in 1995.

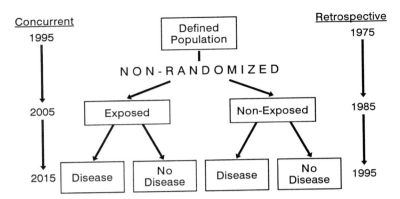

Figure 8–8. Time frames for a hypothetical concurrent and a hypothetical retrospective cohort study begun in 1995.

cohort studies is the Framingham Study of cardiovascular disease, which was begun in 1948.[1] Framingham is a town in Massachusetts, about 20 miles from Boston. It was thought that the characteristics of its population (just under 30,000) would be appropriate for such a study and would facilitate follow-up of participants.

Residents were considered eligible if they were between 30 and 62 years of age. The rationale for using this age range was that people younger than 30 years would generally be unlikely to manifest the cardiovascular end-points being studied during the proposed 20-year follow-up period. Many persons older than 62 years would already have established coronary disease, and it would therefore not be rewarding to study persons in this age group for incidence of coronary disease.

The investigators sought a sample size of 5,000. Table 8–3 shows how the final study population was derived. It consisted of 5,127 men and women between ages 30 and 62 years at the time of entry who were free of cardiovascular disease at that time. In this study many "exposures" were defined, including smoking, obesity, elevated blood pressure, ele-

vated cholesterol levels, low levels of physical activity, and other factors.

New coronary events were identified by examining the study population every 2 years and by daily surveillance of hospitalizations at the only hospital in Framingham.

The study was designed to test the following hypotheses:

- Incidence of CHD increases with age. It occurs earlier and more frequently in males.
- Persons with hypertension develop CHD at a greater rate than those who are normotensive.
- Elevated blood cholesterol level is associated with an increased risk of CHD.
- Tobacco smoking and habitual use of alcohol are associated with an increased incidence of CHD.
- Increased physical activity is associated with a decrease in development of CHD.
- An increase in body weight predisposes a person to CHD.
- An increased rate of development of CHD occurs in patients with diabetes mellitus.

When we examine this list today, we might wonder why such obvious and well-known relationships

Table 8–3. Derivation of the Framingham Study Population

	No. of Men	No. of Women	Total
Random sample	3,074	3,433	6,507
Respondents	2,024	2,445	4,469
Volunteers	312	428	740
Respondents free of CHD	1,975	2,418	4,393
Volunteers free of CHD	307	427	734
Total free of CHD: The Framingham Study Group	2,282	2,845	5,127

From Dawber TR, Kannel WB, Lyell LP: An approach to longitudinal studies in a community: The Framingham Study. Ann NY Acad Sci 107:539–556, 1993.

should have been examined in such an extensive study. The danger of this "hindsight" approach should be kept in mind; it is primarily *because* of the Framingham Study, a classic cohort study that made fundamental contributions to our understanding of the epidemiology of cardiovascular disease, that these relationships are well known today.

This study employed the second method described earlier in the chapter for selecting a study population for a cohort study: A defined population was selected on the basis of location of residence or other factors not related to the exposure(s) in question. The population was then observed over time to determine which individuals developed or already had the "exposure(s)" of interest and, later on, to determine which ones developed the cardiovascular outcome(s) of interest. This approach offered an important advantage: It permitted the investigators to study multiple "exposures," such as hypertension, smoking, obesity, cholesterol levels, and other factors, as well as the complex interactions among the exposures, by using multivariate techniques. Thus, whereas a cohort study that begins with an exposed and an unexposed group focuses on the specific exposure, a cohort study that begins with a defined population can explore the roles of many exposures.

Example 2: Breast Cancer Incidence and Progesterone Deficiency

It has long been recognized that breast cancer is more common in women who are older at the time of their first pregnancy. A difficult question is raised by this observation: Is the relation of late age at first pregnancy with risk of breast cancer due to the fact that an early first pregnancy protects against breast cancer (and therefore such protection is missing in women who have a later pregnancy or no pregnancy), or are both a delayed first pregnancy and an increased risk of breast cancer the result of some third factor, such as an underlying hormonal abnormality?

It is difficult to tease apart these two interpretations. However, in 1978, Cowan and co-workers[2] carried out a study designed to determine which of these two explanations was likely to be the correct one (Fig. 8–9). The researchers identified a population of women who were patients at the Johns Hopkins Hospital Infertility Clinic, Baltimore, from 1945 to 1965. Because they were patients at this clinic, the subjects, by definition, all had a late age at first pregnancy. In the course of their diagnos-

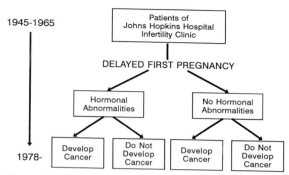

Figure 8–9. Design of Cowan's retrospective cohort study of breast cancer. (Data from Cowan LD, Gordis L, Tonascia JA, Jones GS: Breast cancer incidence in women with progesterone deficiency. Am J Epidemiol 114:209–217, 1981.)

tic evaluations, detailed hormonal profiles were developed for each woman. The researchers were therefore able to separate the women into those with an underlying hormonal abnormality, including progesterone deficiency (exposed), and those without such a hormonal abnormality (non-exposed) who had another cause for infertility, such as a problem with tubal patency or a husband's low sperm count. Both groups of women were then followed up for subsequent development of breast cancer.

How could the results of this study design clarify the relationship of late age at first pregnancy to risk of breast cancer? If the explanation for the association of late age at first pregnancy and increased risk of breast cancer is that an early first pregnancy protects against breast cancer, we would not expect any difference in breast cancer incidence between the women who have a hormonal abnormality and those who do not. However, if the explanation for the increased risk of breast cancer is that the underlying hormonal abnormality predisposes to breast cancer, we would expect to find a higher incidence of breast cancer in women with the hormonal abnormality than in those without this abnormality.

The study found that when the development of breast cancer was considered for the entire group, there was a 1.8 times greater incidence in women with hormonal abnormalities than in women without such abnormalities, but the finding was not statistically significant. However, when the occurrence of breast cancers was divided into categories of premenopausal and postmenopausal incidence, a 5.4 times greater risk for premenopausal occurrence of breast cancer was found in women with hormonal abnormalities; no difference was seen for postmenopausal occurrence of breast cancer. It is not clear whether this lack of a difference for postmenopausal breast cancer incidence represents the true absence of a difference or whether it can be attributed to the small number of women in this population who had reached menopause at the time the study was conducted.

What type of study design is this? Clearly, it is a cohort design, because it compares exposed and non-exposed persons. Furthermore, because the study was carried out in 1978 and the investigator utilized a roster of patients who had been seen at the Infertility Clinic from 1945 to 1965, it is a retrospective cohort design.

POTENTIAL BIASES IN COHORT STUDIES

A number of potential biases must be either avoided or taken into account in conducting cohort studies. The major biases include the following:

1. *Bias in assessment of the outcome:* If the person who decides whether or not disease has developed in each subject also knows whether or not that subject was exposed, and if that person is aware of the hypothesis being tested, that person's judgment as to whether or not the disease developed may be biased by that knowledge. This problem can be addressed by blinding (masking) the person who is making the disease assessment and also by checking on whether or not this person was, in fact, aware of each subject's exposure status.
2. *Information bias:* If the quality and extent of information obtained is different for exposed people than for non-exposed people, a significant bias can be introduced. This is particularly likely to occur in historical cohort studies in which information is obtained from past records. As we discussed in regard to randomized trials, it is essential in any cohort study that the quality of the information obtained be comparable in both exposed and non-exposed individuals.
3. *Biases from non-response and losses to follow-up:* As was discussed in connection with randomized trials, non-participation and non-response can introduce major biases that can complicate interpretation of the study findings. Similarly, loss to follow-up can be a serious

problem: If people with the disease are selectively lost to follow-up, the incidence rates calculated in the exposed and non-exposed groups will clearly be difficult to interpret.

4. *Analytic bias:* As in any study, if the epidemiologists and statisticians who are analyzing the data have strong preconceptions, they may unintentionally introduce their biases into their data analyses and into their interpretation of the study findings.

WHEN IS A COHORT STUDY WARRANTED?

When we carry out a cohort study, we begin with an exposed group and a non-exposed group. It is clear, therefore, that to carry out such a study we must have some idea of which exposures are suspected as a possible cause of a disease, and which are therefore worth investigating. Consequently, a cohort study is indicated when good evidence suggests an association of a disease with a certain exposure or exposures (evidence obtained either from clinical observations or from case-control or other types of studies).

Because cohort studies often involve follow-up of populations over a long period, the cohort approach is particularly good when we are able to minimize attrition (loss to follow-up) of the study population. Consequently, such studies are generally easier to conduct when the interval between the exposure and the development of disease is short. An example of an association in which the interval between exposure and outcome is short is the relation of rubella infection during pregnancy to development of congenital malformations in the offspring.

Several considerations often make the cohort design impractical. Often, strong evidence does not exist to justify mounting a large and expensive study for in-depth investigation of the role of a specific risk factor in the etiology of a disease. Even when such evidence is available, a cohort of exposed and of non-exposed persons often cannot be identified. Generally, we do not have appropriate past records or other sources of data that enable us to conduct a retrospective cohort study; as a result, a long study is necessitated by the need for extended follow-up of the population after exposure. Furthermore, many of the diseases that are of interest today occur at very low rates. Consequently, very large cohorts must be enrolled in a study to ensure that enough cases develop by the end of the study period to permit valid analysis and conclusions.

In view of these considerations, an approach other than a cohort design is often needed—one that will surmount many of the difficulties enumerated above. Chapter 9 presents such a study design—the case-control study. A third study design, the cross-sectional study, is also described. Chapters 10 and 11 discuss the use of these study designs in estimating any increased risk associated with an exposure, and the characteristics of both cohort and case-control studies are reviewed in Chapter 12.

References

1. Kannel WB: CHD Risk Factors: A Framingham Study Update. Hosp Pract 25:93–104, 1990.
2. Cowan LD, Gordis L, Tonascia JA, Jones GS: Breast cancer incidence in women with progesterone deficiency. Am J Epidemiol 114:209–217, 1981.

Review Questions

1. It is essential in cohort studies of the role of a suspected factor in etiology of a disease that:
   a. There be equal numbers of persons in both study groups
   b. At the beginning of the study, those with the disease and those without the disease have equal risks of having the factor
   c. The study group with the factor and the study group without the factor be representative of the general population
   d. The exposed and unexposed groups under study be as similar as possible with regard to possible confounding factors
   e. Both *b* and *c*

2. Which of the following is *not* an advantage of a concurrent cohort study?
   a. It can usually be done more cheaply than a case-control study
   b. Precise measurement of exposure is possible
   c. Incidence rates can be calculated
   d. Recall bias is minimized compared with a case-control study
   e. Many disease outcomes can be studied simultaneously

3. Retrospective cohort studies are characterized by all of the following *except:*
   a. The study groups are exposed and non-exposed
   b. Incidence rates may be computed

   c. The required sample size is smaller than that needed for a concurrent cohort study
   d. The required sample size is similar to that needed for a concurrent cohort study
   e. They are useful for rare exposures

4. A major problem resulting from the lack of randomization in a cohort study is:
   a. The possibility that a factor that led to the exposure rather than the exposure itself might have caused the disease
   b. The possibility that a greater proportion of people in the study may have been exposed
   c. The possibility that a smaller proportion of people in the study may have been exposed
   d. That without randomization the study may take longer to carry out
   e. Planned crossover is more likely

5. In conducting a cohort study, the advantage of starting by selecting a defined population for study before any of its members become exposed, rather than starting by selecting exposed and non-exposed individuals, is that:
   a. The study can be completed more rapidly
   b. A number of outcomes can be studied simultaneously
   c. A number of exposures can be studied stimultaneously
   d. The study will be cheaper to carry out
   e. *a* and *d*

CHAPTER 9

Case-Control and Cross-sectional Studies

Suppose you are a clinician and that you have seen a few patients with a certain type of cancer, almost all of whom report that they have been exposed to a particular chemical. You hypothesize that the exposure is related to the risk of developing this type of cancer. How would you go about confirming or refuting your hypothesis?

Consider two real-life examples:

In the early 1940s, Alton Ochsner, a surgeon in New Orleans, observed that virtually all of the patients on whom he was operating for lung cancer gave a history of cigarette smoking.[1] Although this relationship is accepted and well recognized today, it was new and controversial at the time that Ochsner made his observation. He hypothesized that cigarette smoking was linked to lung cancer. Based only on his observations in cases of lung cancer, was this conclusion valid?

A second example:

Again in the 1940s, Sir Norman Gregg, an Australian ophthalmologist, observed a number of infants and young children in his ophthalmology practice who presented with an unusual form of cataract.[2] Gregg noted that these children had been in utero during the time of a rubella (German measles) outbreak. He suggested that there was an association between prenatal rubella exposure and the development of the unusual cataracts. Keep in mind that at that time there was no knowledge that a virus could be teratogenic. Thus, he proposed his hypothesis solely on the basis of observational data, the equivalent of data from ambulatory or bedside practice today.

Let us suppose that Gregg had observed that 90% of these infants had been in utero during the rubella outbreak. Would he have been justified in concluding that rubella was associated with the cataracts? Clearly, the answer is no. For although such an observation would be interesting, it would be difficult to interpret without data for a comparison group of children without cataracts. It is possible, for ex-

ample, that 90% of *all* mothers in that community—both mothers of children with the cataracts and mothers of children with no cataracts—had been pregnant during the outbreak of rubella. In such a case, the exposure history would be no different for mothers of children with cataracts than for mothers of controls. The question was, therefore, whether the prevalence of rubella exposure (i.e., having been in utero during the outbreak) was greater in infants with cataracts than in a group of children without cataracts.

To determine the significance of such observations in a group of cases, a comparison or control group is needed. Without such a comparison, Ochsner's or Gregg's observations would only constitute a case series. The observations would have been intriguing, but no conclusion is possible without comparative observations in a series of *noncases*. Comparison is an essential component of epidemiologic investigation and is well exemplified by the case-control study design.

DESIGN OF A CASE-CONTROL STUDY

Figure 9–1 shows the design of a *case-control study*. To examine the possible relation of an exposure to a certain disease, we identify a group of

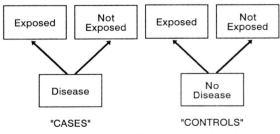

Figure 9–1. Design of a case-control study.

Table 9–1. Design of Case-Control Studies

		First, Select:	
		Cases (With Disease)	Controls (Without Disease)
Then, Measure Past Exposure:	Were exposed	a	b
	Were not exposed	c	d
	Total	a + c	b + d
	Proportions exposed	$\dfrac{a}{a + c}$	$\dfrac{b}{b + d}$

individuals with that disease (called *cases*) and, for purposes of comparison, a group of people without that disease (called *controls*). We determine what proportion of the cases were exposed and what proportion were not. We also determine what proportion of the controls were exposed and what proportion were not. In the example of the children with cataracts, the cases would consist of children with cataracts and the controls would consist of children without cataracts. For each child, it would then be necessary to ascertain whether or not the mother was exposed to rubella during her pregnancy with that child. We anticipate that if the exposure (rubella) is in fact related to the disease (cataracts), the prevalence of history of exposure among the cases—children with cataracts—will be greater than that among the controls—children with no cataracts. Thus, in a case-control study, if there is an association of an exposure with a disease, the prevalence of history of exposure should be higher in persons who have the disease (cases) that in those who do not (controls).

Table 9–1 presents a hypothetical schema of how a case-control study is conducted. We begin by selecting cases with the disease and controls without the disease, and then measure past exposure by interview and by review of medical or employee records or of results of chemical or biologic assays of blood, urine, or tissues. If exposure is dichotomous—that is, exposure has either occurred (yes) or not occurred (no)—breakdown into four groups is possible: There are *a* cases who were exposed and *c* cases who were not exposed. Similarly, there are *b* controls who were exposed and *d* controls who were not exposed. Thus the total number of cases is *a* + *c* and the total number of controls is *b* + *d*. If exposure is associated with disease, we would expect the proportion of the

cases who were exposed, or $\dfrac{a}{a + c}$, to be greater than the proportion of the controls who were exposed, or $\dfrac{b}{b + d}$.

A hypothetical example of a case-control study is seen in Table 9–2. We are conducting a case-control study of the relationship of smoking to coronary heart disease (CHD). We start with 200 people with CHD (cases) and compare them to 400 people without CHD (controls). If there is a relationship between smoking and CHD we would anticipate that a greater proportion of the CHD cases than of the controls would have been smokers (exposed). We find that of the 200 CHD cases, 112 were smokers and 88 were non-smokers. Of the 400 controls, 176 were smokers and 224 were non-smokers. Thus 56% of CHD cases were smokers compared to 44% of the controls. This calculation is only a first step. Further calculations to determine whether or not there is an association of the exposure with the disease will be discussed in Chapters 10 and 11. This chapter focuses on issues of design in case-control studies.

Parenthetically, it is of interest to note that if we use only the data from a case-control study, we cannot estimate the prevalence of the disease. In this example we had 200 cases and 400 controls,

Table 9–2. Hypothetical Example of a Case-Control Study of CHD and Cigarette Smoking

	CHD	Controls
Smoke cigarettes	112	176
Do not smoke cigarettes	88	224
Total	200	400
% Smoking cigarettes	56.0	44.0

but this does not imply that the prevalence is 33%, or $\frac{200}{200 + 400}$. The decision as to the number of controls to select per case in a case-control study is in the hands of the investigator, and it is an arbitrary decision. In this example, the investigator could have selected, for example, 200 cases and 200 controls (1 control per case), or 200 cases and 800 controls (4 controls per case). Because the proportion of the entire study population that consists of cases is determined by the ratio of controls per case, and this proportion is determined by the investigator, it clearly does not reflect the true prevalence of the disease in the population.

At this point, we should emphasize that *the hallmark of the case-control study is that it begins with people with the disease (cases) and compares them to people without the disease (controls)*. This is in contrast to the design of a cohort study, discussed in Chapter 8, which begins with a group of exposed people and compares them to a non-exposed group. Some people have the erroneous impression that the distinction between the two types of study design is that cohort studies go forward in time and case-control studies go backward in time. Such a distinction is not correct; in fact, it is unfortunate that the term *retrospective* has been used for case-control studies, as the term incorrectly implies that calendar time is the characteristic that distinguishes case-control from cohort design. As was shown in the previous chapter, a retrospective cohort study also utilizes data obtained in the past. Thus, calendar time is not the characteristic that distinguishes a case-control from a cohort study. What distinguishes the two study designs is whether the study begins with diseased and non-diseased people (case-control study) or with exposed and non-exposed people (cohort study).

Table 9–3 presents the results of a case-control study of the use of artificial sweeteners and bladder cancer. This study included 3,000 cases with bladder cancer and 5,776 controls without bladder cancer. Why the unusual number of controls? The most likely explanation is that the investigation planned for two controls per case (i.e., 6,000 controls), and that some of the controls did not participate. Of the 3,000 cases, 1,293 had used artificial sweeteners (43.1%), and of the 5,776 controls, 2,455 had used artificial sweeteners (42.5%). The proportions are very close, and the investigators in this study did not confirm the findings that had been reported in animal studies, which had caused considerable controversy and had major policy implications for government regulation.

One of the earliest studies of cigarette smoking and lung cancer was conducted by Sir Richard Doll and Bradford Hill. (Sir Richard Doll is an internationally known epidemiologist who was knighted for his scientific work, an honor that comes all too infrequently to epidemiologists!) Table 9–4 presents data from this study for 1,357 males with lung cancer and 1,357 controls according to the average number of cigarettes smoked per day in the 10 years preceding the present illness.[3]

We see that there are fewer heavy smokers among the controls and very few non-smokers among the lung cancer cases, a finding strongly suggestive of an association between smoking and lung cancer. In contrast to the previous example, exposure in this study is not just dichotomized (exposed or not exposed), but the exposure data are further stratified in terms of dose, as measured by the number of cigarettes smoked per day. Because many of the environmental exposures about which we are concerned today are not all-or-nothing exposures, the possibility of doing a study and analysis

Table 9–3. History of Use of Artificial Sweeteners in Bladder Cancer Cases and Controls

Artificial Sweetener Use	Cases	Controls
Ever	1,293	2,455
Never	1,707	3,321
Total	3,000	5,776

From Hoover RN, Strasser PH: Artificial sweeteners and human bladder cancer: Preliminary results. Lancet 1:837–840, 1980.

Table 9–4. Distribution of 1,357 Male Lung Cancer Patients and a Male Control Group According to Average Number of Cigarettes Smoked Daily Over the 10 Years Preceding Onset of the Present Illness

Average Daily Cigarettes	Lung Cancer Patients	Control Group
0	7	61
1–4	55	129
5–14	489	570
15–24	475	431
25–49	293	154
50 +	38	12
Total	1,357	1,357

From Doll R, Hill AB: A study of the aetiology of carcinoma of the lung. Br Med J 2:1271–1286, 1952.

that takes into account the dose of the exposure is very important.

SELECTION OF CASES AND CONTROLS

Selection of Cases

In a case-control study, cases can be selected from a variety of sources, including hospital patients, patients in physicians' practices, or clinic patients. Many communities maintain registries of patients with certain diseases, such as cancer, and such registries can serve as valuable sources of cases for such studies.

Several problems must be kept in mind in selecting cases for a case-control study. If cases are selected from a single hospital, any risk factors that are identified may be unique to that hospital as a result of referral patterns or other factors, and the results may not be generalizable to all patients with the disease. Consequently, if hospitalized cases are to be used, it is desirable to select the cases from several hospitals in the community. Furthermore, if the hospital from which the cases are drawn is a tertiary care facility, which selectively admits severely ill patients, any risk factors identified in the study may be risk factors only in persons with severe forms of the disease. In any event, it is essential that in case-control studies, just as in randomized trials, the criteria for eligibility be carefully specified in writing.

Incident or Prevalent Cases

An important consideration in case-control studies is whether to use incident cases of a disease— that is, newly diagnosed cases—or prevalent cases of the disease—that is, people who may have had the disease for some time. The problem with use of incident cases is that we must often wait for new cases to be diagnosed; whereas if we use prevalent cases, which have already been diagnosed, a larger number of cases is often available for study. Despite this practical advantage of using prevalent cases, however, it is generally preferable to use incident cases of the disease in case-control studies of disease etiology. The reason is that any risk factors we may identify in a study using prevalent cases may be related more to *survival* with the disease than to the development of the disease (*incidence*). If, for example, most people who develop the disease die soon after diagnosis, they will be underrepresented in a study that uses prevalent cases, and such a study is more likely to include longer-term survivors. This would constitute a highly nonrepresentative group of cases, and any risk factors identified with this nonrepresentative group may not be a general characteristic of patients with the disease, but only of survivors.

Even if we include only *incident* cases (patients who have been newly diagnosed with the disease) in a case-control study, we will of course be excluding any patients who may have died before the diagnosis was made. There is no easy solution to this problem or to certain other problems in case selection, but it is important that we keep these issues in mind when we finally interpret the data and derive conclusions from the study. At that time, it is critical to take into account possible selection biases that may have been introduced by the study design and by the manner in which the study was conducted.

Selection of Controls

In 1929, Raymond Pearl, Professor of Biostatistics at Johns Hopkins University, Baltimore, conducted a study to test the hypothesis that tuberculosis protected against cancer.[4] From 7,500 consecutive autopsies at Johns Hopkins Hospital, Pearl identified 816 cases of cancer. He then selected a control group of 816 from among the others on whom autopsies had been carried out at Johns Hopkins and determined the percent of the cases and of the controls who had findings of tuberculosis on autopsy. Pearl's findings are seen in Table 9–5.

Of the 816 autopsies of patients with cancer, 54 had tuberculosis (6.6%), whereas of the 816 controls with no cancer, 133 had tuberculosis (16.3%). From the finding that the prevalence of tuberculosis was considerably higher in the control group (no cancer findings) than in the case group (cancer diagnoses), Pearl concluded that tuberculosis had an antagonistic or protective effect against cancer.

Table 9–5. Summary of Data From Pearl's Study of Cancer and Tuberculosis

	Cases (With Cancer)	Controls (Without Cancer)
Total no. of autopsies	816	816
No. (%) of autopsies with tuberculosis	54 (6.6)	133 (16.3)

From Pearl R: Cancer and tuberculosis. Am J Hyg 9:97–159, 1929.

Was Pearl's conclusion justified? The answer to this question depends on the adequacy of his control group. If the prevalence of tuberculosis in the *non-cancer* patients was similar to that of all people who were free of cancer, his conclusion would be valid. But that was not the case. At the time of the study, tuberculosis was one of the major reasons for hospitalization at Johns Hopkins Hospital. Consequently, what Pearl had inadvertently done in choosing the cancer-free control group was to select a group in which many of the patients had been diagnosed with and hospitalized for tuberculosis. Pearl thought that the control group's rate of tuberculosis would represent the level of tuberculosis expected in the general population; but because of the way he selected the controls, they came from a pool that was heavily weighted with tuberculosis patients, which did not represent the general population. He was, in effect, comparing the prevalence of tuberculosis in a group of patients with cancer with the prevalence of tuberculosis in a group of patients in which many had already been diagnosed with tuberculosis. Clearly, his conclusion was not justified on the basis of these data.

How could Pearl have overcome this problem in his study? Instead of comparing his cancer patients with a group selected from all other autopsied patients, he could have compared the patients with cancer to a group of patients admitted for some specific diagnosis other than cancer (and not tuberculosis). In fact, some years later Carlson and Bell[5] repeated Pearl's study but compared the patients who died of cancer to patients who died of heart disease at Johns Hopkins. They found no difference in the prevalence of tuberculosis at autopsy between the two groups. (It is of interest, however, that despite the methodologic limitations of Pearl's study, bacille Calmette-Guérin [BCG] is used today as a form of immunotherapy in several types of cancer.)

The problem with Pearl's study exemplifies the challenge of selecting appropriate controls for case-control studies. This is one of the most difficult problems in epidemiology. The challenge is this: If we conduct a case-control study and find more exposure in the cases than in the controls, we would like to be able to conclude that there is an association between the exposure and the disease in question. The way the controls were selected is a major determinant of whether such a conclusion is valid.

A fundamental conceptual issue relating to selection of controls is whether the controls should be similar to the cases in all respects other than having the disease in question, or whether they should be representative of all persons without the disease in the population from which the cases are selected. This question has stimulated considerable discussion, but in actuality, the characteristics of the non-diseased people in the population from which the cases are selected are often not known, because the reference population may not be well defined.

Consider, for example, a case-control study using hospitalized cases. We want to identify the reference population that is the source of the cases so that we can then sample this reference population to select controls. Unfortunately, it is usually either not easy or not possible to identify such a reference population for hospitalized patients. Patients admitted to a hospital may come from the surrounding neighborhood, may live further away in the same city, or may, through a referral process, come from another city or other country. Under these circumstances it is virtually impossible to define a specific reference population from which the cases emerged and from which we might select controls. Nevertheless, we want to design our study so that when it is finished, we can be reasonably certain that if we find a difference in exposure history between cases and controls, there are not likely to be any other important differences between them that might limit the inferences we may derive.

Sources of Controls

Controls may be selected from non-hospitalized persons living in the community or from hospitalized patients admitted for diseases other than that for which the cases were admitted.

Non-hospitalized Persons as Controls

Non-hospitalized controls may be selected from several sources in the community. Ideally, a probability sample of the total population might be selected, but as a practical matter, this is rarely possible. Other sources include school rosters, selective service lists, and insurance company lists. Another option is to select, as a control for each case, a resident of a defined area, such as the neighborhood in which the case lives. Such *neighborhood controls* have been used for many years. In this approach, interviewers are instructed to identify the home of a case as a starting point, and from there walk past a specified number of houses in a specified direction and seek the first household that contains an eligible control. Because of increasing problems of security in urban areas of the United States, however, many people will no longer open their doors to interviewers. Nevertheless, in many other countries, particularly in developing countries, the door-to-door approach to obtaining controls may be ideal.

Because of the difficulties in many cities in the United States in obtaining neighborhood controls using the door-to-door approach, an alternate method for selecting such controls is to use random-digit dialing. Because telephone exchanges generally match neighborhood boundaries, a case's seven-digit telephone number, of which the first three digits are the exchange, can be used to select a control telephone number, in which the terminal four digits of the phone number are randomly selected and the same three-digit exchange is used. In many developing countries this approach is impractical, as only government offices and business establishments are likely to have telephones.

Another approach to control selection is to use a *best friend control*. A case is asked for the name of a best friend who, in principle, is more likely to participate in the study knowing that his or her friend is also participating. A control obtained in this fashion may be likely to be similar to the case in age and in many other demographic and social characteristics. Sometimes a spouse or sibling control may be useful; a sibling may provide some control over genetic differences between cases and controls.

Hospitalized Patients as Controls

Hospital inpatients are often selected as controls because of the extent to which they are a "captive population" and are clearly identified; it should therefore be relatively more economical to carry out a study using such controls. However, as just discussed, they represent a sample of an ill-defined reference population that generally cannot be characterized. Moreover, hospital patients differ from people in the community. For example, the prevalence of cigarette smoking is known to be higher in hospitalized patients than in community residents; many of the diagnoses for which people are admitted to the hospital are smoking related.

Given that we generally cannot characterize the reference population from which hospitalized cases come, there is a conceptual attractiveness to comparing hospitalized cases to hospitalized controls from the same institution, who would presumably tend to come from the same reference population (Fig. 9–2): that is, whatever selection factors in the

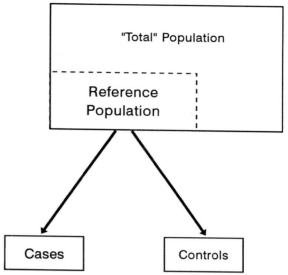

Figure 9–2. Whatever selection factors in the referral system affected cases' admission to a certain hospital would also affect hospital controls.

referral system affected the cases' admission to a particular hospital would also pertain to the controls. However, referral patterns at the same hospital may differ for various clinical services, and such an assumption may be questionable.

In using hospital controls, the question arises of whether to use a sample of all other patients admitted to the hospital (other than those with the cases' diagnosis) or whether to select a specific "other diagnosis." If we wish to choose specific diagnostic groups, on what basis do we select those groups, and on what basis do we exclude others? The problem is that although it is attractive to choose as hospitalized controls a disease group that is obviously unrelated to the putative causative factor under investigation, such controls are unlikely to be representative of the general reference population. As a result, it will not be clear whether it is the cases or the controls who differ from the general population.

The issue of which diagnostic groups would be eligible for use as controls and which would be ineligible (and would therefore be excluded) is very important. Let us say we are conducting a case-control study of lung cancer and smoking: we select as cases patients who have been hospitalized with lung cancer, and as controls we select patients who have been hospitalized with emphysema. What problem would this present? Because we know that there is a strong relationship between smoking and emphysema, our controls, the emphysema patients, would include a high number of smokers. Consequently, any relationship of smoking to lung cancer would not be detectable in this study, because we would have selected as controls persons who also have a greater-than-expected prevalence of smoking. We might therefore want to exclude from our control group persons with many smoking-related diagnoses, such as CHD, bladder cancer, pancreatic cancer, and emphysema. Such exclusions might yield a control group with a lower-than-expected prevalence of smoking; however, the exclusion process becomes complex. One alternative is to not exclude any groups from selection as controls in the design of the study, but to analyze the study data separately for different diagnostic subgroups that constitute the control group.

PROBLEMS IN CONTROL SELECTION

The following example demonstrates the problem of exclusions in the process of control selection.

In 1981, MacMahon and co-workers[6] reported a case-control study of cancer of the pancreas. The cases were patients with histologically confirmed diagnoses of pancreatic cancer in 11 Boston and Rhode Island hospitals from 1974 to 1979. Controls were selected from all patients who were hospitalized at the same time as the cases, and they were selected from other inpatients hospitalized by the attending physicians who had hospitalized the cases. One finding in this study that the investigators presented was an apparent dose-response relationship between coffee consumption and cancer of the pancreas, particularly in women (Table 9–6).

When such a relationship is observed, it is difficult to know whether the disease is *caused* by the coffee consumption or is caused by some factor closely related to the coffee consumption. Because smoking is a known risk factor for cancer of the pancreas, and because coffee consumption is closely related to cigarette smoking (it is rare to find a smoker who does not drink coffee), did MacMahon and others observe an association of coffee consumption with pancreatic cancer because the coffee caused the pancreatic cancer, or because coffee consumption is related to cigarette smoking, and cigarette smoking is known to be a risk factor for cancer of the pancreas? Recognizing this problem, the authors analyzed the data after stratifying for smoking history. The relationship with coffee consumption held both for current smokers and for those who had never smoked (Table 9–7).

This report aroused great interest in both the scientific and lay communities, particularly among coffee manufacturers. Given the widespread exposure of human beings to coffee, if the reported relationship were true, it would have major public health implications.

Let us examine the design of this study. The cases were white patients with cancer of the pancreas at 11 Boston and Rhode Island hospitals. The controls are of particular interest: They were patients with other diseases who were hospitalized by the same physicians who had hospitalized the cases. That is, when a case had been identified, the attending physician was asked if another of his or her patients who was hospitalized at the same time for another condition could be interviewed as a control. This unusual method of control selection had a practical advantage: One of the major obstacles in obtaining participation of hospital controls in case-

Table 9–6. Distribution of Cases and Controls by Coffee-Drinking Habits and Estimates of Risk Ratios

| Sex | Category | Coffee Consumption (Cups/Day) | | | | |
		0	*1–2*	*3–4*	*≥5*	Total
M	No. of cases	9	94	53	60	216
	No. of controls	32	119	74	82	307
	Adjusted relative risk*	1.0	2.6	2.3	2.6	2.6
	95% Confidence interval	—	1.2–5.5	1.0–5.3	1.2–5.8	1.2–5.4
F	No. of cases	11	59	53	28	151
	No. of controls	56	152	80	48	336
	Adjusted relative risk*	1.0	1.6	3.3	3.1	2.3
	95% Confidence interval	—	0.8–3.4	1.6–7.0	1.4–7.0	1.2–4.6

*Chi-square (Mantel extension) with equally spaced scores, adjusted over age in decades: 1.5 for men, 13.7 for women. Mantel-Haenszel estimates of risk ratios, adjusted over categories of age in decades. In all comparisons, the referent category was subjects who never drank coffee.

From MacMahon B, Yen S, Trichopoulos D, et al: Coffee and cancer of the pancreas. N Engl J Med 304:630–633, 1981.

Table 9–7. Estimates of Relative Risk*
of Cancer of the Pancreas Associated
With Use of Coffee and Cigarettes

Cigarette Smoking Status	Coffee Drinking (Cups/Day)			
	0	1–2	≥3	Total†
Never smoked	1.0	2.1	3.1	1.0
Ex-smokers	1.3	4.0	3.0	1.3 (0.9–1.8)
Current smokers	1.2	2.2	4.6	1.2 (0.9–1.8)
Total*	1.0	1.8 (1.0–3.0)	2.7 (1.6–4.7)	

*The referent category is the group that uses neither cigarettes nor coffee. Estimates are adjusted for sex and age in decades.

†Values are adjusted for the other variable, in addition to age and sex, and are expressed in relation to the lowest category of each variable. Values in parentheses are 95% confidence intervals of the adjusted estimates.

From MacMahon B, Yen S, Trichopoulos D, et al: Coffee and cancer of the pancreas. N Engl J Med 304:630–633, 1981.

control studies is that permission to contact the patient is requested of the attending physician. The physicians are often not motivated to have their patients serve as controls, because the patients do not have the disease that is the focus of the study. By asking physicians who had already given permission for patients with pancreatic cancer to participate, the likelihood was increased that permission would be granted for patients with other diseases to participate as controls.

Did that practical decision introduce any problems? The underlying question that the investigators wanted to answer was whether patients with cancer of the pancreas drank more coffee than did people without cancer of the pancreas in the same population. What MacMahon and co-workers found was that the level of coffee consumption in cases was greater than the level of coffee consumption in controls (Fig. 9–3).

The investigators would like to be able to establish that the level of coffee consumption observed in the controls is what would be expected in the general population without pancreatic cancer, and that cases therefore demonstrate *excessive* coffee consumption. But the problem is this: Which physicians are most likely to admit patients with cancer of the pancreas to the hospital? Gastroenterologists are often the admitting physicians. Many of their other hospitalized patients (who served as controls) also have gastrointestinal problems, such as esophagitis and peptic ulcer. So in this study, the persons who served as controls may very well have reduced their intake of coffee, either because of a

physician's instructions or because of their own realization that reducing their coffee intake could relieve their symptoms. We cannot assume that the controls' levels of coffee consumption are representative of the level of coffee consumption expected in the general population; their rate of coffee consumption may be abnormally low. Thus, the observed difference in coffee consumption between pancreatic cancer cases and controls may not necessarily have been the result of cases drinking more coffee than expected, but rather of the controls drinking less coffee than expected (Fig. 9–4).

MacMahon and his colleagues subsequently repeated their analysis, but separated controls with gastrointestinal illness from controls with other conditions. They found that the risk associated with coffee consumption was indeed higher when the comparison was with controls with gastrointestinal illness, but that the relationship between coffee consumption and pancreatic cancer persisted, albeit at a lower level, even when the comparison was with controls with other illnesses. Several years later, Hsieh and co-workers reported a new study that attempted to replicate these results; it did not support the original findings.[7]

In summary, when a difference in exposure is observed between cases and controls, we must ask whether the level of exposure observed in the controls is really the expected level in the population in which the study was carried out, or whether—perhaps given the manner of selection—the controls may have a particularly low level of exposure that might not be representative of the level in the population in which the study was carried out.

MATCHING

A major concern in conducting a case-control study is that cases and controls may differ in charac-

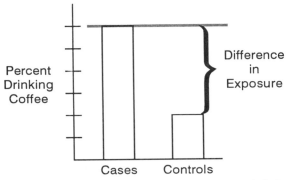

Figure 9–3. Interpreting the results of a case-control study of coffee-drinking and pancreatic cancer.

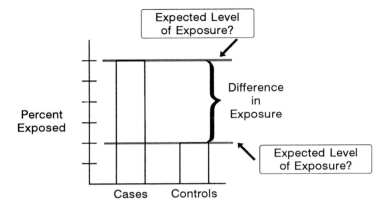

Figure 9–4. Interpreting the results of case-control studies: What is the expected level of exposure?

teristics or exposures other than the one that has been targeted for study. If more cases than controls are found to have been exposed, we may be left with the question of whether the observed association could be due to differences between the cases and controls in factors other than the exposure being studied. For example, if more cases are found to have been exposed than have controls, and if most of the cases are poor and most of the controls are affluent, we would not know whether the factor determining development of disease is exposure to the factor being studied or another characteristic associated with being poor. To avoid such a situation, we would like to ensure that the distribution of the cases and controls by socioeconomic status is similar, so that a difference in exposure will likely constitute the critical difference, and the presence or absence of disease is not likely to be attributable to a difference in socioeconomic status.

One approach to dealing with this problem in the design and conduct of the study is to match the cases and controls for factors about which we may be concerned, such as income in the preceding example. *Matching* is defined as the process of selecting the controls so that they are similar to the cases in certain characteristics, such as age, race, sex, socioeconomic status, and occupation. Matching may be of two types: (1) group matching and (2) individual matching.

Group Matching

Group matching (or *frequency matching*) consists of selecting the controls in such a manner that the proportion of controls with a certain characteristic is identical to the proportion of cases with the same characteristic. Thus, if 25% of the cases are married, the controls will be selected so that 25%

of that group is also married. This type of selection generally requires that all of the cases be selected first. After calculations are made of the proportions of certain characteristics in the group of cases, then a control group, in which the same characteristics occur in the same proportions, is selected.

Individual Matching

A second type of matching is *individual matching* (or *matched pairs*). In this approach, for each case selected for the study, a control is selected who is similar to the case in terms of the specific variable or variables of concern. For example, if the first case enrolled in our study is a 45-year-old white woman, we will seek a 45-year-old white female control. If the second case is a 24-year-old black man, we will select a control who is also a 24-year-old black man. This type of control selection yields matched case-control pairs; that is, each case is individually matched to a control. The implications of this method of control selection for the estimation of excess risk are discussed in the Chapter 10.

Individual matching is often used in case-control studies that use hospital controls. The reason for this is more practical than conceptual. Let us say that sex and age are considered important variables, and it is thought to be important that the cases and the controls be comparable in terms of these two characteristics. There is generally no practical way to dip into a pool of hospital patients to select a group with certain sex and age characteristics. Rather, it is easier to identify a case and then to choose the next hospital admission that matches the case for sex and age. Thus individual matching is most expedient in studies using hospital controls.

What are the problems with matching? The problems with matching are of two types: practical and conceptual.

1. *Practical Problems With Matching:* If an attempt is made to match according to too many characteristics, it may prove difficult or impossible to identify an appropriate control. For example, suppose it is decided to match each case for race, sex, age, marital status, number of children, zip code of residence, and occupation. If the case is a 48-year-old black woman who is married, has four children, lives in zip code 21209, and works in a photo-processing plant, it may prove difficult or impossible to find a control who is similar to the case in all of these characteristics. Therefore, the more variables that we choose to match, the more difficult it will be to find a suitable control.

2. *Conceptual Problems With Matching:* Perhaps a more important problem is the conceptual one: *Once we have matched controls to cases according to a given characteristic, we cannot study that characteristic.* For example, suppose we are interested in studying marital status as a risk factor for breast cancer. If we match the cases (breast cancer) and the controls (no breast cancer) according to marital status, we can no longer study whether or not marital status is a risk factor for breast cancer. Why not? Because in matching according to marital status we have artificially established an identical proportion in cases and controls: if 35% of the cases are married, and through matching we create a control group in which 35% are also married, we have artificially ensured that the proportion of married subjects will be identical in both groups. By using matching to impose comparability for a certain factor, we ensure the same prevalence of that factor in the cases and in the controls. Clearly, we will then not be able to ask whether cases differ from controls in the prevalence of that factor. We would therefore not want to match on the variable of marital status in this study. Indeed, we do not want to match on any variable that we may wish to explore in our study.

It is also important to recognize that unplanned matching may inadvertently occur in case-control studies. For example, if we use neighborhood controls, we are in effect matching for socioeconomic status as well as for cultural and other characteristics of a neighborhood. If we use best-friend controls, it is likely that the case and his or her best friend share many lifestyle characteristics, which in effect produces a match for these characteristics.

For example, in a study of oral contraceptive use and cancer in which best-friend controls were considered, there was concern that if the case used oral contraceptives it might well be that her best friend would also be likely to be an oral contraceptive user. The result would be an unplanned matching on oral contraceptive use, so that this variable could no longer be investigated in this study.

In carrying out a case-control study, therefore, we only match on variables that we are convinced are risk factors for the disease, characteristics that we are not interested in investigating in this study. Matching on variables other than these, in either a planned or inadvertent manner, is called *overmatching*.

PROBLEMS OF RECALL

A major problem in case-control studies is that of recall. Recall problems are of two types: (1) limitations of recall and (2) recall bias.

Limitations in Human Recall

Much of the information relating to exposure in case-control studies often involves collecting data from subjects by interviews. Because virtually all human beings are limited to varying degrees in their ability to recall information, limitations in recall are an important issue in such studies. A related issue that is somewhat different from limitations in recall is that persons being interviewed may simply not have the information being requested.

This was demonstrated years ago in a study carried out by Lilienfeld and Graham.[8] At that time, considerable interest centered on the observation that cancer of the cervix was highly unusual in two groups of women: Jewish women and nuns. This observation suggested that an important risk factor for cervical cancer could be sexual intercourse with an uncircumcised man, and a number of studies were carried out to confirm this hypothesis. However, the authors were skeptical about the validity of the responses regarding circumcision status. To address this question they asked a group of men whether or not they had been circumcised. The men were then examined by a physician. As seen in Table 9–8, of the 56 men who stated they were circumcised, 19, or 33.9%, were found to be uncircumcised. Of the 136 men who stated they were not circumcised, 47, or 34.6%, were found to be circumcised. These data demonstrate that the find-

Table 9–8. Comparison of Patients' Statements With Examination Findings Concerning Circumcision Status, Roswell Park Memorial Institute, Buffalo, New York

Examination Finding	Patients' Statements Regarding Circumcision			
	Yes		No	
	No.	%	No.	%
Circumcised	37	66.1	47	34.6
Not circumcised	19	33.9	89	65.4
Total	56	100.0	136	100.0

Adapted from Lilienfeld AM, Graham S: Validity of determining circumcision status by questionnaire as related to epidemiologic studies of cancer of the cervix. J Natl Cancer Inst 21:713–720, 1958.

ings from studies using interview data may not always be clear-cut.

If a limitation of recall regarding exposure affects all subjects in a study to the same extent, regardless of whether they are cases or controls, no bias is introduced. But a resulting misclassification of exposure status has resulted, so that some of the cases or controls who were actually exposed will be erroneously classified as unexposed, and some who were actually not exposed will be erroneously classified as exposed. This generally results in an underestimate of the true risk of the disease associated with the exposure.

Recall Bias

A more serious potential problem in case-control studies is that of recall bias. Suppose we are studying the possible relationship of congenital malformations to prenatal infections. We conduct a case-control study and interview mothers of children with congenital malformations (cases) and mothers of children without malformations (controls). Each mother is questioned regarding infections she may have had during the pregnancy.

A mother who has had a child with a birth defect often tries to identify some unusual event that occurred during her pregnancy with that child. She wants to know whether the abnormality was caused by something she did. Why did it happen? Such a mother may even recall an event, such as a mild respiratory infection, that a mother of a child without a birth defect may not even notice or may have forgotten entirely. This type of bias is known as *recall* bias; it has also been called "rumination bias" by Wynder.

In the study just mentioned, let us assume that the true infection rate during pregnancy in mothers of malformed infants and in mothers of normal infants is 15%—that is, there is no difference in infection rates. Suppose that mothers of malformed infants recall 60% of any infections they had during pregnancy and mothers of normal infants recall only 10% of infections they had during pregnancy. As seen in Table 9–9, the *apparent* infection rate estimated from this case-control study using interviews would be 9% for mothers of malformed infants and 1.5% for mothers of control infants. Thus the *differential recall* between cases and controls introduces a recall bias into the study that could artifactually suggest a relation of congenital malformations and prenatal infections. Although a potential for recall bias is self-evident in case-control studies, in point of fact it is difficult to find actual examples to demonstrate that recall bias has been a major problem in case-control studies and has resulted in erroneous conclusions regarding associations. Nevertheless, the potential problem cannot be disregarded, and the possibility for such bias must always be kept in mind.

USE OF MULTIPLE CONTROLS

Early in the chapter we referred to the fact that the investigator can determine how many controls will be used per case in a case-control study; multiple controls for each case are frequently used. Such controls may be either (1) *controls of the same type,* or (2) *controls of different types,* such as hospital

Table 9–9. Example of Artificial Association Resulting From Recall Bias: A Study of Maternal Infections During Pregnancy and Congenital Malformations

	Cases (With Congenital Malformations)	Controls (Without Congenital Malformations)
Assume That:		
True incidence of infection (%)	15	15
Infections recalled (%)	60	10
Result Will Be:		
Infection rate as ascertained by interview (%)	9.0	1.5

Figure 9–5. Study groups in Gold's study of brain tumors in children. (Data from Gold EB, Gordis L, Tonascia J, Szklo M: Risk factors for brain tumors in children. Am J Epidemiol 109:309–319, 1979.)

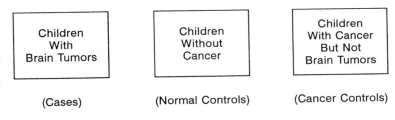

Children With Brain Tumors	Children Without Cancer	Children With Cancer But Not Brain Tumors
(Cases)	(Normal Controls)	(Cancer Controls)

and neighborhood controls, or controls with different diseases.

Controls of the Same Type

Multiple controls *of the same type*, such as two controls or three controls for each case, are used to increase the power of the study. Practically speaking, a noticeable increase in power is gained only up to a ratio of about 1 case to 4 controls. One might ask, Why use multiple controls for each case? Why not keep the ratio of controls to cases at 1:1 and just increase the number of cases? The answer is that for many of the relatively infrequent diseases we study, there may be a limit to the number of potential cases available for study. A clinic may see only a certain number of patients with a given cancer or with a certain connective tissue disorder each year. Because the number of cases cannot be increased without either extending the study in time to enroll more cases or developing a collaborative multi-centered study, the option of increasing the number of controls per case is often chosen. These controls are of the same type; only the ratio of controls to cases has changed.

Multiple Controls of Different Types

In contrast, we may choose to use *multiple controls of different types*. For example, we may be concerned that the exposure of the hospital controls used in our study may not represent the rate of exposure that is "expected" in a population of non-diseased persons—that is, the controls may be a highly selected subset of non-diseased individuals and may have a very different exposure experience. We mentioned earlier that hospitalized patients smoke more than people living in the community, and we are concerned because we do not know what the prevalence level of smoking in hospitalized controls represents or how to interpret a comparison of these rates with those of the cases. To address this problem, we may choose to use an additional control group, such as neighborhood con-

trols. The hope is that the results obtained when cases are compared with hospital controls will be similar to the results obtained when cases are compared with neighborhood controls. If the findings differ, the reason for the discrepancy should be sought. In using multiple controls of different types, the investigator should ideally decide which comparison will be considered the "gold standard of truth" before embarking on the actual study.

In 1979 Gold and co-workers published a case-control study of brain tumors in children.[9] They used two types of controls: children with no cancer (called *normal controls,* or NC) and children with cancers other than brain tumors (called *cancer controls,* or CC) (Fig. 9–5). What was the rationale for these two control groups?

Let us consider the question, Did mothers of children with brain tumors have more prenatal radiation exposure than control mothers? Some possible results are seen in Figure 9–6.

If the radiation exposure of mothers of children with brain tumors is found to be greater than that of mothers of normal controls, and the radiation exposure of mothers of children with other cancers is also found to be greater than that of mothers of

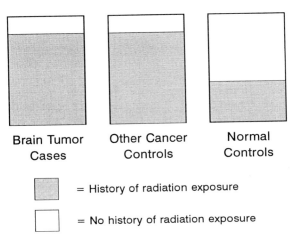

Brain Tumor Cases	Other Cancer Controls	Normal Controls

☐ = History of radiation exposure

☐ = No history of radiation exposure

Figure 9–6. Rationale of brain tumor study: I. (Data from Gold EB, Gordis L, Tonascia J, Szklo M: Risk factors for brain tumors in children. Am J Epidemiol 109:309–319, 1979.)

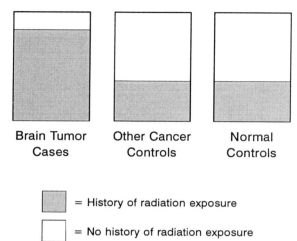

Figure 9–7. Rationale of brain tumor study: II. (Data from Gold EB, Gordis L, Tonascia J, Szklo M: Risk factors for brain tumors in children. Am J Epidemiol 109:309–319, 1979.)

normal children, what are the possible explanations? One conclusion might be that prenatal radiation is a risk factor both for brain tumors and for other cancers; that is, its effect is that of a carcinogen that is not site-specific. Another explanation to consider is that the findings could have resulted from recall bias, and that mothers of children with any type of cancer recall any prenatal radiation exposure better than do the mothers of normal children.

Consider another possible set of findings shown in Figure 9–7.

If mothers of children with brain tumors have a greater radiation exposure history than do both mothers of normal controls and mothers of children with other cancers, the findings might suggest that prenatal radiation is a specific carcinogen for the brain. These findings would also reduce the likelihood that recall bias is playing a role, as it would seem implausible that mothers of children with brain tumors would recall prenatal radiation better than mothers of children with other cancers. Thus, multiple controls of different types can be valuable for exploring alternate hypotheses and for taking into account possible potential biases, such as recall bias.

Despite the issues raised in this chapter, case-control studies are invaluable in exploring the etiology of disease. For example, in October 1989, three patients with eosinophilia and severe myalgia who had been taking L-tryptophan were reported to the Health Department in New Mexico. This led to

recognition of a distinct entity, the eosinophilia-myalgia syndrome (EMS). To confirm the apparent association of EMS with L-tryptophan ingestion, a case-control study was conducted.[10] Eleven cases and 22 matched controls were interviewed for information on symptoms and other clinical findings and on use of L-tryptophan–containing products. All 11 cases were found to have used L-tryptophan compared to only 2 of the controls. These findings led to a nationwide recall of over-the-counter L-tryptophan preparations in November 1989.

A subsequent case-control study in Oregon compared the brand and source of L-tryptophan used by 58 patients with EMS with the brand and source of L-tryptophan used by 30 asymptomatic controls.[11] A single brand and lot of L-tryptophan manufactured by a single Japanese petrochemical company was used by 98% of the cases compared with 44% of the controls. In a case-control study in Minnesota, 98% of cases had ingested L-tryptophan from that manufacturer compared with 60% of the controls.[12] The findings of both studies indicated that a contaminant introduced during the manufacturing of L-tryptophan or some alteration of L-tryptophan in the manufacturing process was responsible for the outbreak of EMS.

NESTED CASE-CONTROL STUDIES

A study design that has been used increasingly in recent years is the *nested case-control study*—a hybrid design in which a case-control study is nested in a cohort study. This design is shown schematically in Figure 9–8.

In this type of study, a population is identified

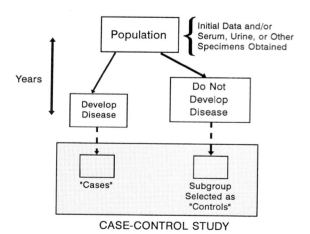

CASE-CONTROL STUDY
Figure 9–8. Diagram of a nested case-control study.

and followed over time. At the time the population is identified, baseline data are obtained from interviews, blood or urine tests, etc. The population is then followed up over a period of years, and for most of the diseases that are studied, a small percent manifest the disease, whereas most do not. As seen in Figure 9–8, a case-control study is then carried out using persons in whom the disease developed (cases) and a sample of those in whom the disease did not develop (controls).

What are the advantages of this type of study design? First, because interviews are performed at the beginning of the study (at baseline), the data are obtained before any disease has developed. Consequently, the problem of possible recall bias is eliminated. Second, if abnormalities in biologic characteristics are found, because the specimens were obtained years before the development of clinical disease, it is more likely that these findings represent risk factors or other pre-morbid characteristics than a manifestation of early, subclinical disease. When such abnormalities are found in the traditional case-control study, we do not know whether they preceded the disease or were a result of the disease. Third, such a study is often more economical to conduct. One might ask, why perform a nested case-control study? Why not perform a regular concurrent cohort study? The answer is that in a cohort study of, say, 10,000 people, laboratory analyses of all the specimens obtained would have to be carried out, often at great cost, to define *exposed* and *non-exposed* groups. In a nested case-control study, however, the specimens obtained are frozen; only after the disease has developed in some subjects is a case-control study begun and the specimens from the relatively small number of people in the case-control study thawed and analyzed. Thus, the laboratory burden and costs are dramatically reduced. For all of these reasons, the nested case-control study is an extremely useful type of study design.

CROSS-SECTIONAL STUDIES

Let us assume we are interested in the possible relationship of increased serum cholesterol level (the *exposure*) to electrocardiographic (ECG) evidence of CHD (the *disease*). We survey a population; for each participant we determine the serum cholesterol level and perform an ECG for evidence of CHD.

This type of study design is called a *cross-sec-tional study* because both exposure and disease outcome are determined *simultaneously* for each subject; it is as if we were viewing a snapshot of the population at a certain point in time. Another way to describe a cross-sectional study is to imagine that we have sliced through the population, capturing levels of cholesterol *and* evidence of coronary heart disease at the same time. Note that in this type of approach, the cases of disease that we identify are *prevalent* cases of the disease in question, because we know that they existed at the time of the study but do not know their duration. For this reason, this design is also called a *prevalence study*.

The general design of such a cross-sectional or prevalence study is seen in Figure 9–9. We define a population and determine presence or absence of exposure and presence or absence of disease for each individual. Each subject then can be categorized into one of four possible subgroups.

The findings can be viewed in a 2 × 2 table as seen in Figures 9–10 and 9–11, which also shows the two approaches to interpreting the findings from such studies.

We identify a population of *n* persons for study, and determine presence or absence of exposure and disease for each subject. As seen in Figures 9–10 and 9–11, there will be *a* persons—who have both been exposed and have the disease, *b* persons—who have been exposed but do not have the disease, *c* persons—who have the disease but have not been exposed, and *d* persons—who have neither been exposed nor have the disease. To determine whether there is an association between exposure and disease, we have two choices: (1) We can calculate the *prevalence of disease* in persons with the exposure $\left(\frac{a}{a+b}\right)$ and compare it with the prevalence of disease in persons without the exposure $\left(\frac{c}{c+d}\right)$; or (2) we can compare the *prevalence of exposure* in persons with the disease $\left(\frac{a}{a+c}\right)$ to the prevalence of exposure in persons without the disease $\left(\frac{b}{b+d}\right)$.

If we determine in such a study that there appears to be an association between increased cholesterol level and CHD, we are left with several problems. First, in this cross-sectional study, we are identifying prevalent cases of CHD rather than incident (new) cases; such prevalent cases may not be representative of all cases of CHD that have developed

Begin with:
Defined Population
Gather Data on Exposure and Disease
Four Groups Are Possible:
Exposed; Have Disease
Exposed; Do Not Have Disease
Not Exposed; Have Disease
Not Exposed; Do Not Have Disease

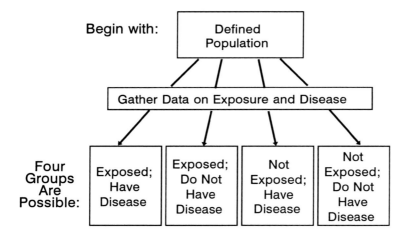

Figure 9–9. Design of a cross-sectional study: I.

Disease
No Disease
Exposed
Not Exposed
a
b
c
d

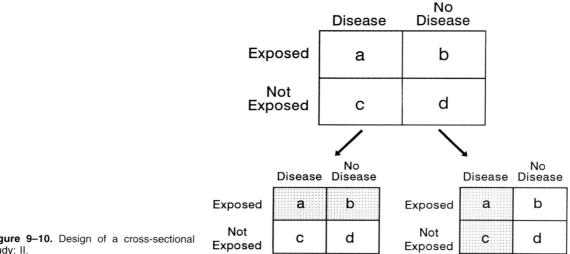

Figure 9–10. Design of a cross-sectional study: II.

Disease
No Disease
Exposed
Not Exposed
a
b
c
d
Prevalence of disease compared in exposed and non-exposed
$\frac{a}{a+b}$ vs. $\frac{c}{c+d}$
OR
Prevalence of exposure compared in diseased and non-diseased
$\frac{a}{a+c}$ vs. $\frac{b}{b+d}$

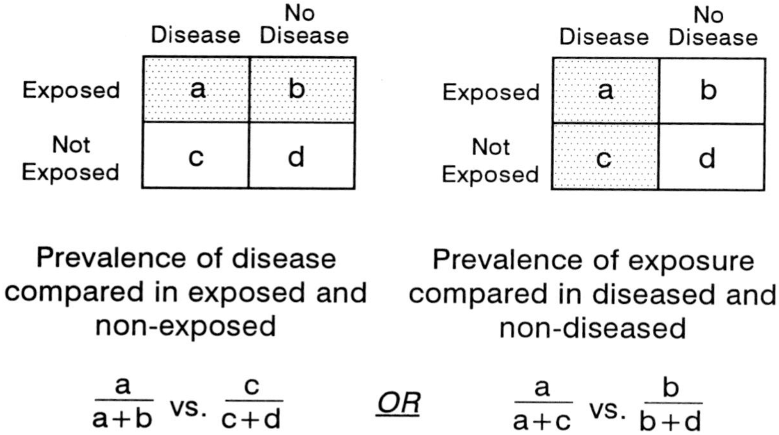

Figure 9–11. Design of a cross-sectional study: III.

Table 9–10. Finding Your Way in the Terminology Jungle

Case-control study	=	Retrospective study
Cohort study	= Longitudinal study =	Prospective study
Concurrent cohort study	= Prospective cohort study =	Concurrent prospective study
Retrospective cohort study	= Historical cohort study =	Non-concurrent prospective study
Randomized trial	=	Experimental study
Cross-sectional study	=	Prevalence survey

in this population. For example, identifying only prevalent cases would exclude those who died after the disease developed but before the study was carried out. Therefore, even if an association of exposure and disease is observed, the association may be with *survival* after CHD rather than with the risk of *development* of CHD. Second, because the presence or absence of both exposure and disease was determined at the same time in each subject in the study, it is often not possible to establish a temporal relationship between the exposure and the onset of disease. Thus, in the example given at the beginning of this section, it is not possible to tell whether the increased cholesterol level *preceded* the development of CHD. Without information on temporal relationships, it is conceivable that the increased cholesterol level could have occurred as a result of the coronary heart disease, or perhaps both may have occurred as a result of another factor. If it turns out that the exposure did not precede the development of the disease, the association cannot reflect a causal relationship.

Consequently, although a cross-sectional study can be very suggestive of a possible risk factor or factors for a disease, when an association is found in such a study, given the limitations in establishing a temporal relationship between exposure and outcome, we rely on cohort and case-control studies for establishment of etiologic relationships.

CONCLUSION

We have now reviewed the basic study designs used in epidemiologic investigations and clinical research. Unfortunately, a variety of different terms are used in the literature to describe different study

designs, and it is important to be familiar with them. Table 9–10 is designed to help guide you through the often confusing terminology.

The purpose of all these types of studies is to identify associations between exposures and diseases. If such associations are found, the next step is to determine whether they are likely to be causal. These topics, starting with estimating risk, are addressed in Chapters 10 through 14.

References

1. Ochsner A, DeBakey M: Carcinoma of the lung. Arch Surg 42:209–258, 1941.
2. Gregg NM: Congenital cataract following German measles in the mother. Trans Ophthalmol Soc Aust 3:35–46, 1941.
3. Doll R, Hill AB: A study of the aetiology of carcinoma of the lung. Br Med J 2:1271–1286, 1952.
4. Pearl R: Cancer and tuberculosis. Am J Hyg 9:97–159, 1929.
5. Carlson HA, Bell ET: Statistical study of occurrence of cancer and tuberculosis in 11,195 post-mortem examinations. J Cancer Res 13:126–135, 1929.
6. MacMahon B, Yen S, Trichopoulos D, et al: Coffee and cancer of the pancreas. N Engl J Med 304:630–633, 1981.
7. Hsieh CC, MacMahon B, Yes S, Trichopoulos D, et al: Coffee and pancreatic cancer (Chapter 2) [Letter]. N Engl J Med 315:587–589, 1986.
8. Lilienfeld AM, Graham S: Validity of determining circumcision status by questionnaire as related to epidemiologic studies of cancer of the cervix. J Natl Cancer Inst 21:713–720, 1958.
9. Gold EB, Gordis L, Tonascia J, Szklo M: Risk factors for brain tumors in children. Am J Epidemiol 109:309–319, 1979.
10. Edison M, Philen RM, Sewell CM, et al: L-Tryptophan and eosinophilia-myalgia syndrome in New Mexico. Lancet 335:645–648, 1990.
11. Slutsker L, Hoesly FC, Miller L, et al: Eosinophilia-myalgia syndrome associated with exposure to tryptophan from a single manufacturer. JAMA 264:213–217, 1990.
12. Belongia EZ, Hedberg CW, Gleich GJ, et al: An investigation of the cause of the eosinophilia-myalgia syndrome associated with tryptophan use. N Engl J Med 232:357–365, 1990.

Review Questions

1. A case-control study is characterized by all of the following *except*:
   a. It is relatively inexpensive compared with most other epidemiologic study designs
   b. Cases with the disease are compared to controls without the disease
   c. Incidence rates may be computed directly
   d. Assessment of past exposure may be biased
   e. Definition of cases may be difficult

2. Residents of three villages with three different types of water supply were asked to participate in a survey to identify cholera carriers. Because several cholera deaths had occurred in the recent past, virtually everyone present at the time submitted to examination. The proportion of residents in each village who were carriers was computed and compared. Classify this study:
   a. Cross-sectional study
   b. Case-control study
   c. Concurrent cohort study
   d. Non-concurrent cohort study
   e. Experimental study

3. Which of the following is a case-control study?
   a. Study of past mortality or morbidity trends to permit estimates of the occurrence of disease in the future
   b. Analysis of previous research in different places and under different circumstances to permit establishment of hypotheses based on cumulative knowledge of all known factors
   c. Obtaining histories and other information from a group of known cases and a comparison group to determine the relative frequency of a characteristic or exposure under study
   d. Study of the incidence of cancer in men who have quit smoking
   e. Both *a* and *c*

4. In a study begun in 1965, a group of 3,000 adults in Baltimore were asked about alcohol consumption. The occurrence of cases of cancer was studied in this group between 1981 and 1995. This is an example of a:

   a. Cross-sectional study
   b. Concurrent cohort study
   c. Retrospective cohort study
   d. Clinical trial
   e. Case-control study

Question 5 is based on the information given below:

In a small pilot study, 12 women with endometrial cancer (cancer of the uterus) and 12 women with no apparent disease were contacted and asked whether they had ever used estrogen. Each woman with cancer was matched by age, race, weight, and parity to a woman without disease.

5. What kind of study design is this?
   a. Concurrent cohort
   b. Retrospective cohort
   c. Case-control
   d. Cross-sectional
   e. Experimental

6. The physical examination records of the entire incoming freshman class of 1935 at the University of Minnesota were examined in 1977 to see if their recorded height and weight at the time of admission to the university was related to their chance of developing coronary heart disease by 1986. This is an example of a:
   a. Cross-sectional study
   b. Case-control study
   c. Concurrent cohort study
   d. Retrospective cohort study
   e. Experimental study

7. In a case-control study, which of the following is(are) true?
   a. The proportion of cases with the exposure is compared with the proportion of controls with the exposure
   b. Disease rates are compared for people with the factor of interest and for people without the factor of interest
   c. The investigator may choose to have multiple comparison groups
   d. Recall bias is a potential problem
   e. *a, c,* and *d*

CHAPTER 10

Estimating Risk: Is There an Association?

In the previous three chapters we have discussed the three basic study designs that are used in epidemiologic investigations. These are shown diagrammatically in Figures 10–1 through 10–3.

Recall that the fundamental difference between a randomized trial and a cohort study is that in a cohort study, subjects are not randomly assigned to be exposed or to remain non-exposed, because randomization to exposure to possibly toxic or carcinogenic agents would clearly not be acceptable. Consequently, cohort studies are used in many studies of etiology, because this study design enables us to capitalize on populations that have had a certain exposure, and to compare them with populations that have not had that exposure. Case-control studies are also used to address questions of etiology. Regardless of which design is employed, the objective is to determine whether there is an excess risk (incidence), or perhaps a reduced risk, of a certain disease in association with a certain exposure or characteristic.

Before describing these comparative approaches, we will introduce the concept of *absolute risk.*

ABSOLUTE RISK

The incidence of a disease in a population is termed the *absolute risk*. Absolute risk can indicate the magnitude of the risk in a group of people with a certain exposure, but because it does not take into consideration the risk of disease in unexposed individuals, it does not indicate whether or not the exposure is associated with an increased risk of the disease. Comparison is fundamental to epidemiology. Nevertheless, absolute risk may have important implications in both clinical and public health policy: For example, a woman who contracts rubella in the first trimester of pregnancy and asks her physician, "What is the risk that my child will be malformed?" is given a certain number as an answer. On the basis of this information, she may decide to abort her pregnancy. She is not explicitly given comparative data, but an implicit comparison is generally being made: The woman is wondering not only what her risk is, but she is wondering how that risk compares with what it would have been

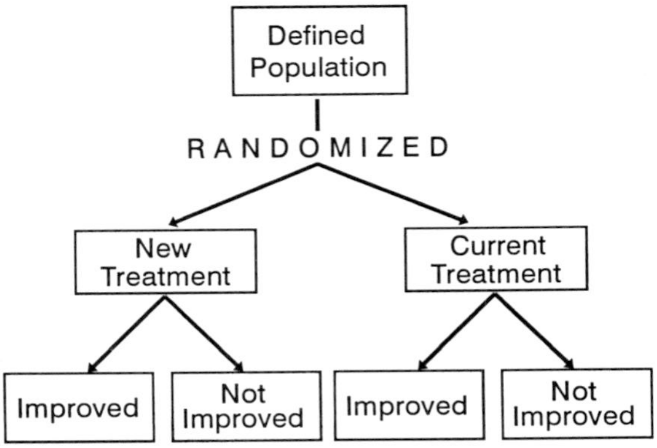

Figure 10–1. Design of a randomized clinical trial.

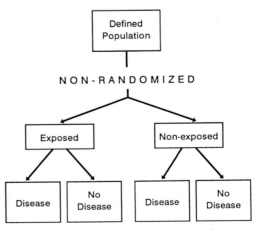

Figure 10–2. Design of a cohort study.

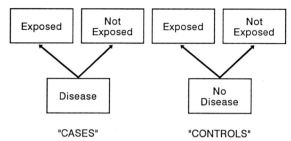

Figure 10–3. Design of a case-control study.

had she not contracted rubella. So although absolute risk does not stipulate any explicit comparison, an implicit comparison is often made whenever we look at the incidence of a disease. However, to address the question of association, we must utilize approaches that involve explicit comparisons.

HOW DO WE DETERMINE WHETHER A CERTAIN DISEASE IS ASSOCIATED WITH A CERTAIN EXPOSURE?

To determine whether such an association exists we must determine, using data obtained in case-control and cohort studies, whether there is an excess risk of the disease in persons who have been exposed to a certain agent. Let us consider the results of a hypothetical investigation of a food-borne disease outbreak. The suspect foods were identified, and for each food, the attack rate (or incidence rate) of the disease was calculated for those who ate the food (exposed) and for those who did not eat the food (non-exposed), as shown in Table 10–1.

How can we determine whether an excess risk is associated with each of the food items? One approach, shown in column C of Table 10–2, is to

Table 10–1. A Foodborne Disease Outbreak: I. Percent of People Sick Among Those Who Ate and Those Who Did Not Eat Specific Foods

Food	Ate (% Sick)	Did Not Eat (% Sick)
Egg salad	83	30
Macaroni	76	67
Cottage cheese	71	69
Tuna salad	78	50
Ice cream	78	64
Other	72	50

calculate the *ratio* of the attack rate in those who ate each food to the attack rate in those who did not eat the food. An alternate approach for identifying any excess risk in exposed individuals is shown in column D; we can subtract the risk in those who did not eat the food from the risk in those who did eat the food, with the *difference* representing the excess risk in those who were exposed.

Thus, as seen in this foodborne outbreak, to determine whether a certain exposure is associated with a certain disease, we must determine whether there is an excess risk of disease in exposed populations by comparing the risk of disease in exposed populations to the risk of disease in non-exposed populations. We have just seen that such an excess risk can be calculated in the two following ways:

1. The ratio of the risks (or of the incidence rates):

$$\frac{\text{Disease risk in exposed}}{\text{Disease risk in non-exposed}}$$

2. The *difference* in the risks (or in the incidence rates):

(Disease risk in exposed) − (disease risk in non-exposed)

Does the method that we choose to calculate excess risk make any difference? Let us consider a hypothetical example of two communities, A and B, seen in Table 10–3.

In community A, the incidence in exposed persons is 40% and the incidence in non-exposed persons is 10%. Is there an excess risk associated with exposure? As in the food poisoning example, we can calculate the ratio of the rates or the difference between the rates. The *ratio* of the incidence rates is 4.0. If we calculate the *difference* in incidence rates it is 30%. In community B, the incidence in exposed persons is 90% and the incidence in non-exposed persons is 60%. If we calculate the *ratio* of the incidence of exposed to non-exposed persons in population B, it is 90/60, or 1.5. If we calculate the *difference* in the incidence in exposed and non-exposed persons in community B it is, again, 30%.

What do these two measures tell us? Is there a difference in what we learn from the ratio of the incidence rates compared to the difference in the incidence rates? This question is the theme of this chapter and of Chapter 11.

RELATIVE RISK

The Concept of Relative Risk

Both case-control and cohort studies are designed to determine whether there is an association be-

Table 10–2. A Foodborne Disease Outbreak: II. Ways of Calculating Excess Risk

Food	(A) Ate (% Sick)	(B) Did Not Eat (% Sick)	(C) (A)/(B)	(D) (A) − (B) (%)
Egg salad	83	30	2.77	53
Macaroni	76	67	1.13	9
Cottage cheese	71	69	1.03	2
Tuna salad	78	50	1.56	28
Ice cream	78	64	1.21	14
Other	72	50	1.44	22

tween exposure to a factor and development of a disease. If an association exists, how strong is it? If we carry out a cohort study, we can put the question another way: What is the ratio of the risk of disease in exposed individuals to the risk of disease in non-exposed individuals? This ratio is called the *relative risk*.

$$\text{Relative risk} = \frac{\text{Risk in exposed}}{\text{Risk in non-exposed}}$$

Interpreting the Relative Risk

How do we interpret the value of a relative risk? There are three possibilities (Table 10–4):

If the relative risk is equal to 1, the numerator equals the denominator, and the risk in exposed persons equals the risk in non-exposed persons. Therefore, no evidence exists for any increased risk in exposed individuals or for any association of the disease with the exposure in question.

If the relative risk is greater than 1, the numerator is greater than the denominator, and the risk in exposed persons is greater than the risk in non-exposed persons. This is evidence of a positive association, and may be causal (this is discussed in Chapter 13).

If the relative risk is less than 1, the numerator is less than the denominator, and the risk in exposed persons is less than the risk in non-exposed persons.

This is evidence for a negative association, and it may be indicative of a protective effect. Such a finding can be observed in people who are given an effective vaccine ("exposed" to the vaccine).

Calculating the Relative Risk in Cohort Studies

In a *cohort* study the relative risk can be calculated *directly*. Recall the design of a cohort study seen in Table 10–5.

In this table, we see that the incidence in exposed individuals is $\frac{a}{a+b}$ and the incidence in non-exposed individuals is $\frac{c}{c+d}$. We calculate the relative risk as follows:

$$\text{Relative risk} = \frac{\text{Incidence in exposed}}{\text{Incidence in non-exposed}} = \frac{\frac{a}{a+b}}{\frac{c}{c+d}}$$

Table 10–6 shows a hypothetical cohort study of 3,000 smokers and 5,000 non-smokers to investigate the relation of smoking to the development of coronary heart disease (CHD) over a 1-year period.

In this example:

$$\text{Incidence among the exposed} = \frac{84}{3,000} = 28.0 \text{ per } 1,000$$

and

Table 10–3. An Example Comparing Two Ways of Calculating Excess Risk

	Population A	Population B
Incidence (%)		
In exposed	40	90
In non-exposed	10	60
Difference in incidence rates (%)	30	30
Ratio of incidence rates	4.0	1.5

Table 10–4. Interpreting Relative Risk (RR) of a Disease

If RR = 1 Risk in exposed equal to risk in unexposed (no association)
If RR > 1 Risk in exposed greater than risk in unexposed (positive association; possibly causal)
If RR < 1 Risk in exposed less than risk in unexposed (negative association; possibly protective)

Table 10–5. Risk Calculations in a Cohort Study

		Then Follow to See Whether			
		Disease Develops	Disease Does Not Develop	Totals	Incidence Rates of Disease
First Select	Exposed	a	b	$a+b$	$\dfrac{a}{a+b}$
	Not exposed	c	d	$c+d$	$\dfrac{c}{c+d}$
	$\dfrac{a}{a+b}$ = Incidence in exposed		$\dfrac{c}{c+d}$ = Incidence in non-exposed		

$$\text{Incidence among the non-exposed} = \frac{87}{5,000} = 17.4 \text{ per } 1,000$$

Consequently,

$$\text{Relative risk} = \frac{\text{Incidence in exposed}}{\text{Incidence in non-exposed}} = \frac{28.0}{17.4} = 1.61$$

A similar expression of risks is seen in Table 10–7, which shows data from the first 12 years of the Framingham Study relating risk of coronary disease to age, sex, and cholesterol level.

First, direct your attention to the upper part of the table, which shows incidence rates per 1,000 by age, sex, and serum cholesterol level. In men, the relation of risk to cholesterol level seems dose related; risk increases for both age groups with increases in cholesterol level. However, the relationship is not as consistent in women.

In the lower half of the table, the values have been converted to relative risks. The authors have taken the incidence rate of 38.2 in younger men with low cholesterol levels and assigned it a risk of 1.0; these subjects are considered "non-exposed." All other risks in the table are expressed in relation to this risk of 1.0. For example, the incidence of

157.5 in younger men with a cholesterol level greater than 250 mg/100 mL is compared to the 38.2 incidence rate; by dividing 157.5 by 38.2 we obtain a relative risk of 4.1. Using these relative risks, it is easier to compare the risks and to identify any trends. Although the lowest risk in men has been chosen as the standard and set at 1.0, the authors could have chosen to set any of the values in the table at 1.0 and to make all others relative to it. One reason for choosing a low value as the standard is that most of the other values will be above 1.0; for most people, the table is easier to read when few values are completely to the right of the decimal.

Table 10–7. Relationship Between Serum Cholesterol Levels and Risk of CHD by Age and Sex: Framingham Study During First 12 Years

Serum Cholesterol (mg/100 mL)	Men		Women	
	30–49 yr	50–62 yr	30–49 yr	50–62 yr
	Incidence Rates (per 1,000)			
<190	38.2	105.7	11.1	155.2
190–219	44.1	187.5	9.1	88.9
220–249	95.0	201.1	24.3	96.3
250+	157.5	267.8	50.4	121.5
	Relative Risks*			
<190	1.0	2.8	0.3	4.1
190–219	1.2	4.9	0.2	2.3
220–249	2.5	5.3	0.6	2.5
250+	4.1	7.0	1.3	3.2

*Incidence for each subgroup is compared with that of males 30 to 49 years of age, and with serum cholesterol levels less than 190 mg/dL (risk = 1.0).

From Truett J, Cornfield J, Kannel W: A multivariate analysis of the risk of coronary heart disease in Framingham. J Chronic Dis 20:511–524, 1967.

Table 10–6. Smoking and CHD: A Hypothetical Cohort Study of 3,000 Cigarette Smokers and 5,000 Non-smokers

	Develop CHD	Do Not Develop CHD	Totals	Incidence per 1,000 per Year
Smoke cigarettes	84	2,916	3,000	28.0
Do not smoke cigarettes	87	4,913	5,000	17.4

Figure 10–4 shows data on 2,282 middle-aged men followed-up for 10 years in the Framingham Study and 1,838 middle-aged men followed-up for 8 years in Albany, New York. The data relate smoking, cholesterol level, and blood pressure to risk of myocardial infarction and death from CHD. The authors have assigned a value of 1 to the lowest of the risks in each of the two parts of the figure, and the other risks are calculated relative to this value. On the left is shown the risk in non-smokers with low cholesterol levels (which has been set at 1) and the risk in non-smokers with high cholesterol levels; risks for smokers with low and high cholesterol levels are each calculated relative to risks for non-smokers with low cholesterol levels. Note that the risk is higher with high cholesterol levels, and that this holds both in smokers and in non-smokers (although the risk is higher in smokers even when cholesterol levels are low). Thus both smoking and elevated cholesterol levels contribute to the risk of myocardial infarction and death from coronary heart disease. A comparable analysis with blood pressure and smoking is shown on the right.

THE ODDS RATIO (RELATIVE ODDS)

We have seen that in order to calculate a relative risk, we must have values for the incidence of the disease in the exposed and the incidence in the non-exposed, as can be obtained from a cohort study. In a *case-control* study, however, we do not know the incidence in the exposed population or the incidence in the non-exposed population because we start with diseased people (cases) and non-diseased people (controls). Hence, in a case-control study we *cannot* calculate the relative risk directly. In this

section we shall see how another measure of association, the *odds ratio*, can be obtained from either a cohort or a case-control study and can be used instead of the relative risk. We will also see that even though we cannot calculate a relative risk from a case-control study, under many conditions, we can obtain a very good *estimate* of the relative risk from a case-control study using the odds ratio.

Defining the Odds Ratio in Cohort and in Case-Control Studies

In previous chapters we discussed the *proportion* of the exposed population in whom disease develops and the *proportion* of the non-exposed population in whom disease develops in a cohort study. Similarly, in case-control studies, we have discussed the *proportion* of the cases who were exposed and the *proportion* of the controls who were exposed (Table 10–8).

An alternate approach is to utilize the concept of *odds*. Suppose we are betting on a horse named Epi Beauty, which has a 60% probability of winning the race (*P*). Epi Beauty therefore has a 40% probability of losing (1 − *P*). If these are the probabilities, what are the *odds* that the horse will win the race? To answer this we must keep in mind that *the odds of an event can be defined as the ratio of the number of ways the event can occur to the number of ways the event cannot occur.*

Consequently, the odds of Epi Beauty winning, as defined above, are as follows:

$$\text{Odds} = \frac{\text{Probability that Epi Beauty will win the race}}{\text{Probability that Epi Beauty will lose the race}}$$

Recall that if *P* is the probability that Epi Beauty will win the race, 1 − *P* equals the probability that

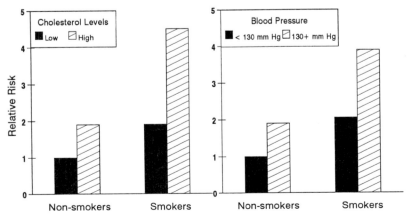

Figure 10–4. Relative risk for myocardial infarction and coronary heart disease death in men aged 30 to 62 years by serum cholesterol and blood pressure levels in relation to cigarette smoking. High cholesterol levels are defined as 220 mg/100 mL or greater. (Adapted from Doyle JT, Dawber TR, Kannel WB, et al: The relationship of cigarette smoking to coronary heart disease. JAMA 190: 886, 1964.)

Table 10–8. Calculation of Proportions Exposed in a Case-Control Study

		First, Select	
		Cases (With Disease)	Controls (Without Disease)
Then, Measure Past Exposure { Were exposed		a	b
Were not exposed		c	d
Totals		$a + c$	$b + d$
Proportions exposed		$\dfrac{a}{a + c}$	$\dfrac{b}{b + d}$

Epi Beauty will lose the race. Consequently the *odds* of Epi Beauty winning are:

$$\text{Odds} = \frac{P}{1 - P} \text{ or } \frac{60\%}{40\%} = 1.5{:}1 = 1.5$$

It is important to keep in mind the distinction between probability and odds. In the above example:

$$\text{Probability of winning} = 60\%$$

and

$$\text{Odds of winning} = \frac{60\%}{40\%} = 1.5$$

The Odds Ratio in Cohort Studies

Let us examine how the concept of odds can be applied to both cohort and case-control studies. Let us first consider the cohort study design shown in Table 10–5. Our first question is, What is the *probability* (P) that the disease will develop in an exposed person? The answer to this is the incidence of the disease in the top row (exposed persons), which equals $\frac{a}{a + b}$. Next let us ask, What are the *odds* that the disease will develop in an exposed person? Again, looking only at the top row in Figure 10–5, we see that there are $a + b$ exposed persons; the odds that the disease will develop in them are $a{:}b$ or $\frac{a}{b}$. (Recall $\frac{P}{1 - P}$ from the Epi Beauty example.) Similarly, looking only at the bottom row of this table, there are $c + d$ non-exposed persons; the probability that the disease will develop in non-exposed persons is $\frac{c}{c + d}$ and the odds of the disease developing in these non-exposed persons are $c{:}d$ or $\frac{c}{d}$.

Just as the ratio of the incidence in the exposed to the incidence in the non-exposed can be used to measure an association of exposure and disease, we can also look at the ratio of the odds that the disease will develop in an exposed person to the odds that it will develop in a non-exposed person. Either measure of association is valid in a cohort study.

In a cohort study, to answer the question of whether there is an association between the exposure and the disease, we can either use the relative risk discussed in the previous section or we can use the odds ratio (also called the *relative odds*). In a *cohort study,* the odds ratio is defined as the *ratio of the odds of development of disease in exposed persons to the odds of development of disease in non-exposed persons,* and it can be calculated as follows:

$$\frac{\dfrac{a}{b}}{\dfrac{c}{d}} = \frac{ad}{bc}$$

The Odds Ratio in a Case-Control Study

As just discussed, in a *case-control study,* we cannot calculate the relative risk directly to determine whether there is an association between the exposure and the disease, because having started with cases and controls rather than with exposed and non-exposed persons, we do not have information about the incidence of disease in exposed persons and the incidence of disease in non-exposed persons. We can, however, use the odds ratio as a measure of association of exposure and disease in a case-control study, but we ask different questions: What are the odds that a case was exposed? Looking at the lefthand column in Table 10–8, we see that the *odds* of a case having been exposed are $a{:}c$

or $\frac{a}{c}$. Next we ask, what are the odds that a control was exposed? Looking at the righthand column we see that the *odds* of a control having been exposed are *b:d* or $\frac{b}{d}$.

We can then calculate the odds ratio, which in a *case-control study* is defined as *the ratio of the odds that the cases were exposed to the odds that the controls were exposed.* This is calculated as follows:

$$\frac{\frac{a}{c}}{\frac{b}{d}} = \frac{ad}{bc}$$

Thus, interestingly, $\frac{ad}{bc}$ represents the odds ratio (or relative odds) in *both* cohort and case-control studies. In both types of studies the odds ratio is an excellent measure of whether a certain exposure is associated with a specific disease (see Fig. 10–5). The *odds ratio* is also known as the *cross-products ratio,* because it can be obtained by multiplying both diagonal cells in a 2 × 2 table and then dividing $\frac{ad}{bc}$, as seen in Figure 10–5.

Interpreting the Odds Ratio

We interpret the odds ratio just as we interpreted the relative risk. If the exposure is not related to the disease, the odds ratio will equal 1. If the exposure is positively related to the disease, the odds ratio will be greater than 1. If the exposure is negatively related to the disease, the odds ratio will be less than 1.

When Is the Odds Ratio a Good Estimate of the Relative Risk?

In a case-control study, only the odds ratio can be calculated as a measure of association, whereas in a cohort study, either the relative risk or the odds ratio is a valid measure of association. However, many people are more comfortable using the relative risk, and this is the most frequently used measure of association reported in the literature when results of cohort studies are published. Even when the odds ratio is used, people are often interested in knowing how well it approximates the relative risk. Even prestigious clinical journals have been known to publish reports of case-control studies and to label a column of results as *relative risks.* Having read the discussion in this chapter, you are aghast to see such a presentation, because you now know that relative risks cannot be calculated directly from a case-control study! Clearly, what is meant is an *estimate* of relative risks based on the odds ratios that are obtained in the case-control studies.

When is the odds ratio (relative odds) obtained in a case-control study a good approximation of the relative risk in the population? When the following three conditions are met:

1. When the *cases* studied are representative, with regard to history of exposure, of all people with the disease in the population from which the cases were drawn.

Figure 10–5. *A,* Odds ratio in a cohort study. *B,* Odds ratio in a case-control study.

2. When the *controls* studied are representative, with regard to history of exposure, of all people without the disease in the population from which the cases were drawn.
3. When the disease being studied is not one that occurs frequently.

The third condition (that the disease occurrence is not frequent) can be intuitively explained as follows:

Recall that there are $a + b$ exposed persons. Because most diseases with which we are dealing occur infrequently, very few persons in an exposed population will actually develop the disease; consequently, a is very small compared to b, and one can approximate $a + b$ as b, or $(a + b) \cong b$. Similarly, very few non-exposed persons $(c + d)$ develop the disease, and we can approximate $c + d$ as d, or $(c + d) \cong d$. Therefore, we may calculate a relative risk as follows:

$$\frac{\dfrac{a}{a + b}}{\dfrac{c}{c + d}} \cong \frac{\dfrac{a}{b}}{\dfrac{c}{d}}$$

From performing this calculation, we obtain ad/bc, which is the odds ratio. For the committed reader, a neater and more sophisticated derivation is provided in the appendix to this chapter.

Figures 10–6 and 10–7 show two examples of cohort studies that demonstrate how the odds ratio provides a good approximation of the relative risk when the occurrence of a disease is infrequent, but not when it is frequent. In the first example, the occurrence of disease is infrequent and we see that

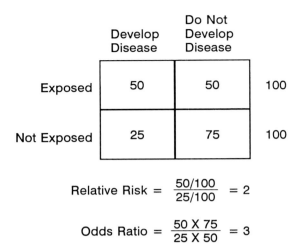

Relative Risk = $\dfrac{50/100}{25/100}$ = 2

Odds Ratio = $\dfrac{50 \times 75}{25 \times 50}$ = 3

Figure 10–7. Example: The odds ratio is *not* a good estimate of the relative risk when a disease is *not* infrequent.

the relative risk is 2. If we now calculate an odds (cross-products) ratio, we find it to be 2.02, which is a very close approximation.

Now let us examine the second example in which the occurrence of disease is frequent. Although the relative risk is again 2.0, the odds ratio is 3.0, which is considerably different from the relative risk.

We therefore see that the odds ratio is in itself a valid measure of association without even considering relative risk. If, however, you choose to use the relative risk as the index of association, you know that when the disease occurrence is infrequent, the odds ratio is a very good approximation of the relative risk.

REMEMBER
- *The relative odds (odds ratio) is a useful measure of association in and of itself, in both case-control and prospective studies.*
- *In a cohort study, the relative risk can be calculated directly.*
- *In a case-control study, the relative risk cannot be calculated directly, so that the relative odds or odds ratio (cross-products ratio) is used as an estimate of the relative risk when the risk of the disease is low.*

Examples of Calculating Odds Ratios in Case-Control Studies

In this section, we will calculate odds ratios in two case-control studies (one in which the controls were *not* matched to the cases, and the other in which they *were* matched). For purposes of these

	Develop Disease	Do Not Develop Disease	
Exposed	200	9800	10,000
Not Exposed	100	9900	10,000

Relative Risk = $\dfrac{200/10,000}{100/10,000}$ = 2

Odds Ratio = $\dfrac{200 \times 9900}{100 \times 9800}$ = 2.02

Figure 10–6. Example: The odds ratio is a good estimate of the relative risk when a disease is infrequent.

examples, let us assume the following: our research budget is small, so we have carried out a case-control study of only 10 cases and 10 controls. N indicates a *non-exposed* individual and E indicates an *exposed* individual.

Calculating the Odds Ratio in an Unmatched Case-Control Study

Let us assume that this case-control study is done without any matching of controls to cases, and that we obtain the results seen in Figure 10–8. Thus, 6 of the 10 cases were exposed and 3 of the 10 controls were exposed. If we arrange these data in a 2 × 2 table, we obtain the following:

	Cases	Controls
Exposed	6	3
Non-exposed	4	7
	10	10

The odds ratio in this *unmatched* study equals the ratio of the cross-products:

$$\text{Odds ratio} = \frac{ad}{bc}$$
$$= \frac{6 \times 7}{4 \times 3} = \frac{42}{12} = 3.5$$

Table 10–9 shows data from a hypothetical unmatched case-control study of smoking and CHD. The letters *a*, *b*, *c*, and *d* have been inserted to identify the cells of the 2 × 2 table that are used for the calculation. The odds ratio as calculated from these data is as follows:

CASES	CONTROLS
E	N
E	E
N	N
E	N
N	E
N	N
E	N
E	E
E	N
N	N

Figure 10–8. A case-control study of ten cases and ten unmatched controls.

$$\text{Odds ratio} = \frac{ad}{bc} = \frac{112 \times 224}{176 \times 88} = 1.62$$

Calculating the Odds Ratio in a Matched Pairs Case-Control Study

As discussed in the previous chapter, in selecting the study population in case-control studies, controls are often selected by matching each control to a case according to variables that are known to be related to disease risk, such as sex, age, or race (individual matching or matched pairs). The results are then analyzed in terms of case-control pairs rather than for individual subjects.

What types of case-control combinations are possible in regard to exposure history? Clearly, if exposure is dichotomous (a person is either exposed or

Table 10–9. Example of Calculating an Odds Ratio From a Case-Control Study

		First, Select	
		CHD Cases	**Controls**
Then, Measure Past Exposure	Smokers	112 (a)	176 (b)
	Non-Smokers	88 (c)	224 (d)
	Total	200	400
	% Smoking cigarettes	56	44
	$\text{Odds ratio} = \dfrac{ad}{bc} = \dfrac{112 \times 224}{176 \times 88} = 1.62$		

not exposed), only the following four types of case-control pairs are possible:

Concordant pairs	1. Pairs in which *both* the case and the control were exposed 2. Pairs in which *neither* the case nor the control was exposed
Discordant pairs	3. Pairs in which the case was exposed but the control was not 4. Pairs in which the control was exposed and the case was not

Note that the case-control pairs that had the same exposure experience are termed *concordant pairs,* and those with different exposure experience are termed *discordant pairs.* These possibilities are shown schematically in the following 2 × 2 table. Note that unlike other 2 × 2 tables that we have examined previously, the figure in each cell represents pairs of subjects (i.e., *case-control pairs*), *not* individual subjects. Thus, the following table contains *a* pairs—in which both the case and the control were exposed; *b* pairs—in which the case was exposed and the control was not; c pairs—in which the case was not exposed and the control was exposed; and *d* pairs—in which neither the case nor the control was exposed.

CONTROL

	Exposed	Not Exposed
CASE Exposed	a	b
Not Exposed	c	d

Calculation of the odds ratio in such a matched-pair study is based on the *discordant pairs* only (*b* and *c*). The concordant pairs (*a* and *d*, in which cases and controls were either both exposed or both not exposed) are ignored, because they do not contribute to our knowledge of how cases and controls differ in regard to past history of exposure.

The *odds ratio for matched pairs* is therefore the ratio of the discordant pairs (i.e., *the ratio of the number of pairs in which the case was exposed and the control was not to the number of pairs in which the control was exposed and the case was not).* The odds ratio for the preceding 2 × 2 table is as follows:

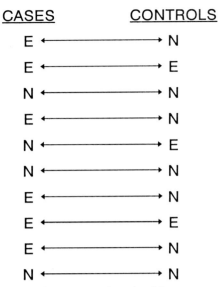

Figure 10–9. A case-control study of ten cases and ten matched controls. (Arrows link matched pairs.)

$$\text{Odds ratio (matched pairs)} = \frac{b}{c}$$

Let us now look at an example of an odds ratio calculation in a matched-pairs case-control study (Fig. 10–9). Let us return to our low-budget study, which included only 10 cases and 10 controls: now our study is designed so that each control has been individually matched to a case, resulting in 10 case-control *pairs* (the horizontal arrows indicate the matching of pairs). If we use these findings to construct a 2 × 2 table for *pairs*, we obtain the following:

CONTROL

	Exposed	Not Exposed
CASE Exposed	2	4
Not Exposed	1	3

Note that there are two pairs in which *both* the case and the control were exposed and three pairs in which *neither* the case *nor* the control was exposed. These concordant pairs are ignored in the analysis of matched pairs.

There are four pairs in which the case was exposed and the control was not and one pair in which the control was exposed and the case was not.

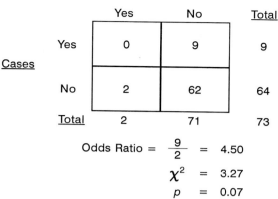

Figure 10–10. Birth weight of index child: Matched pairs comparison of cases and normal controls (8 lb and over vs. under 8 lb). (Data from Gold E, Gordis L, Tonascia J, et al: Risk factors for brain tumors in children. Am J Epidemiol 109:309–319, 1979.)

Figure 10–11. Exposure of index child to sick pets: Matched pairs comparison of cases and normal controls. (Data from Gold E, Gordis L, Tonascia J, et al: Risk factors for brain tumors in children. Am J Epidemiol 109:309–319, 1979.)

Hence, the odds ratio for matched pairs is as follows:

$$\text{Odds ratio} = \frac{b}{c} = \frac{4}{1} = 4$$

Figures 10–10 and 10–11 present data selected from the case-control study of brain tumors in children that was referred to in the previous chapter. Data are shown for two variables. Figure 10–10 presents a matched-pairs analysis for birth weight. A number of studies have suggested that children with higher birth weights are at increased risk for certain childhood cancers. In this analysis, *exposure* is defined as birth weight greater than 8 lb. The result is an odds ratio of 2.57.

In Figure 10–11, a matched-pairs analysis is presented for exposure to sick pets. Many years ago, the Tri-State Leukemia Study found that more of cases of leukemia than controls had family pets. Recent interest in oncogenic viruses has stimulated an interest in exposure to sick pets as a possible source of such agents. Gold and co-workers explored this question in their case-control study,[1] and the results are shown in Figure 10–11. Although the odds ratio was 4.5, the number of discordant pairs was very small.

CONCLUSION

This chapter has introduced the concepts of absolute risk, relative risk, and odds ratio. In Chapter 11 we turn to another important aspect of risk: the attributable risk. We will then review the study designs and indices of risk that have been discussed (Chapter 12) before addressing the use of these concepts in deriving causal inferences (Chapters 13 and 14).

Reference

1. Gold E, Gordis L, Tonascia J, Szklo M: Risk factors for brain tumors in children. Am J Epidemiol 109:309–319, 1979.

Review Questions

1. Of 2,872 persons who had received radiation treatment in childhood because of enlarged thymus, cancer of the thyroid developed in 24 and benign thyroid tumor developed in 52. A comparison group consisted of 5,055 children who had received no such treatment (brothers and sisters of those children who had received radiation treatment). During the follow-up period, none of the comparison group developed thyroid cancer, but benign thyroid tumors developed in 6.

   Calculate the relative risk for benign thyroid tumors: _____

2. In a study of a disease in which all cases that developed were ascertained, if the relative risk for the association between a factor and the disease is *equal to or less than* 1.0, then:
   a. There is no association between the factor and the disease
   b. The factor protects against development of the disease
   c. Either matching or randomization has been unsuccessful
   d. The comparison group used was unsuitable and a valid comparison is not possible
   e. There is either no association or a negative association between the factor and the disease

Questions 3 and 4 are based on the information given below:

In a small pilot study, 12 women with uterine cancer and 12 with no apparent disease were contacted and asked whether they had ever used estrogens. Each women with cancer was matched by age, race, weight, and parity to a woman without disease. The results are shown below.

Pair Number	Women with Uterine Cancer	Women Without Uterine Cancer
1	Estrogen user	Estrogen non-user
2	Estrogen non-user	Estrogen non-user
3	Estrogen user	Estrogen user
4	Estrogen user	Estrogen user
5	Estrogen user	Estrogen non-user
6	Estrogen non-user	Estrogen non-user
7	Estrogen user	Estrogen non-user
8	Estrogen user	Estrogen non-user
9	Estrogen non-user	Estrogen user
10	Estrogen non-user	Estrogen user
11	Estrogen user	Estrogen non-user
12	Estrogen user	Estrogen non-user

3. What is the *estimated* relative risk of cancer when analyzing this study as a matched pairs study?
   a. 0.25
   b. 0.33
   c. 1.00
   d. 3.00
   e. 4.20

4. Unmatch the pairs. What is the *estimated* relative risk of cancer when analyzing this as an unmatched study design?
   a. 0.70
   b. 1.43
   c. 2.80
   d. 3.00
   e. 4.00

Questions 5 and 6 are based on the information given below:

Rates of Atherosclerotic Heart Disease (ASHD) per 10,000 population, by Age and Sex, Framingham, Mass.

Age at Beginning of Study (yr)	Men		Women	
	ASHD Rates at Initial Exam	Yearly Follow-up Exams (Mean Annual Incidence)	ASHD Rates at Initial Exam	Yearly Follow-up Exams (Mean Annual Incidence)
29–34	76.7	19.4	0.0	0.0
35–44	90.7	40.0	17.2	2.1
45–54	167.6	106.5	111.1	29.4
55–62	505.4	209.1	211.1	117.8

5. The relative risk for developing ASHD subsequent to entering this study *in men as compared to women* is:
   a. Approximately equal in all age groups
   b. Highest in the oldest age group
   c. Lowest in the youngest and oldest age groups, and highest at ages 35–44 and 45–54 years
   d. Highest in the youngest and oldest age groups, and lowest at ages 35–44 and 45–54 years
   e. Lowest in the oldest age group

6. The most likely explanation for the differences in rates of ASHD between the *initial* examination and the yearly *follow-up* examinations in men is:
   a. The prevalence and incidence of ASHD increase with age in men
   b. Case-fatality rates of ASHD are higher at younger ages in men
   c. A classic cohort effect explains these results
   d. The case fatality rate in ASHD is highest in the first 24 hours following a heart attack
   e. The initial examination measures the prevalence of ASHD, whereas the subsequent examinations primarily measure the incidence of ASHD

Questions 7 through 9 are based on the information given below:

Talbot and colleagues carried out a study of sudden unexpected death in women. Data on smoking history are shown in the following table:

Smoking History for Cases of ASHD Sudden Death and Controls (Current Smoker, 1 + Pack/Day (Matched Pairs), Allegheny County, 1980

| | Controls | | |
Cases	Smoking 1+ Pack/Day	Smoking <1 Pack/Day	Total
Smoking 1 + pack/day	2	36	38
Smoking <1 pack/day	8	34	42
Total	10	70	80

7. Calculate the matched-pairs odds ratio for these data. _____

8. Using data from the above table, unmatch the pairs and calculate an unmatched odds ratio. _____

9. What are the odds that controls smoke 1+ pack/day? _____

Appendix

Derivation of the relationship of the odds ratio and the relative risk can be demonstrated by the following algebra. Recall that:

$$\text{Relative risk (RR)} = \frac{\frac{a}{a+b}}{\frac{c}{c+d}}$$

$$\text{The odds ratio (OR)} = \frac{ad}{bc}$$

The relationship of the relative risk to the odds ratio can therefore be expressed as the ratio of the RR to the OR:

(1) $$\frac{RR}{OR} = \frac{\left(\frac{\frac{a}{a+b}}{\frac{c}{c+d}}\right)}{\frac{ad}{bc}}$$

$$= \frac{\frac{a}{a+b}}{\frac{c}{c+d}} \times \frac{bc}{ad}$$

$$= \frac{\frac{abc}{a+b}}{\frac{cad}{c+d}} = \frac{\frac{b}{a+b}}{\frac{d}{c+d}}$$

Since

$$\frac{b}{a+b} = \frac{a+b-a}{a+b} = \frac{a+b}{a+b} - \frac{a}{a+b} = 1 - \frac{a}{a+b}$$

and

$$\frac{d}{c+d} = \frac{c+d-c}{c+d} = \frac{c+d}{c+d} - \frac{c}{c+d} = 1 - \frac{c}{c+d}$$

The relationship of the relative risk to the odds ratio can therefore be reduced to the following equation:

$$\frac{RR}{OR} = \frac{1 - \dfrac{a}{a + b}}{1 - \dfrac{c}{c + d}}$$

Or, by multiplying through by the OR:

$$RR = \frac{1 - \dfrac{a}{a + b}}{1 - \dfrac{c}{c + d}} \times OR$$

If the disease is rare, both $a/(a + b)$ and $c/(c + d)$ will be very small, so that the term in parentheses in formula (1) will be approximately 1, and the odds ratio will then approximate the relative risk.

It also is of interest to examine this relationship in a different form. Recall the definition of *odds*—that is, the ratio of the number of ways the event can occur to the number of ways the event cannot occur:

$$O = \frac{P}{1 - P}$$

where O is the *odds* of developing the disease and P is the *risk* of developing the disease.

Note that as P becomes smaller, the denominator $1 - P$ approaches 1, with the result that:

$$\frac{P}{1 - P} \sim \frac{P}{1} = P$$

that is, the *odds* become a good approximation of the *risk*. Thus, if the risk is low (the disease is rare), the *odds* of developing the disease are a good approximation of the *risk* of developing the disease.

Now consider an exposed group and a non-exposed group: if the risk of a disease is very low, the *ratio* of the *odds* in the exposed to the *odds* in the non-exposed, closely approximates the *ratio* of the *risk* in the exposed to the *risk* in the non-exposed *(the relative risk):*

That is, when P is very small:

$$\frac{O_{exp}}{O_{non\text{-}exp}} \cong \frac{P_{exp}}{P_{non\text{-}exp}}$$

where:

O_{exp} is the odds of the exposed population developing the disease,

$O_{non\text{-}exp}$ is the odds of the non-exposed population developing the disease,

P_{exp} is the probability (or risk) of the exposed population developing the disease, and

$P_{non\text{-}exp}$ is the probability (or risk) of the non-exposed population developing the disease.

This ratio of odds is the odds ratio or relative odds.

CHAPTER 11

More on Risk: Estimating the Potential for Prevention

ATTRIBUTABLE RISK

Our discussion in the previous chapter focused on the relative risk and on the odds ratio, which is often used as a surrogate for the relative risk in a case-control study. The *relative risk* is important as a measure of *the strength of the association,* which (as Chapter 13 demonstrates) is a major consideration in deriving causal inferences. In this chapter, we turn to a different question: *How much of the disease that occurs can be attributed to a certain exposure?* This is answered by another measure of risk, the *attributable risk,* which is defined as the amount or proportion of disease incidence (or disease risk) that can be attributed to a specific exposure. For example, how much of the lung cancer risk experienced by smokers can be attributed to smoking? Whereas the relative risk is important in establishing etiologic relationships, the attributable risk is in many ways more important in clinical practice and public health, because it addresses a different question: How much of the risk (incidence) of disease can we hope to prevent if we are able to eliminate exposure to the agent in question?

We can calculate the attributable risk for exposed persons (e.g., the attributable risk of lung cancer in smokers), or the attributable risk for the total population, which includes both exposed and non-exposed persons (e.g., the attributable risk of lung cancer in a total population, which consists both of smokers and non-smokers). These calculations and their uses and interpretations are discussed in this chapter.

Attributable Risk for the Exposed Group

Figure 11–1 offers a schematic introduction to this concept. Consider two groups: one exposed and the other not exposed. In Figure 11–1A, the total risk of the disease in the exposed group is indicated by the full height of the bar on the left, and the total risk of disease in the non-exposed group is indicated by the full height of the bar on the right. As seen here, the total risk of the disease is higher in the exposed group than in the non-exposed group. We can ask the following question: In the exposed persons, how much of the total risk of disease is actually due to exposure (e.g., in a group of smokers, how much of the risk of lung cancer is due to smoking?)

How can this question be answered? Let us consider non-exposed persons, designated by the bar on the right. Although they are not exposed, they have some risk of disease (albeit at a much lower level than that of the exposed persons). That is, the risk of the disease is not zero even in non-exposed persons. For instance, in this example of smoking and lung cancer, even non-smokers have some risk (albeit a low risk) of lung cancer, possibly due to environmental chemical carcinogens or other factors. This risk is termed *background risk.* Every person shares the background risk regardless of whether or not he or she has had the specific exposure in question (in this case, smoking) (see Fig. 11–1B). Thus, both non-exposed and exposed persons have this background risk in addition to any risk they may have as a consequence of exposure. Therefore, the total risk of the disease in exposed individuals is the sum of the background risk that any person has and the risk due to the exposure in question. If we want to know how much of the total risk in *exposed* persons is *due to the exposure,* we should subtract the background risk from the total risk (see Fig. 11–1C). Because the risk in the non-exposed group is equal to the background risk, we can calculate the risk in the exposed group that is a result of the specific exposure by subtracting the

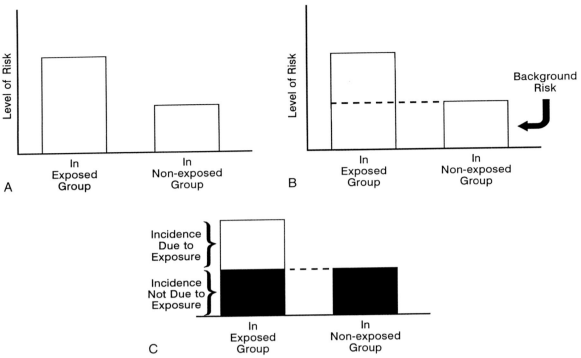

Figure 11–1. *A*, Total risks in exposed and non-exposed groups. *B*, Background risk. *C*, Incidence attributable to exposure and incidence not attributable to exposure.

risk in the non-exposed group (the background risk) from the total risk in the exposed group.

Thus, the incidence of a disease that is attributable to the exposure in the exposed group can be calculated as follows:

Formula 11.1

$$\left(\begin{array}{c}\text{Incidence in}\\\text{exposed group}\end{array}\right) - \left(\begin{array}{c}\text{Incidence in}\\\text{non-exposed group}\end{array}\right)$$

We could instead ask, What *proportion* of the risk in exposed persons is due to the exposure? We could then express the attributable risk as the *proportion* of the total incidence in the exposed group that is attributable to the exposure by simply dividing formula 11.1 by the incidence in the exposed group, as follows:

Formula 11.2

$$\frac{\left(\begin{array}{c}\text{Incidence in}\\\text{exposed group}\end{array}\right) - \left(\begin{array}{c}\text{Incidence in}\\\text{non-exposed group}\end{array}\right)}{\text{Incidence in exposed group}}$$

The attributable risk expresses the most that we can hope to accomplish in reducing the risk of the disease if we completely eliminate the exposure. If all smokers were induced to stop smoking, how much of a reduction could we anticipate in lung cancer rates? From a practical programmatic standpoint, the attributable risk may be more relevant than the relative risk. The relative risk is a measure of the strength of the association and the possibility of a causal relationship, but the attributable risk indicates the potential for prevention if the exposure could be eliminated.

The practicing clinician is mainly interested in the attributable risk *in the exposed group*: for example, when a physician advises a patient to stop smoking, she is in effect telling the patient that stopping smoking will reduce the risk of coronary heart disease (CHD). Implicit in this advice is the physician's estimate that the patient's risk will be reduced by a certain proportion if he stops smoking; the risk reduction is motivating the physician to give that advice. Although the physician often does not have a specific value in mind for the attributable risk, she is in effect relying on an attributable risk for an exposed group (smokers) to which the patient belongs. The physician is implicitly addressing the question: In a population of smokers, how much of the CHD that they experience is due to smoking, and, consequently, how much of the CHD could be prevented if they did not smoke? Thus attributable risk tells us the potential for prevention.

If all the incidence of a disease were the result of a single factor, the attributable risk for that disease would be 100%. However, this is rarely if ever the case. Both the concept and the calculation of attributable risk imply that not all of the disease incidence is due to a single specific exposure, as the disease even develops in some non-exposed individuals.

The diagram at the bottom of the page recapitulates this concept.

Attributable Risk for the Total Population

Let us turn to a somewhat different question relating to attributable risk. Assume that we know how to eliminate smoking. We tell the mayor that we have a highly effective way to eliminate smoking in the community and we want her to provide the funds to support such a program. The mayor responds that she is delighted to hear the news, but asks: "What will the impact of your smoking cessation program be on lung cancer incidence rates in our city?" This question differs from that which was just discussed. For if we talk about lung cancer rates in the entire population of a city, and not just in exposed individuals, we are talking about a population that is composed of both smokers and non-smokers. The mayor is not asking what impact we will have on smokers in this city, but rather what impact will we have on the entire population of the city, which includes both smokers and non-smokers.

Let us consider this question further. In addition to the assumption that we have a terrific smoking cessation program, let us also assume that everyone in the city smokes. (Heaven forbid!) We now want to calculate the attributable risk. Clearly, because everyone in the city smokes, the attributable risk for the entire population of the city would equal the attributable risk for an exposed population. If everybody smokes, the attributable risk for the exposed group tells us what we can hope to accomplish with a smoking cessation program in the total population.

Now let us assume that an ideal situation exists and that nobody in the city smokes. What will be the potential for preventing lung cancer by use of the completely effective smoking cessation program that we wish to apply to the population of the city? The answer is zero; as there are no exposed people in the city, a program to eliminate the exposure would have no effect on the risk of lung cancer. So we have a spectrum of potential impact that runs from a maximum (if everybody smokes) to zero (if nobody smokes). Of course, in reality the answer is generally somewhere in between, because some members of the population smoke and some do not. The latter group (all non-smokers) will clearly not benefit from a smoking cessation program regardless of how effective it is.

To this point we have discussed the concept and calculation of attributable risk *for an exposed group*. For example, in a population of smokers, how much of the lung cancer that they experience is due to smoking and, consequently, how much of the lung cancer could be prevented if they did not smoke? However, to answer the mayor's question as to what effect the smoking cessation program will have on the city's population as a whole, we need to calculate *the attributable risk for the total population:* What proportion of the disease incidence in a *total population* (both exposed and non-exposed) can be attributed to a specific exposure? What would be the total impact of a prevention program on the community? If we want to calculate the attributable risk in the total population, the calculation is similar to that for exposed people, but we begin with the *incidence in the total population* and again subtract the background risk, or the incidence in the non-exposed population. The incidence in the total population that is due to the exposure* can be calculated as shown in Formula 11.3 (next page).

---

*The incidence in the population that is due to the exposure can also be calculated as follows: (Attributable risk for the exposed group) × (Proportion of the population exposed).

| Incidence in Exposed Group | = | Incidence Not Due to the Exposure (Background Incidence) | + | Incidence Due to the Exposure |

| Incidence in Non-exposed Group | = | Incidence Not Due to the Exposure (Background Incidence) |

Formula 11.3

$$\left(\begin{array}{c} \text{Incidence in} \\ \text{total population} \end{array}\right) - \left(\begin{array}{c} \text{Incidence in} \\ \text{non-exposed group} \\ \text{(background risk)} \end{array}\right)$$

Again, if we prefer to express this as the *proportion* of the incidence in the *total population* that is attributable to the exposure, formula 11.3 can be divided by the incidence in the total population:

Formula 11.4

$$\frac{\left(\begin{array}{c} \text{Incidence in} \\ \text{total population} \end{array}\right) - \left(\begin{array}{c} \text{Incidence in} \\ \text{non-exposed group} \end{array}\right)}{\text{Incidence in total population}}$$

The attributable risk for the total population is a valuable concept for the public health worker. The question addressed is: What *proportion* of lung cancer in the total population can be attributed to smoking? This question could be reworded as follows: If smoking were eliminated, what *proportion* of the incidence of lung cancer in the total population (which consists of both smokers and non-smokers) would be prevented? The answer is: the attributable risk *in the total population* (as discussed earlier).*

From a public health standpoint, this is often both the critical issue and the question that is raised by policy-makers and by those responsible for funding preventive programs. They may want to know what the proposed program is going to do for the community. How is it going to change the burden on the health care system or the burden of suffering in the entire community, not just in exposed individuals? For example, if all smokers in the community stopped smoking, what would the impact of this change be on the incidence of lung cancer in the total community population (which includes both smokers and non-smokers)?

An Example of an Attributable Risk Calculation for the Exposed Group

This section presents a step-by-step calculation of attributable risk in both an exposed group and in a total population. We will use the example previously presented of a prospective study of smoking and CHD. The data are again shown in Table 11–1.

The incidence of CHD in the exposed group (smokers) which is attributable to the exposure is calculated according to formula 11.1:

Formula 11.1

$$\left(\begin{array}{c} \text{Incidence in} \\ \text{exposed group} \end{array}\right) - \left(\begin{array}{c} \text{Incidence in} \\ \text{non-exposed group} \end{array}\right)$$
$$= \frac{28.0 - 17.4}{1,000} = \frac{10.6}{1,000}$$

What does this mean? It means that 10.6 of the 28/1,000 incident cases in smokers are attributable to the fact that these people smoke. Stated another way, if we had an effective smoking cessation campaign, we could hope to prevent 10.6 of the $\frac{28}{1,000}$ incident cases of CHD that smokers experience.

If we prefer, we can express this as a *proportion*. The proportion of the total incidence in the exposed group that is attributable to the exposure can be calculated by dividing formula 11.1 by the incidence in the exposed group (formula 11.2):

---

*Another way to calculate the attributable risk for the total population is to use Levin's formula, which is given in the appendix to this chapter.

Table 11–1. Smoking and Coronary Heart Disease (CHD): A Hypothetical Cohort Study of 3,000 Cigarette Smokers and 5,000 Non-smokers

	Develop CHD	Do Not Develop CHD	Total	Incidence per 1,000 per Year
Smoke cigarettes	84	2,916	3,000	28.0
Do not smoke cigarettes	87	4,913	5,000	17.4

$$\text{Incidence among smokers} = \frac{84}{3,000} = 28.0 \text{ per 1,000}$$

$$\text{Incidence among non-smokers} = \frac{87}{5,000} = 17.4 \text{ per 1,000}$$

Formula 11.2

$$\frac{\left(\begin{array}{c}\text{Incidence in} \\ \text{exposed group}\end{array}\right) - \left(\begin{array}{c}\text{Incidence in} \\ \text{non-exposed group}\end{array}\right)}{\text{Incidence in exposed group}}$$

$$= \frac{28.0 - 17.4}{28.0} = \frac{10.6}{28.0} = 0.379 = 37.9\%$$

Thus, 37.9% of the morbidity from CHD among smokers may be attributable to smoking and could presumably be prevented by eliminating smoking.

An Example of an Attributable Risk Calculation in the Total Population

Using the same example let us calculate the attributable risk for the total population: The question we are asking is: What can we hope to accomplish with our smoking cessation program *in the total population* (i.e., the entire community, which consists of both smokers and non-smokers)?

Remember that in the total population, the incidence that is due to smoking (the exposure) can be calculated by subtracting the background risk (i.e., the incidence in the non-smokers, or non-exposed) from the incidence in the total population:

Formula 11.3

$$\left(\begin{array}{c}\text{Incidence in} \\ \text{total population}\end{array}\right) - \left(\begin{array}{c}\text{Incidence in} \\ \text{non-exposed group}\end{array}\right)$$

To calculate formula 11.3, we must know *either* the incidence of the disease (CHD) in the total population (which we often do not know) *or* all of the following three values, from which we can then calculate the incidence in the total population:

1. The incidence among smokers
2. The incidence among non-smokers
3. The proportion of the total population that smokes

In this example we know that the incidence among the smokers is 28.0 per 1,000 and the incidence among the non-smokers is 17.4 per 1,000. However, we do not know the incidence in the total population. Let us assume that from some other source of information we know that the proportion of smokers in the population is 44% (and therefore the proportion of non-smokers is 56%). The incidence in the total population can then be calculated as follows:

$$\left(\begin{array}{c}\text{Incidence} \\ \text{in smokers}\end{array}\right)\left(\begin{array}{c}\% \text{ smokers} \\ \text{in population}\end{array}\right) + \left(\begin{array}{c}\text{Incidence in} \\ \text{non-smokers}\end{array}\right)\left(\begin{array}{c}\% \text{ non-smokers} \\ \text{in population}\end{array}\right)$$

(We are simply weighting the calculation of the incidence in the total population, taking into account the proportion of the population that smokes and the proportion of the population that does not smoke).

So in this example, the incidence in the total population can be calculated as follows:

$$\left(\frac{28.0}{1,000}\right)(.44) + \left(\frac{17.4}{1,000}\right)(.56) = \frac{22.1}{1,000}$$

We now have the values needed for using formula 11.3 to calculate the attributable risk in the total population:

Formula 11.3

$$\left(\begin{array}{c}\text{Incidence in} \\ \text{total population}\end{array}\right) - \left(\begin{array}{c}\text{Incidence in} \\ \text{non-exposed group}\end{array}\right)$$

$$= \frac{22.1}{1000} - \frac{17.4}{1000} = \frac{4.7}{1,000}$$

What does this tell us? How much of the total risk of CHD in this population (which consists of both smokers and non-smokers) is attributable to smoking? If we had an effective prevention program (smoking cessation) in this population, how much of a reduction in CHD incidence could we anticipate, at best, in the total population (of both smokers and non-smokers)?

If we prefer to calculate the *proportion* of the incidence in the *total population* that is attributable to the exposure, this can be accomplished by dividing formula 11.3 by the incidence in the total population (formula 11.4):

Formula 11.4

$$\frac{\left(\begin{array}{c}\text{Incidence in} \\ \text{total population}\end{array}\right) - \left(\begin{array}{c}\text{Incidence in} \\ \text{non-exposed group}\end{array}\right)}{\text{Incidence in total population}}$$

$$= \frac{22.1 - 17.4}{22.1}$$

$$= 21.3\%$$

Thus, 21.3% of the incidence of CHD in this total population can be attributed to smoking, and if an effective prevention program eliminated smoking, the best we could hope to achieve would be a reduction of 21.3% in the incidence of CHD in the total population (consisting of both smokers and non-smokers).

Attributable risk is a critical concept in virtually any area of public health and in clinical practice. It is also of interest that in the legal arena, in which toxic tort litigation has become increasingly common, the concept of attributable risk has taken on great importance. One of the legal criteria used in finding a company responsible for an environmental injury, for example, is whether it is "more likely than not" that the company caused the injury. It has been suggested that an attributable risk of greater than 50% might represent a quantitative determination of the legal definition of "more likely than not."

COMPARISON OF RELATIVE RISK AND ATTRIBUTABLE RISK

Chapters 10 and 11 have reviewed several measures of risk and of excess risk. The relative risk and odds ratio are important as measures of the strength of the association, which is an important consideration in deriving a causal inference. The attributable risk is a measure of how much of the disease risk is attributable to a certain exposure. Consequently, the attributable risk is useful in answering the question of how much disease can be prevented if we have an effective means of eliminating the exposure in question. Thus, the relative risk is valuable in etiologic studies of disease, whereas the attributable risk has major applications in clinical practice and public health.

Table 11–2 shows an example from a study by Doll and Peto[1] that relates mortality from lung cancer and CHD in smokers and non-smokers and provides an illuminating comparison of relative risk and attributable risk in the same set of data.

Let us first examine the data for lung cancer. (Note that in this example we are using mortality as a surrogate for risk.) We see that the mortality risk is 140 for smokers and 10 for non-smokers. We can calculate the relative risk as $\frac{140}{10} = 14$.

Now let us look at the data for CHD. The CHD mortality rate is 669 in smokers and 413 in non-smokers. The relative risk can be calculated as $\frac{669}{413} = 1.6$. Thus, the relative risk is much higher for smoking and lung cancer than it is for smoking and CHD.

Now let us turn to the attributable risks in smokers. How much of the total risk in smokers can we attribute to smoking? To calculate the attributable risk, we subtract the background risk—the risk in the non-exposed group (non-smokers)—from the risk in the exposed group (smokers). Using the data for lung cancer, $(140 - 10) = 130$.

To calculate the attributable risk for CHD and smoking, we subtract the risk in the non-exposed group (non-smokers) from the risk in the exposed group (smokers), $(669 - 413) = 256$. That is, of the total 669 deaths per 100,000 in smokers, 256 can be attributed to smoking.

If we prefer to express the attributable risk for lung cancer and smoking as a proportion (i.e., the proportion of the lung cancer risk in smokers that can be attributed to smoking) we divide the attributable risk by the risk in smokers: $(140 - 10)/140 = 92\%$.

If we prefer to express the attributable risk of CHD and smoking as a proportion (i.e., the proportion of the CHD risk in smokers that can be attributed to smoking) we divide the attributable risk $(669 - 413)$ by the risk in smokers, $(669 - 413)/669 = 38\%$.

What does this table tell us? First we see a tremendous difference in the relative risks for lung cancer and for CHD in relation to smoking—14.0 for lung cancer compared with 1.6 for CHD (i.e., a much stronger association exists for smoking and lung cancer than for smoking and CHD). However, the attributable risk is almost twice as high (256) for CHD as it is for lung cancer (130). If we choose to express the attributable risk as a proportion, we find that 92% of lung cancer deaths in smokers can be attributed to smoking (and are potentially

Table 11–2. Lung Cancer and CHD Mortality in Male British Physicians: Smokers vs. Non-smokers

	Age-Adjusted Death Rates per 100,000		Relative Risk	Attributable Risk	% Attributable Risk
	Smokers	Non-smokers			
Lung cancer	140	10	14.0	130	92
Coronary heart disease	669	413	1.6	256	38

From Doll R, Peto R: Mortality in relation to smoking: Twenty years' observations on male British doctors. Br Med J 2:1525–1536, 1976.

Table 11–3. Summary of Attributable Risk Calculations

	In Exposed Group	In Total Population
Incidence attributable to exposure	$\left(\begin{array}{c}\text{Incidence in}\\\text{exposed group}\end{array}\right) - \left(\begin{array}{c}\text{Incidence in}\\\text{non-exposed group}\end{array}\right)$	$\left(\begin{array}{c}\text{Incidence in}\\\text{total population}\end{array}\right) - \left(\begin{array}{c}\text{Incidence in}\\\text{non-exposed group}\end{array}\right)$
Proportion of incidence attributable to exposure	$\dfrac{\left(\begin{array}{c}\text{Incidence in}\\\text{exposed group}\end{array}\right) - \left(\begin{array}{c}\text{Incidence in}\\\text{non-exposed group}\end{array}\right)}{\left(\begin{array}{c}\text{Incidence in}\\\text{exposed group}\end{array}\right)}$	$\dfrac{\left(\begin{array}{c}\text{Incidence in}\\\text{total population}\end{array}\right) - \left(\begin{array}{c}\text{Incidence in}\\\text{non-exposed group}\end{array}\right)}{\left(\begin{array}{c}\text{Incidence in}\\\text{total population}\end{array}\right)}$

preventable by eliminating smoking) compared with only 38% of deaths from CHD in smokers that can be attributed to smoking.

Thus, the relative risk is much higher for lung cancer than for CHD, and the attributable risk expressed as a proportion is also much higher for lung cancer. However, if an effective smoking cessation program were available today and smoking were eliminated, would the preventive impact be greater on mortality from lung cancer or from CHD? If we examine the table we see that if smoking were eliminated, 256 deaths per 100,000 from CHD would be prevented in contrast to only 130 from lung cancer, despite the fact that the relative risk is higher for lung cancer and despite the fact that the proportion of deaths attributable to smoking is greater for lung cancer. Why is this so? This is a result of the fact that the baseline mortality level is much higher for CHD than for lung cancer (669 compared to 140) and that the attributable risk (the difference between total risk in smokers and background risk) is much greater for CHD than for lung cancer.

SUMMARY

In this chapter we have introduced the concept of attributable risk and described how it is calculated and interpreted. Attributable risk is summarized in the four calculations shown in Table 11–3.

The concepts of relative risk and attributable risk are essential for understanding causation and the potential for prevention. Several measures of risk have now been discussed: (1) absolute risk, (2) relative risk, (3) odds ratios, and (4) attributable risk. In the next chapter we shall briefly review study designs and concepts of risk before proceeding to a discussion of how to use estimates of excess risk to derive causal inferences.

References

1. Doll R, Peto R: Mortality in relation to smoking: Twenty years' observations on male British doctors. Br Med J 2:1525–1536, 1976.
2. Levin ML: The occurrence of lung cancer in man. Acta Intern Cancer 9:531, 1953.
3. Leviton A: Definitions of attributable risk. Am J Epidemiol 98:231, 1973.

Review Questions

1. Several studies have found that approximately 85% of cases of lung cancer are due to cigarette smoking. This measure is an example of:
   a. An incidence rate
   b. An attributable risk
   c. A relative risk
   d. A prevalence risk
   e. A proportionate mortality ratio

Questions 2 and 3 refer to the following information:

Results of a 10-year cohort study of smoking and coronary heart disease (CHD) are shown below:

At Beginning of Study	Outcome After 10 yr	
	Developed CHD	*Did Not Develop CHD*
2,000 Healthy smokers	65	1,935
4,000 Healthy non-smokers	20	3,980

2. The incidence of CHD in smokers that can be attributed to smoking is: _____

3. The proportion of the total incidence of CHD in smokers that is attributable to smoking is: _____

Questions 4 and 5 are based on the information given below:

In a cohort study of smoking and lung cancer, the incidence of lung cancer among smokers was found to be 9/1,000 and the incidence among non-smokers was 1/1,000. From another source we know that 45% of the total population were smokers.

4. The incidence of lung cancer attributable to smoking in the total population is: _____

5. The proportion of the risk in the total population which is attributable to smoking: _____

Appendix

Levin's Formula for the Attributable Risk for the Total Population

Another way to calculate this *proportion* for the *total population* is to use Levin's formula:[2]

$$\frac{p(r-1)}{p(r-1)+1}$$

where p is the proportion of the population with the characteristic or exposure and r is the relative risk (or odds ratio).

Leviton[3] has shown that Levin's formula[2] and the following formula are algebraically identical:

$$\frac{\left(\begin{array}{c}\text{Incidence in} \\ \text{total population}\end{array}\right) - \left(\begin{array}{c}\text{Incidence in} \\ \text{non-exposed group}\end{array}\right)}{\text{Incidence in total population}}$$

CHAPTER 12

A Pause for Review: Comparing Cohort and Case-Control Studies

At this point in our discussion we will pause to review some of the material that has been covered in Section II. Because the presentation proceeds in a stepwise manner, it is important that the reader understand what has been discussed thus far.

First, let us compare the designs of cohort and case-control studies as seen in Figure 12–1. The important distinguishing point between the two types of study design is that in a cohort study, exposed and non-exposed persons are compared, and in a case-control study, persons with the disease (cases) and without the disease (controls) are compared.

Table 12–1 presents a detailed comparison of case-control, concurrent cohort, and retrospective (historical) cohort study designs. If the reader has followed the discussion in Section II to this point, the entries in the table should be easy to understand.

As seen in Table 12–1, case-control studies have a number of advantages: They are relatively inexpensive and require a relatively small number of subjects for study. They are desirable when the disease occurrence is rare, because if a cohort

study were performed in such a circumstance, a tremendous number of people would have to be followed to generate enough cases for study. As seen in Figure 12–2, in a case-control study, because we begin with cases and controls, we are able to study more than one possible etiologic factor and to explore interactions among the factors.

Since case-control studies often require data about past events or exposures, they are often encumbered by the difficulties encountered in using such data (including a potential for recall bias). Furthermore, as has been discussed in some detail, selection of an appropriate control group is one of the most difficult methodologic problems encountered in epidemiology. In addition, in most case-control studies we cannot calculate disease incidence in either the total population or the exposed and non-exposed groups without some supplemental information.

When we begin a cohort study with exposed and non-exposed groups we can study only the specific exposure which distinguishes one group from the

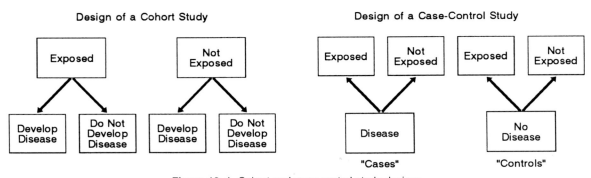

Figure 12–1. Cohort and case-control study designs.

Table 12–1. Comparisons of Case-Control and Cohort Studies

	Case-Control Studies	Cohort Studies — Concurrent	Cohort Studies — Retrospective
A. Study group	Persons with diseases (cases) $(a+c)$	Exposed persons $(a+b)$	Exposed persons $(a+b)$
B. Comparison group	Persons without disease (controls) $(b+d)$	Non-exposed persons $(c+d)$	Non-exposed persons $(c+d)$
C. Outcome measurements	Proportion of cases exposed $\left(\dfrac{a}{a+c}\right)$ and Proportion of controls exposed $\left(\dfrac{b}{b+d}\right)$	Incidence in the exposed $\left(\dfrac{a}{a+b}\right)$ and Incidence in the non-exposed $\left(\dfrac{c}{c+d}\right)$	Incidence in the exposed $\left(\dfrac{a}{a+b}\right)$ and Incidence in the non-exposed $\left(\dfrac{c}{c+d}\right)$
D. Measures of risk	— — Odds ratio Attributable risk*	Absolute risk Relative risk Odds ratio Attributable risk	Absolute risk Relative risk Odds ratio Attributable risk
E. Temporal relationship between exposure and disease	Sometimes hard to establish	Easily established	Sometimes hard to establish
F. Multiple associations	Possible to study associations of a disease with several exposures or factors	Possible to study associations of an exposure with several diseases†	Possible to study associations of an exposure with several diseases†
G. Time required for the study	Relatively short	Generally long because of need to follow-up the subjects	May be short
H. Cost of study	Relatively inexpensive	Expensive	Generally less expensive than a concurrent study
I. Population size needed	Relatively small	Relatively large	Relatively large
J. Potential bias	Assessment of exposure	Assessment of outcome	Susceptible to bias both in assessment of exposure and assessment of outcome
K. Best when	Disease is rare Exposure is frequent among the diseased	Exposure is rare Disease is frequent among exposed	Exposure is rare Disease is frequent among exposed
L. Problems	Selection of appropriate controls often difficult Incomplete information on exposure	Selection of non-exposed comparison group often difficult Changes over time in criteria and methods	Selection of non-exposed comparison group often difficult Changes over time in criteria and methods

*Provided additional information is available.
†Also possible to study multiple exposures when the study population is selected on the basis of a factor unrelated to the exposure.

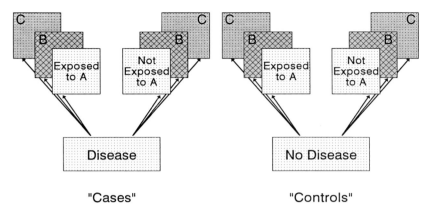

Figure 12–2. Study multiple exposures in a case-control study.

other. But as shown in Figure 12–3, we can study multiple outcomes or diseases in relation to the exposure of interest.

However, it is possible to study multiple exposures in a cohort study when the study population is selected on the basis of a factor unrelated to exposure, such as residence. Thus, in the Framingham Study, it was possible to study many exposures, including weight, blood pressure, cholesterol level, smoking, and physical activity.

In cohort studies incidence in both exposed and non-exposed groups *can* be calculated, and we can therefore directly calculate the relative risk. Less potential for recall and other bias in assessing the exposure and greater validity to the exposure assessments may well exist in concurrent cohort studies. However, in retrospective cohort studies, which require data from the past, these problems may be significant. Cohort studies are desirable when the exposure of interest is rare. In a case-control design, we are unlikely to identify a sufficient number of exposed persons when we are dealing with a rare exposure. In concurrent cohort studies in particular we are likely to have better data on the temporal relationship between exposure and outcome—that is, did the exposure precede the outcome? Among

the disadvantages of cohort studies is that they usually require large populations, and, in general, concurrent cohort studies are especially expensive to carry out because follow-up of a large population over time is required. A greater potential bias for assessing the outcome is present in cohort studies. Finally, cohort studies often become impractical when the disease under study is rare.

The nested case-control design combines elements of both cohort and case-control studies and offers a number of advantages: The possibility of recall bias is eliminated because the data on exposure are obtained before the disease develops. Exposure data are more likely to represent the pre-illness state, as they are obtained years before clinical illness is diagnosed. Finally, costs are reduced compared with those of a cohort study, because laboratory tests need to be done only on specimens from subjects who are later chosen as cases or controls.

Finally, we have discussed the cross-sectional study design, in which data on both exposure and disease outcomes are collected simultaneously from each subject. The data can therefore be analyzed by comparing the prevalence of disease in exposed individuals with that in non-exposed individuals, or by comparing the prevalence of exposure in persons

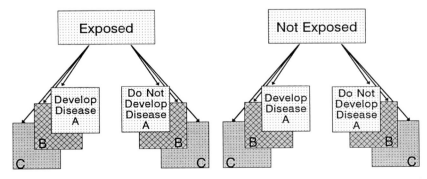

Figure 12–3. Study multiple outcomes in a cohort study.

with the disease with that of persons without the disease. Although cross-sectional data are often obtained in surveys and can be very useful, they often do not permit determination of the temporal relationship between exposure and the development of disease. As a result, their value for deriving causal inferences is limited. However, they can provide important directions for further research employing cohort, case-control, and nested case-control designs.

CHAPTER 13

From Association to Causation: Deriving Inferences From Epidemiologic Studies

In the previous chapters we discussed the designs of epidemiologic studies that are used to determine whether an association exists between an exposure and a disease (Fig. 13–1). We then addressed different types of risk measurement that are used to quantitatively express an excess in risk. If we determine that an exposure is associated with a disease, the next question is whether the observed association reflects a causal relationship (Fig. 13–2). Although Figures 13–1 and 13–2 refer to an environmental exposure, they could just as well have specified a genetic characteristic or characteristics or a specific combination of environmental and genetic factors. As we shall see in Chapter 15, studies of disease etiology generally address the contributions of both genetic and environmental factors and their interactions.

This chapter discusses the derivation of causal inferences in epidemiology. Let us begin by asking: What approaches are available for studying the etiology of disease?

APPROACHES FOR STUDYING DISEASE ETIOLOGY

If we are interested in whether a certain substance is carcinogenic in human beings, a first step in the study of the substance's effect might be to expose animals to the carcinogen in a controlled laboratory environment. Although such *animal* studies afford us the opportunity to control the exposure dose and other environmental conditions precisely, and to keep loss to follow-up to a minimum, at the conclusion of the study we are left with the problem of having to extrapolate data across species, from ani-

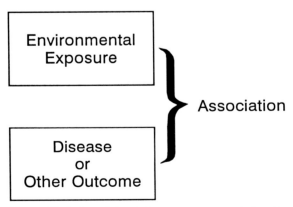

Figure 13–1. Association between exposure and disease.

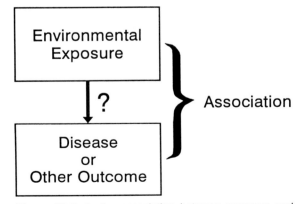

Figure 13–2. Is the association between exposure and disease causal?

mal to human populations. Certain diseases seen in humans have neither occurred nor been produced in animals. It is also difficult to extrapolate animal doses to human doses, and species differ in their responses. Thus, although such toxicologic studies can be very useful, they still leave a gnawing uncertainty as to whether the animal findings can be generalized to human beings.

We can also use *in vitro systems,* such as cell culture or organ culture. However, as these are artificial systems, we are again left with the difficulty of extrapolating from an artificial system to an intact, whole human organism.

In view of these limitations, if we want to be able to draw a conclusion as to whether a substance causes disease in human beings, we need to make *observations in human populations.* Because we cannot ethically or practically randomize human beings to exposure to a suspected carcinogen, we are dependent on non-randomized observations, such as those made in case-control and cohort studies.

Approaches to Etiology in Human Populations

Epidemiology capitalizes on what have been called ''unplanned'' or ''natural'' experiments. (Some think that this phrase is a contradiction in terms, in that the word ''experiment'' implies a planned exposure.) What we mean by *unplanned* or *natural* experiments is that we take advantage of groups who have been exposed for non-study purposes, such as occupational cohorts in specific industries, persons exposed to toxic chemicals (such as those affected by the explosion at Bhopal, India), or persons subjected to other toxic exposures (such as residents of Hiroshima and Nagasaki who were exposed to atomic bomb radiation in 1945). Each of these exposed groups can be compared to a non-exposed group to determine whether there is an increased risk of a certain adverse effect in persons who have been exposed.

In conducting human studies, the sequence shown in Figure 13–3 is frequently followed.

The initial step may consist of *clinical observations* at the bedside. For example, when the surgeon Alton Ochsner observed that virtually every patient on whom he operated for lung cancer gave a history of cigarette smoking, he was among the first to suggest a possible causal relationship.[1] A second step is to try to identify *routinely available data,* the analysis of which might shed light on the ques-

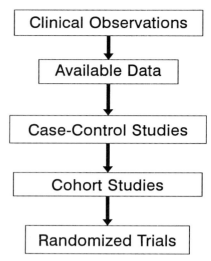

Figure 13–3. A frequent sequence of studies in human populations.

tion. We can then carry out *new studies* such as the cohort and case-control studies discussed in Chapters 8 and 9, which are specifically designed to determine whether there is an association between an exposure and a disease, and whether a causal relationship exists.

The usual first step in carrying out new studies to explore a relationship is often a *case-control study.* For example, if Ochsner had wanted to further explore his suggestion that cigarette smoking may be associated with lung cancer, he would have compared the smoking histories of a group of his lung cancer patients with those of a group of patients without lung cancer—a case-control study.

If a case-control study yields evidence that a certain exposure is suspect, we might next do a *cohort study* (e.g., comparing smokers and non-smokers and determining the rate of lung cancer in each group). Although a randomized trial might be the next step in rare situations, it is generally only used for potentially beneficial agents.

Conceptually, a two-step process is followed in carrying out studies and evaluating the evidence. In practice, this process often becomes interactive and deviates from a fixed sequence:

1. We determine whether there is an association between an exposure or characteristic and the risk of a disease. To do so, we use:
   a. Studies of group characteristics: ecologic studies
   b. Studies of individual characteristics: e.g., case-control and cohort studies
2. If an association is demonstrated, we determine

whether the observed association is likely to be a causal one.

Ecologic Studies

The first approach in determining whether or not an association exists might be to conduct studies of group characteristics, called *ecologic studies.* Figure 13–4 shows the relation between breast cancer incidence and dietary fat consumption by country.[2]

As dietary fat consumption increases, breast cancer incidence increases. We might therefore be tempted to conclude that dietary fat may be a causal factor for breast cancer. What is the problem with this type of study? Consider Switzerland, for example, which has a high breast cancer incidence and a high average consumption of dietary fat. The problem is that we do not know whether the *individuals* in that country in whom breast cancer developed actually had high dietary fat intake. All we have are *average* values of dietary fat consumption for each country and the breast cancer incidence for each country. In fact, one might argue that given the same overall picture, it is conceivable that those who developed breast cancer ate very little dietary fat. Figure 13–4 alone does not reveal whether this might be true; in effect, this characterizes individuals in the country by the average figure for that country. No account is taken of variability between individuals in that country in regard to dietary fat consumption. This is called the *ecologic fallacy*-

–we may be ascribing to members of a group characteristics that they in fact do not possess as individuals. This problem arises in an ecologic study because we only have data for groups; we do not have exposure and outcome data for each individual in the population.

Table 13–1 shows data from a study in northern California exploring a possible relation between prenatal exposure to influenza during an influenza outbreak and the later development of acute lymphocytic leukemia in a child.[3] The data presented in this table show the incidence data for children who were not in utero during a flu outbreak and for children who were in utero—in the first, second, and third trimester of the pregnancy—during the outbreak. Below these figures, the data are presented as relative risks, with the risk being set at 1.0 for those who were not in utero during the outbreak and the other rates being set relative to this. The data indicate a high relative risk for leukemia in children who were in utero during the flu outbreak in the first trimester.

What is the problem? The authors themselves wrote: ''The observed association is between pregnancy during an influenza epidemic and subsequent leukemia in the offspring of that pregnancy. It is not known if the mothers of any of these children actually had influenza during their pregnancy.'' What we are missing are individual data on exposure. One might ask, Why didn't the investigators obtain the necessary exposure data? The likely rea-

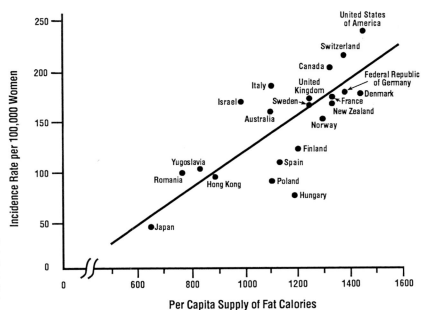

Figure 13–4. Correlation between dietary fat intake and breast cancer by country. (From Prentice RL, Kakar F, Hursting S, et al: Aspects of the rationale for the Women's Health Trial. J Natl Cancer Inst 80:802–814, 1988.)

Table 13–1. Average Annual Crude Incidence Rates and Relative Risks of Acute Lymphocytic Leukemia By Cohort and Trimester of Flu Exposure for Children Younger Than 5 Years, San Francisco/Oakland (1969–1973)

| | No Flu Exposure | Flu Exposure | | | |
| | | Trimester | | | |
		1st	2nd	3rd	Total
Incidence rates per 100,000	3.19	10.32	8.21	2.99	6.94
Relative risks	1.0	3.2	2.6	0.9	2.2

Adapted from Austin DF, Karp S, Dworsky R, Henderson BE: Excess leukemia in cohorts of children born following influenza epidemics. Am J Epidemiol 10:77–83, 1977.

son is that the investigators used birth certificates and data from a cancer registry; both types of data are relatively easy to obtain. This approach did not require follow-up and direct contact with individual subjects. If we were impressed by these ecologic data we might want to carry out a study specifically designed to explore the possible relationship of prenatal flu and leukemia.

In view of the these problems, are ecologic studies of value? Yes, they can suggest avenues of research that may be promising in casting light on etiologic relationships. In and of themselves, however, they do not demonstrate that a causal association exists.

Recognizing the limitations of ecologic studies that use group data, we turn next to studies of individual characteristics: case-control and cohort studies. It has been claimed that because epidemiologists generally show tabulated data and refer to characteristics of groups, the data in all epidemiologic studies are group data. This is not true. For what distinguishes case-control and cohort studies from ecologic studies is that although both of these rely on groups of individuals, for each subject in a case-control or cohort study we have information on both exposure (whether or not and, often, how much exposure occurred) and disease outcome (whether or not the person developed the disease in question). In ecologic studies, we only have data on groups.

TYPES OF ASSOCIATIONS

Real or Spurious Associations

Let us turn next to the types of associations that we might observe in a cohort or case-control study. If we observe an association, the first question is, Is it a true (real) association or a false (spurious) one? For example, if we designed the study to select controls in such a way that they tended to be non-exposed, we might observe an association of exposure with disease (more exposure in cases than in controls), which would not be a true association but only a result of the study design. Recall that this was the issue raised in Chapter 9 regarding a study of coffee consumption and cancer of the pancreas, in which the possibility was suggested that the controls selected for the study had a lower rate of coffee consumption than was found in the general population.

Interpreting Real Associations

If the observed association is real, is it causal? Figure 13–5 shows two possibilities. Figure 13–5A shows a causal association: we observe an association of exposure and disease, as indicated by the bracket, and the exposure induces development of the disease, as indicated by the arrow. Figure 13–5B shows the same observed association of exposure and disease, but they are associated only because they are both linked to a third factor, designated *factor X*. This association is a result of confounding and is non-causal. Confounding is discussed in greater detail in Chapter 14.

In Chapter 9 we discussed this issue in relation to McMahon's study of coffee and cancer of the pancreas. McMahon observed an association of coffee consumption with risk of pancreatic cancer. As seen in Figure 13–6, cigarette smoking was known to be associated with pancreatic cancer, and coffee drinking and cigarette smoking are closely associated (few smokers do not drink coffee). Therefore, was the observed association of coffee drinking and cancer of the pancreas likely to be a causal relationship, or could the association be due to the fact that coffee and cigarette smoking are associ-

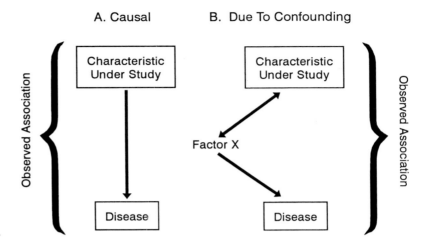

Figure 13–5. Types of associations.

ated, and that cigarette smoking is a known risk factor for cancer of the pancreas?

The same issue is exemplified by the observed association of increased serum cholesterol level and risk of coronary heart disease (CHD), shown in Figure 13–7. Is increased cholesterol a causal factor for increased risk of CHD, or is the observed association due to confounding? That is, are we observing an association of increased cholesterol and CHD because both are associated with a factor X (such as a particular genetic profile), which might cause people to have both increased levels of cholesterol and an increased risk of CHD?

Is this distinction really important? What difference does it make? It makes a tremendous difference from both clinical and public health standpoints. If the relation is causal, we will succeed in lowering the risk of CHD if we lower cholesterol levels. But if the relationship is due to confounding,

then the increased risk of CHD is caused by factor X, and changes in the level of serum cholesterol will have no effect on the risk of CHD. Thus, it is extremely important that we be able to distinguish between an association due to a causal relationship and an association due to confounding (non-causal).

Let us look at another example. For many years it has been known that cigarette smoking by pregnant women is associated with low birth weight in their infants. As seen in Figure 13–8, the effect is not just the result of the birth of a few low–birth-weight babies in this group of women. Rather, the entire weight distribution curve is shifted to the left in the babies born to smokers. The reduction in birth weight is also not a result of shorter pregnancies. As shown in Figure 13–9, the babies of smokers are smaller than those of non-smokers at each gestational age. A dose-response relationship is also seen (Fig. 13–10). The more a woman smokes, the

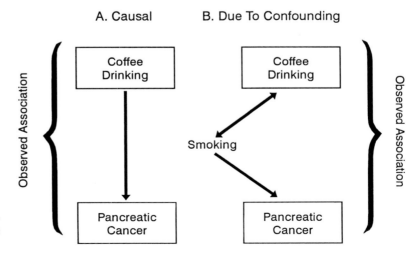

Figure 13–6. Interpreting an observed association between coffee drinking and pancreatic cancer.

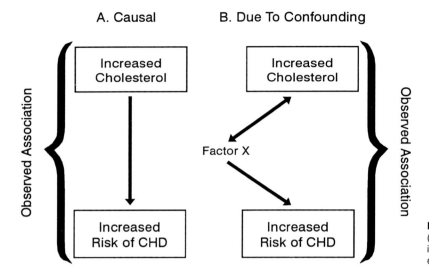

Figure 13–7. Types of associations (example, increased cholesterol and increased risk of coronary heart disease [CHD]).

greater her risk of having a low–birth-weight baby. For many years the interpretation of this association was the subject of great controversy. Many believed the association reflected a causal relation. Others, including a leading statistician, Jacob Yerushalmy, believed the association was due to confounding and was not causal. He wrote as follows:

> A comparison of smokers and non-smokers shows that the two differ markedly along many environmental, behavioral and biologic variables. For example, smokers are less likely to use contraceptives and to plan the pregnancy. Smokers are more likely to drink coffee, beer and whiskey and the non-smoker, tea, milk and wine. The smoker is more

likely than the non-smoker to indulge in these habits to excess. In general, the non-smokers are revealed to be more moderate than the smokers who are shown to be more extreme and carefree in their mode of life. Some biologic differences are also noted between them: Thus smokers have a higher twinning rate only in whites and their age for menarche is lower than for non-smokers.

In view of these many differences between smokers and non-smokers, Yerushalmy believed that it was not the *smoking* that caused the low birth weight, but rather that the low weight was attributable to *other characteristics of the smokers*. It is interesting to examine a study Yerushalmy car-

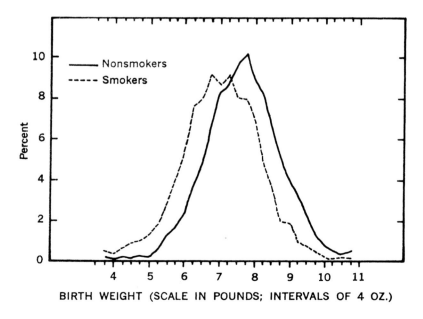

Figure 13–8. Percentage distribution by birth weight of mothers who did not smoke during pregnancy and of those who smoked 1 pack of cigarettes or more per day. (From U.S. Department of Health, Education, and Welfare: The Health Consequences of Smoking. Washington, DC, Public Health Service, 1973, p. 105.)

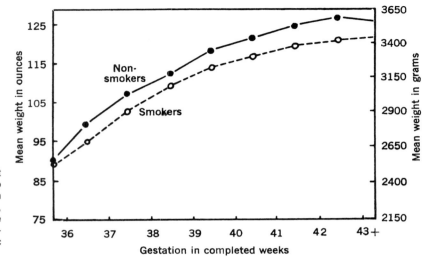

Figure 13–9. Mean birth weight for week of gestation according to maternal smoking habit. (From U.S. Department of Health, Education, and Welfare: The Health Consequences of Smoking. Washington, DC, Public Health Service, 1973, p. 104.)

ried out to support his position at the time (Fig. 13–11).[4]

Yerushalmy examined the results of one pregnancy (the study pregnancy) in a population of women who had had several pregnancies. The rate of low–birth-weight babies in the study pregnancy was 5.3% for women who were non-smokers in *all* of their pregnancies. However, if they were smokers in *all* of their pregnancies, the rate of low birth weight in the study pregnancy was almost 9%. When he examined pregnancies of women who were non-smokers in the study pregnancy, but who later became smokers, he found that their rate of

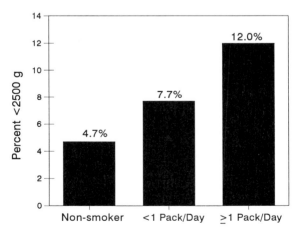

Figure 13–10. Percent of pregnancies (n = 50,267) with infant weighing less than 2500 g, by cigarette smoking category. (Redrawn from Ontario Department of Health: Second Report of the Perinatal Mortality Study in Ten University Teaching Hospitals. Toronto, Ontario Department of Health, Ontario Perinatal Mortality Study Committee, vol I, 1967, p. 275.)

low–birth-weight babies was about equal to that of women who smoked in all pregnancies. When he examined pregnancies of women who were smokers in the study pregnancy, but who subsequently stopped smoking, he found that their rate of low birth weight in the study pregnancy was similar to that of women who were non-smokers in all of their pregnancies.

On the basis of these data, Yerushalmy came to the conclusion that it was not the smoking, but that it was rather a characteristic of the smoker that caused the low birth weight. Today, however, it is virtually universally accepted that smoking is a cause of low birth weight. The causal nature of this relation has also been demonstrated in randomized trials that have reduced the frequency of low birth weight by initiating programs for smoking cessation in pregnant women. Although this issue has now largely been resolved, it is illuminating to review both the controversy and the study, as they exemplify the reasoning that is necessary in trying to distinguish causal from non-causal interpretations of observed associations.

TYPES OF CAUSAL RELATIONS

A causal pathway can be either *direct* or *indirect* (Fig. 13–12). In direct causation, factor A directly causes disease B without any intermediate step. In indirect causation, factor A causes disease B, but only through an intermediate step or steps. In human biology, intermediate steps are virtually always present in any causal process.

If a relationship is causal, four types of causal

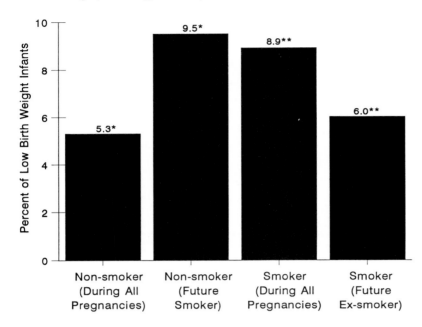

Figure 13–11. Percent of low–birth-weight infants by smoking status of their mothers. *Symbols:* *, P <0.01; **, P <0.02.) (Redrawn from Yerushalmy J: Infants with low-birth weight born before their mothers started to smoke cigarettes. Am J Obstet Gynecol 112:277–284, 1972.)

relations are possible: (1) necessary and sufficient, (2) necessary but not sufficient, (3) sufficient but not necessary, and (4) neither sufficient nor necessary.

Necessary and Sufficient

In the first type of causal relation, a factor is both necessary and sufficient for producing the disease. Without that factor, the disease never develops (the factor is necessary), and in the presence of that factor, the disease always develops (the factor is sufficient) (Fig. 13–13). This situation rarely if ever occurs. For example, in most infectious diseases, a number of people are exposed, some of whom will manifest the disease and others who will not. Members of households of a person with tuberculosis do not uniformly acquire the disease from the index case. If the exposure dose is assumed to be the same, there are likely differences in immune status, genetic susceptibility, or other characteristics that determine who develops the disease and who does not. A one-to-one relationship of exposure to disease, which is a consequence of a necessary and sufficient relationship, rarely if ever occurs.

Necessary but Not Sufficient

Another model consists of each factor being necessary, but not in itself sufficient to cause the disease (Fig. 13–14). Thus, multiple factors are required, often in a specific temporal sequence. For example, carcinogenesis is considered to be a multi-stage process involving both initiation and promotion. For cancer to result, a promoter must act after an initiator has acted. Action of an initiator or a promoter alone will not produce a cancer.

Again, in tuberculosis, the tubercle bacillus is clearly a necessary factor, even though its presence may not be sufficient to produce the disease in every infected individual.

Sufficient but Not Necessary

In this model, the factor can produce the disease, but so can other factors that are acting alone (Fig.

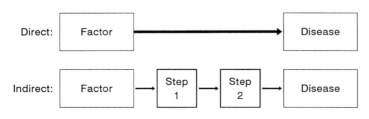

Figure 13–12. Direct vs. indirect causes of disease.

A Factor Is a Necessary and Sufficient Cause:

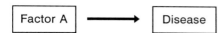

Figure 13–13. Types of causal relationships: I.

13–15). Thus, radiation exposure or benzene exposure can each produce leukemia without the presence of the other. Even in this situation, not everyone who has experienced radiation or benzene exposure has development of cancer, so although both factors are not needed, other co-factors probably are. Thus the criterion of *sufficient* is rarely met by a single factor.

Neither Sufficient Nor Necessary

In the fourth model, a factor by itself is neither sufficient nor necessary (Fig 13–16). This is a more complex model, which probably most accurately represents the causal relationships that operate in most chronic diseases.

EVIDENCE FOR A CAUSAL RELATION

Many years ago, when the major disease problems faced by man were infectious in origin, the question arose as to what evidence would be necessary to prove that an organism causes a disease. In 1840, Henle proposed postulates for causation that were expanded by Koch in the 1880s.[5] The postulates for causation were as follows:

1. The organism is *always* found with the disease.
2. The organism is *not* found with any other disease.
3. The organism, isolated from one who has the disease, and cultured through several genera-

Each Factor Is Sufficient But Not Necessary:

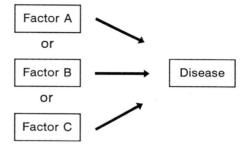

Figure 13–15. Types of causal relationships: III.

tions, produces the disease (in experimental animals).

Koch added that "Even when an infectious disease cannot be transmitted to animals, the 'regular' and 'exclusive' presence of the organism (postulates 1 and 2) proves a causal relationship."[5]

These postulates, though not perfect, proved very useful for infectious diseases. However, as apparently non-infectious diseases assumed increasing importance toward the middle of the 20th century, the issue arose as to what would represent strong evidence of causation in diseases that were generally not of infectious origin. In such disease there was no organism that could be cultured and grown in animals. Specifically, as attention was directed to a possible relationship between smoking and lung cancer, the U.S. Surgeon General appointed an expert committee to review the evidence. The committee developed a set of guidelines,* which have been revised over the years. A modified list

---

*United States Department of Health, Education and Welfare. Smoking and Health: Report of the Advisory Committee to the Surgeon General, Washington, DC, Public Health Service, 1964.

Each Factor Is a Necessary But Not a Sufficient Cause:

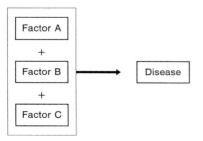

Figure 13–14. Types of causal relationships: II.

Each Factor Is Neither Necessary Nor Sufficient:

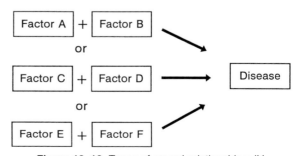

Figure 13–16. Types of causal relationships: IV.

of these guidelines is presented in the following text, with some brief comments.

GUIDELINES FOR JUDGING WHETHER AN ASSOCIATION IS CAUSAL

1. TEMPORAL RELATIONSHIP

It is clear that if a factor is believed to be the cause of a disease, exposure to the factor must have occurred before the disease developed. Figure 13–17 shows the number of deaths per day and the mean concentration of airborne particles in London in early December 1952 (Schwartz, 1994). The pattern of a rise in particle concentration followed by a rise in mortality and a subsequent decline in particle concentration followed by a decline in mortality strongly supported the increase in mortality being due to the increase in air pollution. This example demonstrates the use of ecologic data for exploring a temporal relationship. Further investigation revealed that the increased mortality consisted almost entirely of respiratory and cardiovascular deaths and was highest in the elderly.

It is often easier to establish a temporal relation in a concurrent cohort study than in a case-control study or retrospective cohort study. In the last two types of studies, exposure information may need to be obtained or recreated from past records and the timing may therefore be imprecise.

Not only is the temporal relationship of exposure

and disease important for clarifying the order in which the two occur, but it is also important regarding the length of the interval between exposure and disease. For example, asbestos has been clearly linked to increased risk of lung cancer, but the latent period between the exposure and the appearance of lung cancer is at least 15 to 20 years. Therefore, if lung cancer develops, for example, after a period of only 3 years since the asbestos exposure, it is safe to conclude that the lung cancer was not a result of this exposure.

2. STRENGTH OF THE ASSOCIATION

This is measured by the relative risk (or odds ratio). The stronger the association the more likely it is that the relation is causal.

3. DOSE-RESPONSE RELATIONSHIP

As the dose of exposure increases, the risk of disease also increases. Figure 13–18 shows an example of dose-response for cigarette smoking and lung cancer. If a dose-response relationship is present, it is strong evidence for a causal relationship. However, the absence of a dose-response relationship does not necessarily rule out a causal relationship. In some cases in which a threshold may exist, no disease may develop up to a certain level of exposure (a threshold); above this level, disease may develop.

4. REPLICATION OF THE FINDINGS

If the relationship is causal, we would expect to see it consistently in different studies and in different populations. Replication of findings is particularly important in epidemiology. If an association is observed we would also expect it to be seen consistently within subgroups of the population, unless there is a clear reason to expect different results.

5. BIOLOGIC PLAUSIBILITY

This refers to coherence with the current body of biologic knowledge. Examples may be cited to demonstrate that epidemiologic observations have sometimes preceded biologic knowledge. Thus, as discussed in an earlier chapter, Gregg's observations on rubella and congenital cataracts preceded any knowledge of teratogenic viruses. Similarly, the implication of high oxygen concentration in the causation of retrolental fibroplasia, a form of blindness in premature infants, preceded any biologic knowledge to support such a relationship. Nevertheless, we seek consistency of the epidemiologic findings with existing biologic knowledge, and when this is not the case, interpreting the meaning

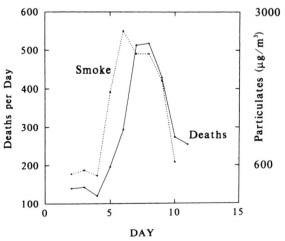

Figure 13–17. The mean concentration of airborne particles (μg/m³) from the four inner monitoring stations in London, and the count of daily deaths in the London Administrative County during the beginning of December 1952. (From Schwartz J: Air pollution and daily mortality: A review and meta analysis. Environ Res 64:36–52, 1994.)

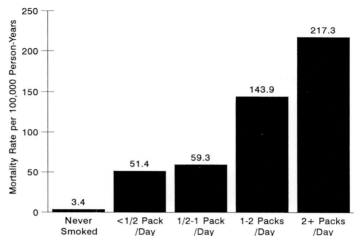

Figure 13–18. Age-standardized death rates due to well-established cases of bronchogenic carcinoma (exclusive of adenocarcinoma) by current amount of smoking. (Adapted from Hammond EC, Horn D: Smoking and death rates: Report on 44 months of follow-up of 187, 783 men: II. Death rates by cause. JAMA 166:1294–1308, 1958.

of the association may be difficult. We may then be more demanding in our requirements about the size and the significance of any differences observed and in having the study replicated by other investigators in other populations.

6. CONSIDERATION OF ALTERNATE EXPLANATIONS

We have discussed the problem in interpreting an observed association in regard to whether a relationship is causal or is the result of confounding. In judging whether a reported association is causal, the extent to which the investigators have taken other possible explanations into account and the extent to which they have ruled out such explanations are important considerations.

7. CESSATION OF EXPOSURE

If a factor is a cause of a disease, we would expect the risk of the disease to decline on reduction or elimination of exposure to the factor. Figure 13–19 shows such data for cigarette smoking and lung cancer.

Eosinophilia myalgia syndrome (EMS), referred to earlier, reached epidemic proportions in 1989. Characterized by severe muscle pain and a high blood eosinophil count, the syndrome was found to be associated with manufactured preparations of L-tryptophan. In November 1989 a nationwide recall by the Food and Drug Administration of over-the-counter preparations of L-tryptophan was followed by dramatic reductions in numbers of cases of EMS reported each month (Fig. 13–20). This is another example of a reduction in incidence being related to cessation of exposure, which adds to the strength of the causal inference regarding the exposure.

When cessation data are available, they provide helpful supporting evidence for a causal association.

However, in certain cases, the pathogenic process may have been irreversibly initiated and the disease occurrence may have been determined by the time the exposure is removed. Emphysema is not reversed with cessation of smoking, but its progression is reduced.

8. SPECIFICITY OF THE ASSOCIATION

This indicates that a specific exposure is associated with only one disease; it is the weakest of all the guidelines and should probably be deleted from the list. Cigarette manufacturers have pointed out that the diseases attributed to cigarette smoking do not meet the requirements of this guideline, as cigarette smoking has been linked to lung cancer, pancreatic cancer, bladder cancer, heart disease, emphysema, and other conditions.

The possibility of such multiple effects from a single factor is not, in fact, surprising: regardless of the tissue that comprises them, all cells have common characteristics, including DNA, RNA, and various subcellular structures, so a single agent could have effects in multiple tissues. Furthermore, cigarettes are not a single factor but constitute a mixture of a large number of compounds; consequently, a large number of effects might be anticipated.

When specificity of an association is found, it provides additional support for a causal inference. However, as with a dose-response relationship, absence of specificity in no way negates a causal relationship.

9. CONSISTENCY WITH OTHER KNOWLEDGE

If a relationship is causal, we would expect the findings to be consistent with other data. For example, Figure 13–21 shows data regarding lung cancer

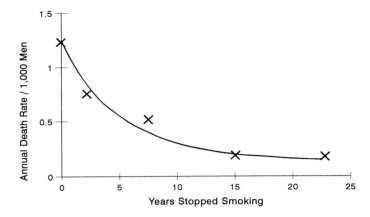

Figure 13–19. Effects of terminating exposure: lung cancer death rates, standardized for age and amount smoked, among men continuing to smoke cigarettes and men who have given up smoking for different time periods. The corresponding rate for non-smokers was 0.07 per 1,000. (Adapted from Doll R, Hill AB: Mortality in relation to smoking: Ten years' observations of British doctors. Br Med J 1:1399–1410, 1964.)

rates in men and women and cigarette smoking in men and women.

We see a consistent direction in the curves, with the increase in lung cancer rates following the increase in cigarette sales in both men and women. These data are consistent with what we would expect if the relationship between smoking and lung cancer is established as a causal one. Although the absence of such consistency would not completely rule out this hypothesis, if we observed rising lung cancer rates following a period of declining cigarette sales, for example, we would have to explain how this observation was consistent with a causal hypothesis.

Although the preceding guidelines do not permit a quantitative estimation of whether or not an association is causal, they can nevertheless be very helpful, as seen in the following example: Peptic

ulcer disease has long been attributed to the effects of gastric acid. Susceptibility to gastric acid has been linked to cigarette smoking, alcohol consumption, and use of non-steroidal anti-inflammatory agents. Therapy has been primarily directed at inhibiting acid secretion and protecting mucosal surfaces from acid.

Beginning in 1982, studies appeared that linked infection with *Helicobacter pylori*—a gram-negative, curved, motile, rod-shaped bacterium—to chronic active gastritis. Additional evidence has now linked this organism to peptic ulcer disease. Table 13–2 categorizes this evidence along the lines of several of the guidelines for causation just discussed.

Thus, as seen here, the guidelines can be extremely helpful regarding the status of the evidence supporting a causal relationship. Although the data

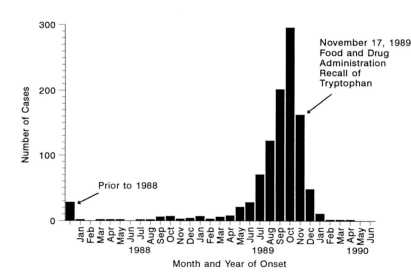

Figure 13–20. Reported dates of illness onset by month and year for cases of eosinophilia-myalgia syndrome, as reported to the Centers for Disease Control and Prevention, Atlanta, as of July 10, 1990. (Adapted from Swygert LA, Maes EF, Sewell LE, et al: Eosinophilia-myalgia syndrome: Results of national surveillance. JAMA 264:1698–1703, 1990.)

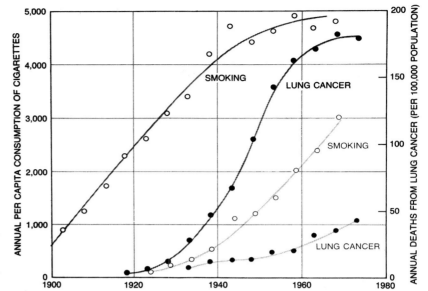

Figure 13–21. Parallel trends between cigarette consumption and lung cancer in men (steeper curves) and in women in England and Wales. (From Cairns J: The cancer problem. Sci Am 235:64–72, 77–78, 1975.)

Table 13–2. Assessment of the Evidence Suggesting *Helicobacter pylori* as a Causative Agent of Duodenal Ulcers

1. Temporal relationship.
   - *H. pylori* is clearly linked to chronic gastritis. About 11% of chronic gastritis patients will go on to develop duodenal ulcers over a 10-year period.
   - In one study of 454 patients who underwent endoscopy 10 years earlier, 34 of 321 patients who had been positive for *H. pylori* (11%) developed duodenal ulcer compared with 1 of 133 *H. pylori*–negative patients (0.8%).
2. Strength of the relationship.
   - *H. pylori* is found in at least 90% of patients with duodenal ulcer. In at least one population reported to lack duodenal ulcers, a northern Australian aboriginal tribe that is isolated from other people, it has never been found.
3. Dose-response relationship.
   - Density of *H. pylori* per square millimeter of gastric mucosa is higher in patients with duodenal ulcer than in patients without duodenal ulcer. Also see item 2 above.
4. Replication of the findings.
   - Many of the observations regarding *H. pylori* have been replicated repeatedly.
5. Biologic plausibility.
   - Although originally it was difficult to envision a bacterium that infects the stomach antrum causing ulcers in the duodenum, it is now recognized that *H. pylori* has binding sites on antral cells and can follow these cells into the duodenum.
   - *H. pylori* also induces mediators of inflammation.
   - *H. pylori*–infected mucosa is weakened and is susceptible to the damaging effects of acid.
6. Consideration of alternate explanations.
   - Data suggest that smoking can increase the risk of duodenal ulcer in *H. pylori*–infected patients but is not a risk factor in patients in whom *H. pylori* has been eradicated.
7. Cessation of exposure.
   - Eradication of *H. pylori* heals duodenal ulcers at the same rate as histamine receptor antagonists.
   - Long-term ulcer recurrence rates were zero after *H. pylori* was eradicated using triple antimicrobial therapy, compared with a 60% to 80% relapse rate often found in patients with duodenal ulcers treated with histamine receptor antagonists.
8. Specificity of the association.
   - Prevalence of *H. pylori* in patients with duodenal ulcers is 90% to 100%. However, it is found in some patients with gastric ulcer and even in asymptomatic individuals.
9. Consistency with other knowledge.
   - Prevalence of *H. pylori* infection is the same in men as in women. The incidence of duodenal ulcer, which in earlier years was believed to be higher in men than in women, has been equal in recent years.
   - Prevalence of ulcer disease is believed to have peaked in latter part of the 19th century, and prevalence of *H. pylori* may have been much higher at that time because of poor living conditions. This reasoning is also based on observations today that *H. pylori* prevalence is much higher in developing countries.

Data from Megraud F, Lamouliatte H: *Helicobacter pylori* and duodenal ulcer: Evidence suggesting causation. Dig Dis Sci 37:769–772, 1992; and DeCross AJ, Marshall BJ: The role of *Helicobacter pylori* in acid-peptic disease. Am J Med Sci 306:381–391, 1993.

Table 13–3. The Process for Using the Evidence in Developing Recommendations on the Effectiveness of Prenatal Interventions

Stage I: Categorizing the Evidence by the Quality of its Source. (In Each Category, studies are listed in Descending Order of Quality.)

1. Trials (planned interventions with contemporaneous assignment of treatment and nontreatment)
   a. Randomized, double-blind, placebo-controlled with sufficient power appropriately analyzed.
   b. Randomized, but blindness not achieved.
   c. Non-randomized trials with good control of confounding, that are well conducted in other respects.
   d. Randomized, but with deficiencies in execution or analysis (insufficient power, major losses to follow-up, suspect randomization, analysis with exclusions).
   e. Non-randomized trials with deficiencies in execution or analysis.
2. Cohort or case-control studies
   a. Hypothesis specified prior to analysis, good data, confounders accounted for.
   b. As above, but hypothesis not specified prior to analysis.
   c. Post hoc, with problem(s) in the data or the analysis.
3. Time-series studies
   a. Analyses that take confounding into account
   b. Analyses that do not consider confounding
4. Case-series studies: Series of case reports without any specific comparison group

Among other issues that must be considered in reviewing the evidence are the precision of definition of the outcome being measured, the degree to which the study methodology has been described, adequacy of the sample size, and the degree to which the characteristics of the population studied and of the intervention being evaluated have been described.

A study can be well designed and carried out in an exemplary fashion (internal validity), but if the population studied is an unusual or highly selected one, the results may not be generalizable (external validity).

Stage II: Guidelines for Evaluating the Evidence of a Causal Relationship. (In Each Category, Studies are Listed in Descending Priority Order.)

1. Major criteria
   a. Temporal relationship: An intervention can be considered evidence of a reduction in risk of disease or abnormality only if the intervention was applied prior to the time the disease or abnormality would have developed.
   b. Biological plausibility: A biologically plausible mechanism should be able to explain why such a relationship would be expected to occur.
   c. Consistency: Single studies are rarely definitive. Study findings that are replicated in different populations and by different investigators carry more weight than those that are not. If the findings of studies are inconsistent, the inconsistency must be explained.
   d. Alternative explanations (confounding): The extent to which alternative explanations have been explored is an important criterion in judging causality.
2. Other considerations
   a. Dose-response relationship: If a factor is indeed the cause of a disease, usually (but not invariably) the greater the exposure to the factor, the greater the risk of the disease. Such a dose-response relationship may not always be seen because many important biologic relationships are dichotomous, and reach a threshold level for observed effects.
   b. Strength of the association: The strength of the association is usually measured by the extent to which the relative risk or odds depart from unity, either above 1 (in the case of disease-causing exposures) or below 1 (in the case of preventive interventions).
   c. Cessation effects: If an intervention has a beneficial effect, then the benefit should cease when it is removed from a population (unless a carryover effect is operant).

Adapted from Gordis L, Kleinman JC, Klerman LV, et al: Criteria for evaluating evidence regarding the effectiveness of prenatal interventions. *In* Merkatz IR, Thompson JE (eds): New Perspectives on Prenatal Care. New York, Elsevier, 1990, pp 31–38.

regarding *H. pylori* and duodenal ulcer are still limited, the available evidence is strongly suggestive of a causal relationship.

A Recent Modification of the Guidelines

In 1986, the U.S. Public Health Service brought together a group of 19 experts to examine the scientific basis of the content of prenatal care and to answer the question: Which measures implemented during prenatal care have actually been demonstrated to be associated with improved outcome? The panel's report was issued in 1989 and served as the basis of a comprehensive report.[7] As the panel began its deliberations, it became clear that questions of causation were at the heart of the panel's task, and that guidelines were needed for assessing the relationship of prenatal measures to health outcomes. A subcommittee reviewed the current guidelines (just enumerated in the preceding text) and defined a process for using evidence that includes (1) categorization of the evidence by the quality of its sources, and (2) evaluation of evidence of a causal relationship using standardized guidelines.[8] These recommendations are excerpted in Table 13–3.

Although the modified guidelines clearly use the original components, they establish reasonable priorities in weighting them. They thus define an approach for looking at causation that may have applicability far beyond questions of the effectiveness of prenatal measures.

CONCLUSION

Although causal guidelines are often referred to as *criteria*, this term does not seem entirely appropriate. Although it may be a desirable goal to place causal inferences on a firm quantitative and structural foundation, at present we generally do not have the information needed for doing so. The preceding list should therefore be considered to be only guidelines which can be of most value when coupled with reasoned judgment in making decisions about causation.

In the next chapter, we address several additional issues that need to be considered in deriving causal inferences from epidemiologic studies.

References

1. DeBakey M, Ochsner A: Primary pulmonary malignancy. Surg Gynecol Obstet 68:562, 1939.
2. Prentice RL, Kakar F, Hursting S, et al: Aspects of the rationale for the Women's Health Trial. J Natl Cancer Inst 80:802–814, 1988.
3. Austin DF, Karp S, Dworsky R, Henderson BE: Excess leukemia in cohorts of children born following influenza epidemics. Am J Epidemiol 101:77–83, 1977.
4. Yerushalmy J: Infants with low birth weight born before their mothers started to smoke cigarettes. Am J Obstet Gynecol 112:227–284, 1972.
5. Evans AS: Causation and Disease: A Chronological Journal. New York, Plenum, 1993, pp 13–39.
6. Schwartz J: Air pollution and daily mortality: A review and meta analysis. Environ Res 64:36–52, 1994.
7. Merkatz IR, Thompson JE (eds): New Perspectives on Prenatal Care. New York, Elsevier, 1990.
8. Gordis L, Kleinman JC, Klerman LV, et al: Criteria for evaluating evidence regarding the effectiveness of prenatal interventions. *In* Merkatz IR, Thompson JE (eds): New Perspectives on Prenatal Care. New York, Elsevier, 1990, pp 31–38.

Review Questions

1. In a large case-control study of pancreatic cancer cases, 17% of the patients were found to be diabetic at the time of diagnosis, compared to 4% of a well-matched control group (matched by age, sex, ethnic group, and several other characteristics) that was examined for diabetes at the same time as the cases were diagnosed.

   It was concluded that the diabetes played a causal role in the pancreatic cancer. This conclusion:
   a. Is correct
   b. May be incorrect because there is no control or comparison group
   c. May be incorrect because of failure to establish the time sequence between onset of the diabetes and pancreatic cancer
   d. May be incorrect because of less complete ascertainment of diabetes in the pancreatic cancer cases
   e. May be incorrect because of more complete ascertainment of pancreatic cancer in nondiabetic persons

2. An investigator examined cases of fetal death in 27,000 pregnancies and classified mothers according to whether they had experienced sexual intercourse within 1 month before delivery. It was found that 11% of the mothers of fetuses that died and 2.5% of the mothers of fetuses that survived had had sexual intercourse during the period.

   It was concluded that intercourse during the month preceding delivery caused the fetal deaths. This conclusion:
   a. May be incorrect because mothers who had intercourse during the month before childbirth may differ in other important characteristics from those who did not
   b. May be incorrect because there is no comparison group
   c. May be incorrect because prevalence rates are used where incidence rates are needed
   d. May be incorrect because of failure to achieve a high level of statistical significance
   e. Both *b* and *c*

3. All of the following are important criteria when making causal inferences *except*:
   a. Consistency with existing knowledge
   b. Dose-response
   c. Consistency of association in several studies
   d. Strength of association
   e. Predictive value

4. Ecologic fallacy refers to:
   a. Assessing exposure in large groups rather than in many small groups

b. Assessing outcome in large groups rather than in many small groups

c. Ascribing the characteristics of a group to every individual in that group

d. Examining correlations of exposure and outcomes rather than time trends

e. Failure to examine temporal relations between exposures and outcomes

Questions 5 and 6 are based on the following:

Factor A, B, or C can each individually cause a certain disease without the other two factors, but only when followed by exposure to factor X. Exposure to factor X alone is not followed by the disease, but the disease never occurs in the absence of exposure to factor X.

5. Factor X is:

a. A necessary and sufficient cause

b. A necessary but not sufficient cause

c. A sufficient but not necessary cause

d. Neither necessary nor sufficient

e. None of the above

6. Factor A is:

a. A necessary and sufficient cause

b. A necessary but not sufficient cause

c. A sufficient but not necessary cause

d. Neither necessary nor sufficient

e. None of the above

CHAPTER 14

More on Causal Inferences: Bias, Confounding, and Interaction

In this chapter, we continue the discussion of causation that was begun in Chapter 13. Our discussion here focuses on three important issues in deriving causal inferences: bias, confounding, and interaction.

BIAS

Bias has been addressed in many of the previous chapters because it is a major issue in virtually any type of epidemiologic study design. Therefore, only a few additional comments are made here.

What do we mean by bias? Bias has been defined as "any systematic error in the design, conduct or analysis of a study that results in a mistaken estimate of an exposure's effect on the risk of disease."[1]

What types of bias do we encounter in epidemiologic studies? The first is *selection bias*. If the way in which cases and controls, or exposed and non-exposed individuals, were selected is such that an apparent association is observed—even if, in reality, exposure and disease are not associated—the apparent association is the result of selection bias.

If a population is monitored over a period of time, disease ascertainment may be better in the monitored population than in the general population, and may introduce a *surveillance bias*, which leads to an erroneous estimate of the relative risk or odds ratio. For example, some years ago a great deal of interest centered on the possible relationship of oral contraceptive use and thrombophlebitis. It was suggested that physicians monitored patients given oral contraceptives much more closely than they monitored their other patients. As a result, they were more apt to identify cases of thrombophlebitis among those patients who were taking oral contraceptives (and who were therefore being more closely monitored) than among other patients who were not as well monitored. As a result, just through better ascertainment of thrombophlebitis in women receiving oral contraceptives, an apparent association of thrombophlebitis with oral contraceptive use may be observed, even if no true association exists.

Given the inaccuracies in methods of data acquisition, we may at times misclassify subjects and thereby introduce a *misclassification bias*. For example, in a case-control study, some people who have the disease (cases) may be misclassified as controls, and some without the disease (controls) may be misclassified as cases. This may result, for example, from limited sensitivity and specificity of the diagnostic tests involved or from inadequacy of information derived from medical or other records. Another possibility is that we may misclassify a person's exposure status: we may believe the person was exposed when this was not, in fact, the case, or we may believe that the person was not exposed when, in fact, exposure did occur. If exposure data are based on interview, for example, a subject may either not be aware of exposure or may erroneously think that it did not occur. If ascertainment of exposure is based on old records, data may be incomplete or inaccurate.

Misclassification may occur in two forms: differential and non-differential. In *differential misclassification*, the rate of misclassification differs in different study groups. For example, misclassification of exposure may occur such that cases are misclassified as being exposed more often than controls are. This was seen in the example of recall bias in the discussion of case-control studies (Chapter 9). Women who had had a baby with a malformation tended to remember more mild infections during their pregnancies than did mothers of normal infants. Thus, there was a tendency for differential misclassification in regard to prenatal infection, in that more unexposed cases were misclassified as exposed than were unexposed controls. The result was an apparent association of malformations with infections, even though none existed. So a differential misclassification bias can lead either to an apparent association even if one does not really exist or to an apparent lack of association when one does exist.

In contrast, *non-differential misclassification* results from the degree of inaccuracy that characterizes how information is obtained from any study group—either cases and controls or exposed and non-exposed persons. Such misclassification is not related to exposure status or to case or control status; it is just a problem inherent in the *data collection methods*. The usual effect of non-differential misclassification is that the relative risk or odds ratio tends to be diluted, and it is shifted toward 1.0. In other words, we are less likely to detect an association even if it really exists.

This can be seen intuitively: Let us say that in reality there is a strong association of an exposure and a disease—that is, people without the disease have much less exposure than do people with the disease. By mistake, we have included some diseased persons in our control group and some non-diseased persons in our case group. We have, in other words, misclassified some of the subjects in regard to diagnosis. In this situation, our controls will not have such a low rate of exposure (because some diseased people have been mistakenly included in this group) and our cases will not have such a high rate of exposure (because some non-diseased people have been mistakenly included in the case group). As a result, a smaller difference in exposure will be found between our cases and our controls than actually exists between diseased and non-diseased people.

Information Bias

Some of the sources of information bias in epidemiologic studies are shown in Table 14–1.

Bias may be introduced in the way information is abstracted from medical, employment or other records or from the manner in which interviewers ask questions. Bias may also result from *surrogate interviews*. What does this mean? Suppose we are carrying out a case-control study of pancreatic can-

Table 14–1. Some Types and Sources of Information Bias

Bias in abstracting records
Recall bias
Interviewer bias
Bias from surrogate interviews
Non-response bias

cer. The case-fatality from this disease is very high and the survival is very short. When we prepare to interview cases, we find that many of them have died and that those who have survived are too ill to be interviewed. We may then approach a family member to obtain information about the case's employment history, other exposures, diet, and other characteristics. The person interviewed is most often a spouse or a child. Several problems arise in obtaining information from such surrogates. First, they may not have accurate information about the case's history. A spouse may not know the work-related exposures of the case. Children often know even less than do spouses. Second, there is evidence that when a wife reports on her husband's work and lifestyle after he dies, she tends to elevate his occupational level and lifestyle: She may ascribe to him a higher occupation category than that in which he was actually engaged. She may also convert him posthumously to a non-drinker and/or non-smoker.

Another type of information bias is that resulting from non-response. Persons who do not respond in a study are generally not a representative group of study subjects. Because no information is obtained from them, this non-response may introduce a serious bias. It is therefore important to keep non-response to a minimum. In addition, any non-respondents should be characterized as much as possible, using whatever information is available, to determine ways in which they differ from respondents and to gauge the likely impact of their non-response on the findings of the study.

Wynder and co-workers[2] coined the term *wish bias* to denote the bias introduced by subjects who have developed a disease and who, in attempting to answer the question, "Why me?", seek to show that the disease is not their fault. Thus, they may deny certain exposures related to lifestyle (such as smoking or drinking); if they are contemplating litigation, they may overemphasize workplace-related exposures.

A point to remember is that *bias is a result of an error in the design and conduct of a study*. Efforts

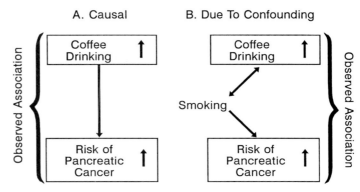

Figure 14–1. The association between coffee drinking and pancreatic cancer.

should therefore be made to reduce or eliminate bias or, at the very least, to recognize it and take it into account when interpreting the findings of a study.

CONFOUNDING

A problem posed in many epidemiologic studies is that we observe a true association and are tempted to derive a causal inference when, in fact, the relationship may not be causal. This brings us to the subject of *confounding*, one of the most important problems in observational epidemiologic studies.

What do we mean by *confounding*? In a study of whether factor A is a cause of disease B, we say that a third factor, factor X is a confounder if the following are true:

1. Factor X is a known risk factor for disease B.
2. Factor X is associated with factor A but is not a result of factor A.

Recall the example we discussed in Chapter 9 of the relationship between coffee and cancer of the pancreas. Smoking was a confounder, because although we were interested in a possible relationship between coffee consumption (factor A) and pancreatic cancer (disease B), the following are true of smoking (factor X):

1. It is a known risk factor for pancreatic cancer.
2. It is associated with coffee drinking but is not a result of coffee drinking.

So if an association is observed between coffee drinking and cancer of the pancreas, it may be (1) that coffee actually causes cancer of the pancreas, or (2) that coffee drinking and cancer of the pancreas may be a result of confounding by cigarette smoking (i.e., we observe the association of coffee

drinking and pancreatic cancer because cigarette smoking is a risk factor for pancreatic cancer and cigarette smoking is associated with coffee drinking) (Fig. 14–1).

When we observe an association we ask whether it is causal (see Fig. 14–1, *left*) or whether it is a result of confounding by a third factor that is both a risk factor for the disease and is associated with the exposure in question (see Fig. 14–1, *right*).

Let us look at a hypothetical example: Table 14–2 shows data from an unmatched case-control study of an exposure and a disease, in which 100 cases and 100 controls were studied.

We calculate an unmatched odds ratio that equals 1.95. The question arises, Is this association of the exposure with the disease a causal one, or could it have resulted from differences in age distributions? (Is the observed relationship confounded by age?) The first question to ask in addressing this issue is whether age is related to being a case or a control. This is answered by the analysis in Table 14–3.

We see that 80% of the controls are younger than 40 years compared with only 50% of the cases. Thus, older age is associated with being a case (having the disease) and younger age with being a control (not having the disease).

Table 14–2. Hypothetical Example of Confounding in an Unmatched Case-Control Study: I. Numbers of Exposed and Not Exposed Cases and Controls

Exposed	Cases	Controls
Yes	30	18
No	70	82
Total	100	100

$$\text{Odds ratio} = \frac{30 \times 82}{70 \times 18} = 1.95$$

Table 14–3. Hypothetical Example of Confounding in an Unmatched Case-Control Study: II. Distribution of Cases and Controls by Age

Age (yr)	Cases	Controls
<40	50	80
≥40	50	20
Total	100	100

Table 14–5. Hypothetical Example of Confounding in an Unmatched Case-Control Study: IV. Calculations of Odds Ratios After Stratifying by Age

Age (yr)	Exposed	Cases	Controls	Odds Ratio
<40	Yes	5	8	$\dfrac{5 \times 72}{45 \times 8} = \dfrac{360}{360} = 1.0$
	No	45	72	
	Total	50	80	
≥40	Yes	25	10	$\dfrac{25 \times 10}{25 \times 10} = \dfrac{250}{250} = 1.0$
	No	25	10	
	Total	50	20	

The next question is whether age is related to whether or not a person has been exposed.

Table 14–4 looks at the relationship of age to exposure for all 200 subjects studied, regardless of their case-control status. We see that 130 people were younger than 40 years (the 50 + 80 in the top row of Table 14-3), and of these, 13 (10%) were exposed. Among the 70 subjects who were older than 40 years, 35 (50%) were exposed. Thus, age is clearly related to exposure. So at this point we know that age is related to being a case (the cases were older than the controls); we also know that being exposed is related to older age.

As shown in Figure 14–2, the question is, Is the association of exposure and disease causal (see Fig. 14–2, *left*), or could we be seeing an association of exposure with disease only because there is an age difference between cases and controls, and age is also related to being exposed (see Fig. 14–2, *right*)? Does exposure cause the disease (i.e., whether a person is a case or a control), or is the observation a result of confounding by a third factor (in this case, age)?

How can we clarify this issue? One approach is seen in Table 14–5. We can carry out a stratified analysis with subjects in two age groups: younger than 40 years and older than 40 years. Within each stratum a 2 × 2 table is created, and an odds ratio is calculated for each. When we calculate the odds ratio separately for the younger and the older subjects, we find the odds ratio to be 1.0 in each stratum. Thus, the only reason we originally had an

odds ratio of 1.95 in Table 14–3 was because there was a difference in age distributions between the cases and the controls. Thus, in this example age is a confounder.

How can we address the problem of confounding? As seen in Table 14–6, the issue of confounding can be addressed either in designing and carrying out a study or in analysis of the data. In *designing and carrying out a study,* we can match the cases to the controls as discussed in Chapter 9 (by either group matching or individual matching for the factor we suspect could be a possible confounder). In this example we could match by age to eliminate any age difference between the cases and the controls. If we then observed an association of exposure and disease, we would know that we could not attribute the association to an age difference.

Alternatively, we can handle the problem of confounding in the *data analysis* in two ways: stratification or adjustment. Let us briefly discuss stratification, which was just demonstrated in the hypothetical example. Let us say we are interested in the relationship of smoking and lung cancer. We want to know whether the observed higher risks of lung cancer in smokers could be a result of confounding by air pollution and/or urbanization.

Table 14–4. Hypothetical Example of Confounding in an Unmatched Case-Control Study: III. Relationship of Exposure to Age

Age (yr)	Total	Exposed	Not Exposed	% Exposed
<40	130	13	117	10
≥40	70	35	35	50

Table 14–6. Approaches to Handling Confounding

In designing and carrying out the study:
1. Individual matching
2. Group matching

In the analysis of data:
1. Stratification
2. Adjustment

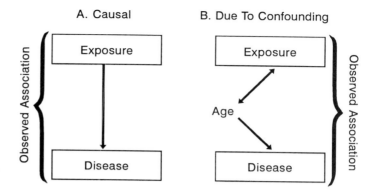

Figure 14-2. Schematic presentation of the issue of potential confounding.

Perhaps we are observing a relationship of smoking and lung cancer not because smoking causes lung cancer, but because air pollution causes lung cancer and smoking is more frequent in polluted areas (i.e., in urban areas). Perhaps smokers just happen to live in the cities.

How can we address this question? One approach would be to stratify the data by degree of urbanization—rural, town, or major city. We then calculate the lung cancer rates in smokers and non-smokers in each urbanization stratum (Table 14-7).

If the relationship of lung cancer to smoking is due to smoking, and not to the confounding effect of pollution and/or urbanization, then *in each stratum of urbanization* the incidence of lung cancer should be higher in smokers than in non-smokers. It would then be clear that the observed association of smoking and lung cancer could not be due to degree of urbanization.

We may prefer not just to dichotomize smoking groups into smokers and non-smokers, but to include in the analysis the number of cigarettes smoked.

In Table 14-8, we have expanded cigarette smoking into categories of amount smoked. Again, we can calculate the incidence in each cell of the table.

If the observed association of cigarette smoking and lung cancer is not due to confounding by urbanization and/or pollution, we would expect to see a dose-response pattern *in each stratum of urbanization.*

Figure 14-3 shows actual age-adjusted lung cancer mortality rates per 100,000 man-years by urban-rural classification and smoking category. For each degree of urbanization, lung cancer mortality rates in smokers are shown by gray bars, and non-smoker mortality rates are indicated by black bars. From these data we see that in every level (or stratum) of urbanization, lung cancer mortality is higher in smokers than in non-smokers. Therefore, the observed association of smoking and lung cancer cannot be attributed to level of urbanization. By examining each stratum separately, we are, in effect, holding urbanization constant, and we still find much higher lung cancer mortality in smokers than in non-smokers.

At the same time, it is interesting to examine the data for non-smokers (shown by the black bars). If we draw a line connecting the tops of the black

Table 14-7. An Example of Stratification: Lung Cancer Rates by Smoking Status and Degree of Urbanization

Degree of Urbanization	Cancer Rates	
	Non-smokers	*Smokers*
None		
Slight		
Town		
City		
Total		

Table 14-8. An Example of Further Stratification: Lung Cancer Rates by Smoking Level and Degree of Urbanization

Degree of Urbanization	Cancer Rates			
		Smokers		
	Non-smokers	*½ Pack/Day*	*1 Pack/Day*	*≥2 Packs/Day*
None				
Slight				
Town				
City				
Total				

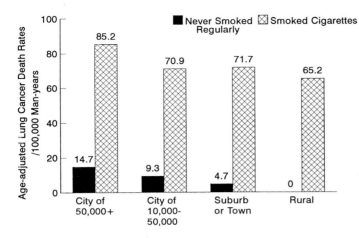

Figure 14–3. Age-adjusted lung cancer death rates per 100,000 man-years by urban-rural classification and by smoking category. (Adapted from Hammond EC, Horn D: Smoking and death rates: report on 44 months of follow-up of 187,783 men: II. Death rates by cause. JAMA 166:1294–1308, 1958.)

bars, we see that the higher the urbanization level the higher the incidence of lung cancer in non-smokers. Thus, there is a dose-response relationship of lung cancer and urbanization in non-smokers. However, as we have seen, this relationship cannot explain the association of lung cancer with smoking as the latter relationship holds within each level of urbanization.

Figure 14–4 shows the relationship among smoking, drinking, and cancer of the esophagus. Four strata (levels) of amount smoked are shown. Within each smoking stratum, the risk of esophageal cancer is plotted in relation to the amount of alcohol consumed.

What do we observe? The more a person smokes,

the higher the levels of esophageal cancer. However, within each stratum of smoking, there is a dose-response relationship of esophageal cancer and the amount of alcohol consumed. Therefore, we cannot attribute to smoking the effects of alcohol consumption on esophageal cancer. Both smoking and alcohol have separate effects on the risk of esophageal cancer.

It is interesting to note that in this presentation of data, we cannot compare smokers to non-smokers or drinkers to non-drinkers because the authors have pooled the group that smokes 0 to 9 g of tobacco per day, and they have also pooled non-drinkers with minimal drinkers. Thus we have no rates for persons who are *non-exposed* to alcohol or

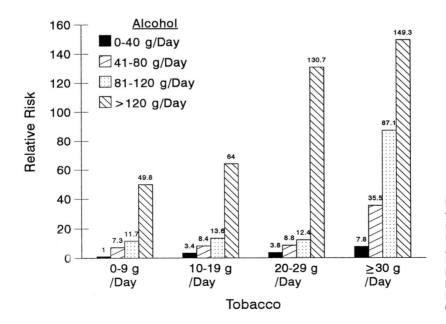

Figure 14–4. Relative risk of developing cancer of the esophagus in relation to smoking and drinking habits. (Adapted from Tuyns AJ, Pequignot G, Jensen OM: Esophageal cancer in Ile-et-Vilaine in relation to levels of alcohol and tobacco consumption: Risks are multiplying. Bull Cancer 64:45–60, 1977.)

tobacco. It would have been preferable to have kept the data for non-exposed persons separate, so that relative risks could have been calculated based on rates in non-exposed persons.

Two final points on confounding: First, when we identify a confounder, we generally consider it a problem and want to find ways to address the issue of confounding. But sometimes finding a confounder can be very useful. We can screen a population for either a risk factor or an etiologic factor for a disease, which enables us to carry out *primary prevention*, or we can screen for confounding factors, which can identify persons at high risk for a disease, factors that do not themselves cause the disease. If we find such a *marker exposure* it can enable us to carry out *secondary prevention*. Thus, even a confounded relationship may be helpful in screening populations even when we do not identify the specific etiologic agent involved.

Second, confounding is not an error in the study, but is rather a true phenomenon that is identified in a study and must be understood. Although bias is a result of an error in the way the study has been carried out, confounding is a valid finding that describes the nature of the relationship among several factors and the risk of disease.

INTERACTION

To this point, the discussion has generally assumed the presence of a single causal factor in the etiology of a disease. Although this approach is useful for discussion purposes, in real life we rarely deal with single causes. In the previous examples of the relationship of lung cancer to smoking and urbanization and the relation of esophageal cancer to drinking and smoking, we have already seen more than one factor involved in disease etiology. In this section, we ask the question: How do multiple factors interact in causing a disease?

What do we mean by *interaction*? MacMahon[3] defined interaction as follows: "When the incidence rate of disease in the presence of two or more risk factors differs from the incidence rate expected to result from their individual effects." The effect can be greater than what we would expect (positive interaction, synergism) or less than what we would expect (negative interaction, antagonism). The problem is to determine what we would *expect* to result from the individual effects of the exposures.

Figure 14–5 shows an algorithm for exploring the possibility of interaction.

In examining our data, the first question is whether an association has been observed between an exposure and a disease. If so, is it due to confounding? If we decide that it is *not* due to confounding—that is, it is causal—then we ask whether the association is equally strong in each of the strata that are formed on the basis of some third variable. For example, is the association of smoking and lung cancer equally strong in strata formed on the basis of degree of urbanization? If the association is equally strong in all strata, there is no interaction. But if the association is of different strengths in different strata formed on the basis of age, for example (if the association is stronger in older people than in younger people), an interaction has been observed between age and exposure in producing the disease. If there were no interaction, we would

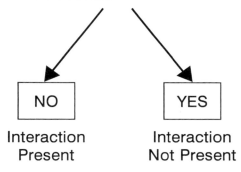

1. Is there an association?

2. If so, is it due to confounding?

3. Is the association equally strong in strata formed on the basis of a third variable?

NO — Interaction Present

YES — Interaction Not Present

Figure 14–5. Questions to ask regarding possible interaction.

Table 14–9. Incidence Rates for Groups Exposed to Neither Risk Factor or to One or Two Risk Factors (Hypothetical Data)

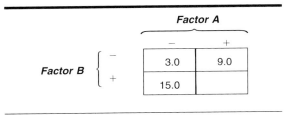

		Factor A	
		−	+
Factor B	−	3.0	9.0
	+	15.0	

expect the association to be of the same strength in each stratum.

Let us look more closely at interaction. Table 14–9 shows the incidence in persons exposed to either one of two risk factors (A and B), to both factors, or to neither factor, in a hypothetical example.

In persons with neither exposure, the incidence is 3.0. In persons exposed to factor A only and not to factor B, the incidence is 9.0. In persons exposed to factor B only and not to factor A, the incidence is 15.0. These are the individual effects of each factor considered separately.

What would we expect the incidence to be in persons who are exposed to both factors A and B (the lower righthand cell in the table) if those people experienced the risk resulting from the independent contributions of both factors? The answer depends on the type of model that we propose. Let us assume that when there are two exposures, the effect of one exposure is *added* to the effect of the second exposure—that is, the model is *additive*. What, then, would we expect to see in the lower righthand cell of the table? Let us use as an example the people who have neither exposure, whose risk in the absence of both exposures is 3.0. How does

exposure to factor A affect their risk? It adds 6.0 to the 3.0 to produce a risk of 9.0. If factor A adds a risk of 6.0 to the risk that exists without factor A, it should have the same effect both in people exposed to factor B and in those not exposed to factor B. Because factor A adds 6.0 to the 3.0, it would also be expected to add 6.0 to the 15.0 rate of people exposed to factor B when they have exposure to A added as well. Thus, we would expect the effects of exposures to both factors to yield an incidence of 21.0.

We can also view this as follows: If factor B adds 12.0 to the 3.0 incidence of people with neither exposure, we would expect it to add 12.0 to any group, including that exposed only to factor A, whose incidence is 9.0. Therefore, the effect of exposure to both A and B would be expected to equal 9.0 added to 12.0, or 21.0. (Remember that the 3.0 is a background risk present in the absence of both A and B. When we calculate the combined effect of factors A and B, we cannot just add 9.0 and 15.0—we must be sure that we do not count the background risk [3.0] twice.) The left side of Table 14–10 shows the completed table from the partial data presented in Table 14–9.

Recall that when we discuss differences in risks, we are talking about *attributable risks*. This is shown on the right side of the table. If we examine persons who have neither exposure, they have a background risk, but the attributable risk—that is the risk attributable to exposure to factor A or B—is 0. As stated earlier, exposure only to factor A adds 6, and exposure only to factor B adds 12. What will the attributable risk be for both exposures? The answer is 18—that is, 18 more than the background risk. The additive model is summarized in Table 14–11.

What if an additive model does not describe correctly the effect of exposure to two independent

Table 14–10. Incidence Rates and Attributable Risks for Groups Exposed to Neither Risk Factor or to One or Two Risk Factors (Hypothetical Data in an Additive Model: I)

		Incidence Rates			Attributable Risks	
		Factor A			Factor A	
		−	+	−	−	+
Factor B	−	3.0	9.0		0	6
	+	15.0	21.0	+	12	

Table 14–11. Incidence Rates and Attributable Risks for Groups Exposed to Neither Risk Factor or to One or Two Risk Factors (Hypothetical Data in an Additive Model: II)

		Incidence Rates		Attributable Risks	
		Factor A		**Factor A**	
		−	+	−	+
Factor B	−	3.0	9.0	0	6
	+	15.0	21.0	12	18

factors? Perhaps a second exposure does not *add* to the effect of the first exposure but instead *multiplies* the effect of the first exposure. If having a certain exposure doubles a person's risk, we might expect it to double that risk regardless of whether or not that person had another exposure. For example, if the effect of alcohol is to double a person's risk for a certain cancer, we might expect it to double that risk for both smokers and non-smokers. The appropriate model for the effects of two independent factors might therefore be a *multiplicative* rather than an additive model.

Let us return to our original data on risk resulting from neither exposure, or from exposure to factor A or B. These data are shown again in Table 14–12.

We see that exposure to factor A triples the risk, compared with that seen when factor A is absent (9.0 compared with 3.0). What would we therefore expect to find in the lower righthand cell of the table when both exposures are present? Since in the absence of factor B, factor A has tripled the risk of 3.0, we would also expect it to triple the risk of 15.0 observed when exposure to factor B is present. If so, the effect from exposure to both factors would

be 45.0. Again, we can calculate this in a different fashion. Factor B multiplies the risk by 5 (15.0 compared to 3.0) when factor A is absent. We would therefore expect it to have the same effect when factor A is present. Because the risk when factor A is present is 9.0, we would expect the presence of factor B to yield a risk of 45.0 (9.0 multiplied by 5) (Table 14–13).

The left side of Table 14–13 shows the completed table. Our discussion of a multiplicative model is, in effect, of a *relative risk model*. This is shown on the right side of the figure. What value would we expect to find in the blank cell?

If we now assign the background risk (3.0) a value of 1, against which to compare the other values in the table, exposure to factor A triples the risk, yielding a relative risk of 3 for factor A in the absence of factor B; factor B multiplies the risk by 5, yielding a relative risk of 5 for exposure to factor B in the absence of factor A. When both factors A and B are operating, we would expect to see a relative risk of 15 (45/3, as shown in the lefthand table) (Table 14–14).

We have considered two models: additive and multiplicative. The question remains, what would we expect to see as a result of the independent effects of two risk factors? Do we expect an additive model or a multiplicative model?

The answer is not obvious. If two factors are operating and the incidence is 21.0, the result is consistent with an additive model. If the incidence is 45.0, the result is consistent with a multiplicative model. If the incidence resulting from two factors is 60.0, for example, even the value for a multiplicative model is clearly exceeded, and an interaction is present—that is, an effect greater than would be expected from the independent effects of the two separate factors.

If, however, the incidence is 30.0, it is less than

Table 14–12. Incidence Rates for Groups Exposed to Neither Risk Factor or to One or Two Risk Factors (Hypothetical Data)

		Factor A	
		−	+
Factor B	−	3.0	9.0
	+	15.0	

Table 14–13. Incidence Rates and Relative Risks for Groups Exposed to Neither Risk Factor or to One or Two Risk Factors (Hypothetical Data in a Multiplicative Model: I)

		Incidence Rates			Relative Risks	
		Factor A			Factor A	
		−	+		−	+
Factor B	−	3.0	9.0	−	1	3
	+	15.0	45.0	+	5	

expected from a multiplicative model and more than expected from an additive model. The question again is, Is this more than we would expect from the independent effects of the two factors? It is difficult to know the answer without more information about the biology of the disease, the mechanisms involved in the pathogenesis of the disease, and how such factors operate at cellular and molecular levels. Most experts accept any effect greater than additive as evidence of positive interaction which is also called *synergism*. However, this opinion is often based on statistical considerations, whereas the validity of the model should ideally be based on biologic knowledge. The model may differ from one disease to another and from one exposure to another.

Let us consider a few examples. In a cohort study of smoking and lung cancer, Hammond and colleagues (1979) studied the risk of lung cancer in 17,800 asbestos workers in the United States and in 73,763 men not exposed to asbestos in relation to their smoking habits. Table 14–15 shows the findings for deaths from lung cancer in relation to exposure. If the relation between smoking and asbestos exposure were an additive one, we would

expect the risk in those exposed to both smoking and asbestos (in the lower right cell) to be 58.4 + 122.6 − 11.3, or 169.7. (The 11.3 background risk is subtracted in order to avoid counting it twice.) Clearly the observed value of 601.6 is much greater than the expected additive value. In fact, the data in this table closely approximate a multiplicative model and strongly suggest a synergism between asbestos exposure and smoking.

A second example is seen in Table 14–16, which shows the relative risk of oral cancer by presence or absence of two exposures: smoking and alcohol consumption. The risk is set at 1.0 for persons with neither exposure. Is there evidence of an interaction? What would we expect the risk to be if the effect was multiplicative? We would expect 1.53 × 1.23, or 1.88. Clearly the observed effect of 5.71 is higher than a multiplicative effect and indicates the presence of interaction.

Let us look at more detailed data for these relationships using dose data for alcohol consumption and for smoking (Table 14–17).

Again, the risk in those who do not drink and do not smoke is set at 1.0. In those with the highest level of alcohol consumption and the highest level

Table 14–14. Incidence Rates and Relative Risks for Groups Exposed to Neither Risk Factor or to One or Two Risk Factors (Hypothetical Data in a Multiplicative Model: II)

		Incidence Rates			Relative Risks	
		Factor A			Factor A	
		−	+		−	+
Factor B	−	3.0	9.0	−	1	3
	+	15.0	45.0	+	5	15

Table 14–15. Deaths From Lung Cancer (per 100,000) Among Individuals With and Without Exposure to Cigarette Smoking and Asbestos

Cigarette Smoking	Asbestos Exposure	
	No	*Yes*
No	11.3	58.4
Yes	122.6	601.6

Adapted from Hammond EC, Selikoff IJ, Seidman H: Asbestos exposure, cigarette smoking and death rates. Ann NY Acad Sci 330:473–490, 1979.

Table 14–17. Relative Risks* of Oral Cancer According to Level of Exposure to Alcohol and Smoking

Alcohol Consumption (oz/Day)	Cigarette Equivalents per Day			
	0	*<20*	*20–39*	*≥40*
0	1.00	1.52	1.43	2.43
<0.4	1.40	1.67	3.18	3.25
0.4–1.5	1.60	4.36	4.46	8.21
>1.5	2.33	4.13	9.59	15.50

*Risks are expressed relative to a risk of 1.00 for persons who neither smoked nor drank.

From Rothman K, Keller A: The effect of joint exposure to alcohol and tobacco on risk of cancer of the mouth and pharynx. J Chron Dis 25:711–716, 1972.

of smoking, the risk is 15.50. Is an interaction evident? The data appear to support this. The highest values in smokers who are non-drinkers and in drinkers who are non-smokers, are 2.43 and 2.33, respectively; the value of 15.5 clearly exceeds the resulting product of 5.66 that would be expected with a multiplicative effect.

However, a problem with these data should be mentioned. Note that each category of smoking or of drinking has upper and lower boundaries except for the highest categories, which have no upper boundaries. So the high risk of 15.5 could result from the presence of one or a few extreme outliers—either extraordinarily heavy smokers or extraordinarily heavy drinkers.

Is there a way to avoid this problem and still use the data shown here? We could ignore the righthand column and the bottom row and look only at the resulting 3 × 3 table. Now all the categories have

both upper and lower limits. If the model was multiplicative we would expect to see 1.43 × 1.60, or 2.29, rather than the 4.46 actually observed. Thus, we still see evidence of interaction, but much weaker evidence than we had seen in the full table with its indefinite high exposure categories. This suggests that the problem of the lack of upper limits of categories was indeed a contributor to the high value of 15.5 seen in the 4 × 4 table.

As we have said, the decision as to whether an additive model or a multiplicative model is most relevant in a given situation should depend on the biology of the disease. Table 14–18 shows interesting data regarding the risks of cancer from radiation and smoking in two different populations: uranium workers (left) and survivors of the atomic bomb (right). Each table shows high and low levels of smoking and high and low levels of radiation.

What kind of model is suggested by the table on the left? Clearly, a multiplicative relationship is

Table 14–16. Relative Risks* of Oral Cancer According to Presence or Absence of Two Exposures: Smoking and Alcohol Consumption

		Smoking	
		No	Yes
Alcohol	No	1.00	1.53
	Yes	1.23	5.71

*Risks are expressed relative to a risk of 1.00 for persons who neither smoked nor drank alcohol.

From Rothman K, Keller A: The effect of joint exposure to alcohol and tobacco on risk of cancer of the mouth and pharynx. J Chron Dis 25:711–716, 1972.

Table 14–18. Relative Risks of Cancer According to Smoking and Radiation Exposure in Two Populations

	Uranium Workers (Smoking Level)		A-Bomb Survivors (Smoking Level)	
	Low	*High*	*Low*	*High*
Radiation level				
Low	1.0	7.7	1.0	9.7
High	18.2	146.8	6.2	14.2

From Blot WJ, Akiba S, Kato H: Ionizing radiation and lung cancer: A review including preliminary results from a case-control study among A-bomb survivors. *In* Prentice RL, Thompson DJ (eds): Philadelphia, Atomic Bomb Survivor Data: Utilization and Analysis. Society for Industrial and Applied Mathematics, 1984, pp 235–248.

suggested; 146.8 is close to the product of 7.7 $\times$ 18.2. The table on the right suggests an additive model; 14.2 is close to the sum of 9.7 + 6.2 − 1.0. So although the data address radiation and smoking in two populations, in one setting the exposures relate in an additive way and in the other they relate in a multiplicative way. It is not known if this is a result of differences in radiation exposure in uranium mines compared with that from atomic bombs. Such a hypothesis is not unreasonable; we know that there was even a difference in the radiation emitted by the atomic bombs at Hiroshima and Nagasaki, and that the dose-response curves for cancer were different in the two cities. In any case, the fact that two exposures that are ostensibly the same (or at least similar) may have different interrelationships in different settings is an intriguing observation that requires further exploration.

Finally, a dramatic example of interaction is seen in the relationship of aflatoxin and chronic hepatitis B infection to the risk of liver cancer (Table 14–19). In this study, hepatitis B infection alone multiplied the risk of liver cancer by 7.3; aflatoxin exposure alone multiplied the risk by 3.4. However, when both exposures were present the relative risk rose to 59.4, far in excess of what we might expect in an additive model. Such an observation of synergy is not only of major clinical and public health interest, but also suggests important directions for further laboratory research into the etiology and pathogenesis of liver cancer.

CONCLUSION

This chapter has reviewed the concepts of bias, confounding, and interaction in relation to the derivation of causal inferences. Biases reflect inadequa-

Table 14–19. Relative Risks* of Liver Cancer for Persons Exposed to Aflatoxin and/or Chronic Hepatitis B Infection: An Example of Interaction

	Aflatoxin Negative	Aflatoxin Positive
HBsAg† negative	1.0	3.4
HBsAg positive	7.3	59.4

*Adjusted for cigarette smoking.
†Abbreviation: HbsAg, hepatitis B surface antigen.
Adapted from Qian GS, Ross RK, Yu MC, et al: A follow-up study of urinary markers of aflatoxin exposure and liver cancer risk in Shanghai, People's Republic of China, Cancer Epidemiology. Biomarkers & Prevention, 3:3–10, 1994.

cies in the design and/or conduct of a study and clearly affect the validity of the findings. Biases therefore need to be assessed and, if possible, eliminated. Confounding and interaction, on the other hand, describe the reality of the interrelationships between certain factors and a certain outcome. Confounding and interaction characterize virtually every situation in which etiology is addressed, because most causal questions involve the relationships of multiple exposures and multiple, possibly etiologic, factors. Such relationships are particularly important in investigating the roles of genetic and environmental factors in disease causation. This subject is discussed in Chapter 15.

References

1. Schlesselman JJ: Case-Control Studies: Design, Conduct, and Analysis. Oxford University Press, New York, 1982.
2. Wynder EL, Higgins IT, Harris RE: The wish bias. J Clin Epidemiol 43:619–621, 1991.
3. MacMahon B: Concepts of multiple factors. *In* Lee DH, Kotin P (eds): Multiple Factors in the Causation of Environmentally Induced Disease. New York, Academic Press, 1972.

Review Questions

1. Which of the following is(are) an approach(es) to handling confounding:
   a. Individual matching
   b. Stratification
   c. Group matching
   d. Adjustment
   e. All of the above

2. It has been suggested that physicians may examine women who use oral contraceptives more often or more thoroughly than women who do not. If so, and if an association is observed between phlebitis and oral contraceptive use, the association may be due to:
   a. Selection bias
   b. Interviewer bias
   c. Surveillance bias
   d. Non-response bias
   e. Recall bias

Questions 3 through 6 are based on the information given below:

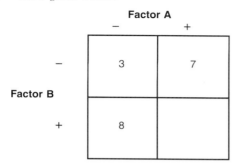

3. Fill in the blank cell above using the additive model of interaction: _____

4. Fill in the blank cell above using the multiplicative model of interaction: _____

Convert the numbers in the above table to attributable risks for the additive model and relative risks for the multiplicative model:

Additive Model

| | Factor A | |
	−	+
Factor B −	0	
+		

Multiplicative Model

| | Factor A | |
	−	+
Factor B −	1	
+		

5. Fill in the bottom right cell for the attributable risk of having both factors A and B (additive model): _____

6. Fill in the bottom right cell for the relative risk of having both factors A and B (multiplicative model): _____

Question 7 is based on the information given below:

A study reported on 50 cases admitted for thyroid cancer and 100 "controls" admitted during the same period for treatment of hernias. Only the cases were interviewed, and 20 of the cases were found to have been exposed to x-ray therapy in the past, based on the interviews and medical records. The controls were not interviewed, but a review of their hospital records when they were admitted for hernia surgery revealed that only 2 controls had been exposed to x-ray therapy in the past.

7. Based on the description given above, what source of bias is *least likely* to be present in this study?
   a. Recall bias
   b. Bias due to controls being nonrepresentative of the non-diseased population
   c. Bias due to use of different methods of ascertainment of exposure in the cases and controls
   d. Bias due to loss of subjects from the control group over time
   e. Selection bias for exposure to x-ray therapy in the past

CHAPTER 15

Identifying the Roles of Genetic and Environmental Factors in Disease Causation

In previous chapters, we have primarily discussed the etiologic role of environmental factors, but to prevent disease, we must look at the interplay of genetic susceptibility and exposure to environmental factors. Human beings clearly differ from one another in physical characteristics, personality, and other factors. They also differ in genetically determined susceptibility to disease. When we investigate the etiology of a disease, we are explicitly or implicitly asking the question: How much of the incidence of the disease is due to genetic factors and how much is due to environmental factors?

Clearly, disease does not necessarily develop in everyone exposed to an environmental risk factor. Even if the relative risk for a specific factor and a disease is very high, the notion of attributable risk conveys the message that not all occurrence of a disease is due only to the specific exposure in question. For example, the relationship of cigarette smoking and lung cancer has been clearly demonstrated. However, lung cancer does not develop in everyone who smokes, and it does develop in some non-smokers. Either another environmental co-factor is needed in addition to cigarette smoking or individuals differ in genetic susceptibility.

People often adopt a fatalistic approach if a disease is primarily genetic in origin. But even in diseases that are primarily of genetic origin, a tremendous amount of environmental interaction often occurs. For example, phenylketonuria is characterized by a genetically determined deficiency of phenylalanine hydroxylase; the affected child cannot metabolize the essential amino acid phenylalanine, and the result of the phenylalanine accumulation is irreversible mental retardation. Can we prevent the genetic abnormality? No, we cannot. Can we reduce the likelihood that a child afflicted with this genetic abnormality will manifest mental

retardation? Yes, we can do so by reducing or eliminating the child's exposure to phenylalanine by providing a diet that is low in phenylalanine. In this example, the adverse effects of a genetic disease can be prevented by controlling the affected person's environment so that the manifestations are not expressed. Thus, from standpoints of both clinical and public health, it is important to keep in mind the interrelationships between genetic and environmental factors in disease causation and expression.

Another example is Down syndrome, in which a trisomy of chromosome 21 occurs in one of two forms: either a non-disjunction occurs—that is, the chromosomes fail to separate during cell division, or a translocation of chromosome 21 is passed on together with a normal chromosome 21 from a balanced carrier. Non-disjunction is more common in older women. Thus non-disjunction Down syndrome is more common in babies born to women who are older than 35 years at the time of pregnancy. Why is there a greater likelihood of non-disjunction in babies of women who are in their late 30s than in those of women who are in their late 20s? Something must happen to cause the increased risk—possibly an accumulation of environmental insults or some other manifestation of biologic aging. To say that Down syndrome is genetic does not account for the age-related change in risk, which may well reflect the interrelation of genetic and environmental factors.

The interaction of genetic and environmental factors was succinctly described many years ago by Lancelot Hogben, who wrote:

> . . . our genes cannot make bricks without straw. The individual differences which men and women display are partly due to the fact that they receive

different genes from their parents and partly due to the fact that the same genes live in different houses.[1]

In this chapter, we discuss some of the approaches used by epidemiologists to distinguish the relative contributions of genetic and environmental factors to disease causation. The discussion covers the use of classical epidemiologic methods and also introduces some of the newer approaches that have been made possible by advances in laboratory genetics and molecular biology.

ASSOCIATION WITH KNOWN GENETIC DISEASES

If we are interested in whether a certain disease has a strong genetic component, one question we can ask is whether the disease is associated with other diseases or conditions that are known to have strong genetic components. For example, children with Down syndrome are known to be at high risk for leukemia. Breast cancer is known to have a high incidence in males with Klinefelter syndrome (XXY syndrome). If we identify such an association between the condition of interest and a disease that has a known genetic etiology, it does not prove that the disease is genetically determined, but it does indicate that at least some components of the causation of the disease or some cases of this disease are likely to be due to genetic factors.

A related approach when a disease occurs in both hereditary and nonhereditary forms is to try and identify genes responsible for the hereditary form in the hope that such identification will provide a clue to the role of genetic factors in nonhereditary cases. A gene that may be responsible for most hereditary breast cancer cases has been designated *BRCA1* (*BR*east *CA*ncer *1*). With the isolation of the candidate gene in 1994 by Miki and co-workers in Skolnick's laboratory, the prospects for improved understanding of the role of genetic factors in sporadic (nonhereditary) cases of breast cancer were greatly enhanced.[2] In 1995, Struewing et al. in Brody's laboratory reported that a specific mutation in the *BRCA1* gene previously detected in high-risk families was present in almost 1% of samples from Ashkenazi Jews.[3] The authors estimated that this mutation may account for 16% of breast cancer in Ashkenazi Jewish women compared to only 4.1% of breast cancer in the non-Ashkenazi population. This finding raised many major ethical and policy issues relating to possible genetic testing.

In 1995 Savitsky and associates, working with others on a team led by Shiloh, discovered the defective gene that causes the serious and rare autosomal recessive disorder, ataxia telangiectasia (AT).[4] The gene called ATM (for AT, mutated) may also be the most important cause of hereditary breast cancer. This possibility is based on epidemiologic evidence from studies of relatives of AT patients that suggest that the risk of breast cancer is increased five-fold in female carriers of the AT gene. Identification of the ATM gene permits study of its role in cases of hereditary breast cancer that have not been linked to other breast cancer genes such as *BRCA1*. Although AT is a rare disease, about 0.5% to 1.4% of the population carry one defective gene, so that the gene could account for up to 8% of all breast cancers.[5]

USE OF GENETIC MARKERS

Genetic markers are genes or gene products that can be evaluated by laboratory methods. Transmission of markers from parent to offspring is observable, and the chromosomal location of genetic markers is often known. A number of types of genetic markers can now be tested in the laboratory as the direct result of revolutionary advances in molecular biology (Table 15–1).

How are associations between diseases and particular genetic markers determined? For example, cancer of the pancreas has been reported to be associated with blood group A. How would we design a study to determine whether cancer of the pancreas is in fact associated with blood group A? We could determine the blood group distribution in a group of patients with cancer of the pancreas (cases), but how do we obtain an "expected rate" of the prevalence of blood group A in the general population from which these cases were drawn? This is again the difficult problem of control selection, as was discussed earlier. Investigators have

Table 15–1. Types and Examples of Genetic Markers Used in Studies of Associations of an Allele and a Disease

A. Analysis of gene products or their phenotypic expression
  1. Blood groups
  2. Human leukocyte antigens (HLA)
  3. Protein polymorphisms
B. Analysis of DNA polymorphisms
  1. Allelic variants of genes
  2. Restriction fragment length polymorphisms (RLFPs)
  3. Variable tandem repeats (VTRs)

Adapted from Khoury MJ, Beaty TH, Cohen BH: Fundamentals of Genetic Epidemiology. New York, Oxford University Press, 1993.

used blood donors at blood banks for comparison, but even 20 years ago there were major selection biases in groups who donated blood and those who did not—the group of persons who donated blood were not representative of the general population. Today, with human immunodeficiency virus (HIV) and acquired immunodeficiency syndrome (AIDS) presenting such a major problem, there is even a greater selection bias in those who donate blood, so that it is even more difficult to interpret the results using such a group for study. However, the problem of selection in using donors for studies of blood groups may not be as relevant for studies of serum proteins or DNA polymorphisms. Another approach for studying the possible association of a certain blood group with cancer of the pancreas is to conduct a case-control study of pancreatic cancer, in which blood group is one of the "exposures" studied. In such a study, the problem of selecting appropriate controls is an important one. When presented with a list of associations with blood groups, we should ask, How were the conclusions regarding such associations arrived at and what comparison groups were used for generating the expected rates?

Considerable interest has also focused on HLA (human leukocyte antigen) types, which are genetically determined. Certain diseases have been shown to be associated with certain HLA antigens, as shown in Table 15–2.

For example, ankylosing spondylitis has a strong association with HLA type B27. Interest in such associations is strong, both because such an association may cast light on the pathogenetic mechanisms involved and because the possibility arises of using HLA as a marker to identify population subsets at increased risk. Furthermore, if ankylosing spondylitis is associated with a certain HLA antigen that is known to be genetically determined, is it because ankylosing spondylitis itself is also genetically determined?

AGE AT ONSET

Epidemiologic observations can be useful in elucidating or confirming biologic mechanisms. An example is age at onset of a disease. Consider retinoblastoma, a tumor of the eye in children. This tumor occurs in two forms: unilateral and bilateral.

Table 15–2. HLA Disease Associations

Disease and HLA Type	Race	Patients (% Positive)	Controls (%)	Odds Ratio*
Ankylosing spondylitis				
B27	White	89	9	69.1
B27	Asian	85	15	207.9
B27	Black	58	4	54.4
Idiopathic hemochromatosis				
A3	White	72	28	6.7
B7	White	48	26	2.9
B14	White	19	6	2.7
Insulin-dependent diabetes mellitus				
B8	White	40	21	2.5
B15	White	22	14	2.1
DR3	White	52	22	3.8
DR4	White	74	24	9.0
DR2	White	4	29	0.1
Rheumatoid arthritis				
DR4	White	68	25	3.8
Celiac disease				
B8	White	68	22	7.6
DR3	White	79	22	11.6
DR7	White	60	15	7.7
Multiple sclerosis				
B7	White	37	24	1.8
DR2	White	51	27	2.7
Narcolepsy				
DR2	White	100	22	129.8
DR2	Asian	100	34	358.1

*Odds ratio values are combined estimates from a number of studies and cannot be directly calculated from the table.
Data from Tiwari JL, Terasaki PI: HLA and Disease Associations. New York, Springer-Verlag, 1985; and from Thomson G, Robinson WP, Kuhner MK, et al: Genetic heterogeneity, modes of inheritance and risk estimates from a joint study of Caucasians with insulin dependent diabetes mellitus. Am J Hum Genet 43:799–816, 1988 (as cited in Thomson G: HLA disease associations: Models for insulin-dependent diabetes mellitus and the study of complex human genetic disorders. Ann Rev Genet 22:31–50, 1988).

The unilateral form (about 60% of cases) generally has a low rate of heritability with little familial pattern, whereas the bilateral form (40%) has a strong familial predisposition and is often transmitted from parents to children.

Children who survive retinoblastoma have an increased risk of developing a second primary tumor at another site, usually osteogenic sarcoma (a tumor of bone). In a large series of patients who survived hereditary retinoblastoma, over 50% developed a second primary tumor during the subsequent 30 years, and most of these tumors were osteogenic sarcomas. Though it was initially suggested that these tumors might be a result of the radiation therapy that had been given, it was subsequently shown that these tumors may occur at sites distant from the field of radiation, which suggests an underlying susceptibility to the development of osteogenic sarcoma. Moreover, some families of retinoblastoma patients include relatives who have osteogenic sarcoma and who have never had retinoblastoma. These observations suggest the presence of a genetically determined pattern of tumor susceptibility that is specific for the type of tumor. Clearly, such issues become very important considerations when we design studies to investigate the etiology of such conditions.

When the ages at onset of familial and nonfamilial tumors are examined, we see that nonfamilial tumors are distributed throughout childhood, with most in early childhood, whereas almost all familial tumors tend to occur in very early childhood only (Fig. 15–1).

This is commonly observed in other diseases: When a disease occurs in both genetic and nongenetic forms, the genetic form develops in patients at much earlier ages than does the nongenetic form.

This observation seems reasonable, for a disease that is not primarily genetic in origin requires an accumulation of environmental insults or exposures that can only build up over time. Consequently, it takes longer for such diseases to develop than for those which are primarily genetic in origin.

Retinoblastoma has been studied extensively. In 1971, Knudson reviewed the clinical and epidemiologic information regarding retinoblastoma—specifically the age distribution of the tumor—and on the basis of a statistical study proposed what has become known as the "two-hit" hypothesis for the development of retinoblastoma[6] (Fig. 15–2).

According to this model, two mutations in the same cell of the retina are required for the development of cancer. In the genetically determined form of retinoblastoma, a child is born with one mutation in the germ cells. Therefore, only one more (somatic) mutation is needed for cancer to develop. In the non-familial form, however, a child is not born with any germ cell mutation. Consequently, for a retinoblastoma to develop, two mutations in a somatic retinal cell are needed. Because these are very rare events, cases of genetically determined retinoblastomas occur at earlier ages than do nongenetic cases. Thus, the epidemiologic observations regarding age at onset can be linked to current hypotheses of biologic mechanisms in the development of cancer.

Retinoblastoma has been shown to be associated with a deletion from a single band on the long arm of chromosome 13 (13q14). Cavenee and co-workers (1983) suggested that homozygosity for a mutant allele in this band is probably needed for development of retinoblastoma; this would in effect constitute a loss of the normal tumor suppressor activity at this locus.[7] A gene responsible for the

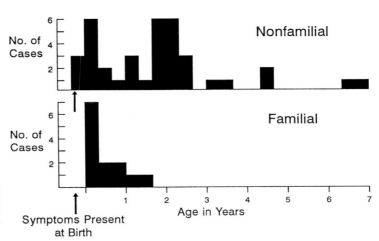

Figure 15–1. Retinoblastoma: age at onset of symptoms. (From Aherne GE, Roberts DF: Retinoblastoma: A clinical survey and its genetic implications. Clin Genet 8:275–290, 1975.)

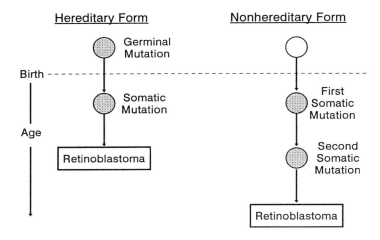

Figure 15–2. Two-hit model for the development of retinoblastoma. (Adapted from Knudson AG Jr: The genetics of childhood cancer. Cancer 35 (suppl 3):1022–1026, 1975.)

development of both retinoblastoma and osteogenic sarcoma was identified and isolated in 1988.[8]

Another example of different age distributions in genetic and nongenetic forms of a disease is shown in Figure 15–3, which indicates the cumulative age distributions for patients with basal or squamous cell skin cancer in the U.S. population and in 94 persons with basal cell cancer who also have a genetically determined condition—xeroderma pigmentosum—in which a defect in DNA repair predisposes them to cancer. The age at onset is clearly earlier in patients with the genetically determined

form of the disease. Childs and Scriver analyzed the age at onset of many genetic and nongenetic diseases and also found a pattern of earlier age at onset of genetic diseases.[9] Presumably, genetically susceptible persons develop their disease relatively rapidly; hence the early age at onset. An accumulation of environmental insults over time is required for development of the remaining diseases.

FAMILY STUDIES

When a disease aggregates in families, what does it tell us about the relative contributions of genetic

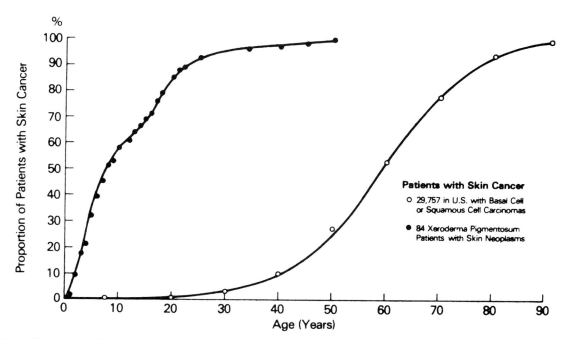

Figure 15–3. Cumulative age distribution of patients with skin cancer. (From Kraemer KH, Lee MN, Scotto J: Early onset of skin and oral cavity neoplasms in xeroderma pigmentosum [letter]. Lancet 1:55, 1982.)

and environmental factors to its causation? Such aggregation could be a result of genetic determination. But could familial aggregation be observed if the disease were environmentally determined? Yes, because certain environmental exposures are also shared by families. Let us examine the methods used to study familial aggregation and the approaches used to interpret the data from such studies.

Risk of the Disease in First-Degree Relatives

When a person with a certain disease is identified, it is valuable to examine his or her first-degree relatives for evidence of a greater-than-expected prevalence of disease. Such an excess in first-degree relatives would suggest, though not prove, a genetic component. It is also possible to examine family pedigrees such as the one shown in Figure 15–4, which shows a family with retinoblastoma in four successive generations. Such pedigrees not only give a visual picture of the familial impact of the disease, but can also be used to estimate the genetic component in the causation of the disease. This pedigree also demonstrates that the disease or susceptibility to it is transmitted by individuals who are not affected themselves because of other factors that may influence expression.

When a person has a disease and there is spousal concordance—that is, husbands and wives of persons with the disease tend also to have the disease—environmental factors are implicated, as spouses are generally not genetically linked (except in unusual inbred populations).

Applying Molecular Biologic Methods to Family Studies

If familial aggregation of disease is observed, the techniques of epidemiology can be coupled with those of molecular biology to determine whether there is a major identifiable gene transmitted from parent to child that is associated with an increased risk of disease. The techniques involve exploring the observed familial aggregation by using segregation analyses and linkage analyses.

Segregation analyses test whether the observed pattern of a disease in families is compatible with a mendelian model of inheritance (e.g., autosomal dominant inheritance). This is done by statistically testing competing models.[10]

Linkage analyses seek to determine whether alleles from two loci segregate together in a family and are passed as a unit from parent to child. Genes that are physically near each other on the same chromosome tend to be transmitted together. Linkage can only be identified through family studies. However, even when linkage is demonstrated, it does not necessarily imply a causal relationship.

The ultimate purpose is to identify and isolate the gene associated with susceptibility to the disease in order to enhance our understanding of disease pathogenesis and to facilitate the development of appropriate preventive strategies. The search for disease-susceptibility genes uses two approaches:

1. Search for an *association* between an allele and a disease using the methods for studying the genetic markers listed in Table 15–1:
   a. Analysis of gene products or their phenotypic expression
   b. Analysis of DNA polymorphisms
   These two steps should be viewed in the context of the progression from genotype to phenotype shown schematically in Figure 15–5. Often, DNA probes may be used even before the specific gene products underlying the disease are known.
2. Use of family studies to identify a *linkage* or co-

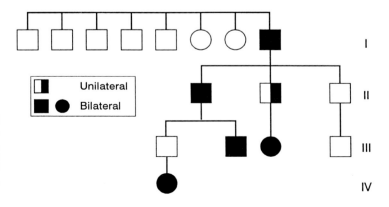

Figure 15–4. Pedigree of family reported with retinoblastoma occurring in four successive generations. *Symbols:* squares, males; circles, females. (From Migdal C: Retinoblastoma occurring in four successive generations. Br J Ophthalmol 60:151–152, 1976.)

Unilateral
Bilateral

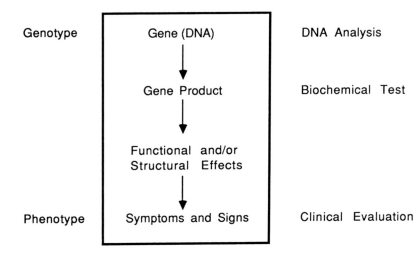

Genotype

Phenotype

DNA Analysis

Biochemical Test

Clinical Evaluation

Figure 15–5. Approaches used for assessing each step from genotype to phenotype. (From Taylor HA, Schroer RJ, Phelan MC, Schwartz CE: Counseling Aids for Geneticists, ed 2. Greenwood, SC, Greenwood Genetic Center, 1989.)

segregation between a certain locus and a possible disease locus.[10] The co-inheritance of genetic markers and disease is used to localize defective genes to a specific chromosome location.

Linkage often casts light on the biologic mechanisms underlying the transmission and pathogenesis of disease. Linkage can be demonstrated using the statistical methods of linkage analysis or various laboratory techniques.

For example, the gene for polycystic kidney dis-

order, an autosomal dominant disease, has been characterized. As seen in the family in Figure 15–6, the 1-allele has been demonstrated to be linked with the appearance of the condition, and is seen in the father and in two of the offspring, all of whom were affected. In the case of cystic fibrosis (Fig. 15–7), an autosomal recessive condition, the 1–4 combination is needed for expression of the disease inherited from both the father and the mother. The disease is thus not seen in either parent, but only in the child who has both alleles.

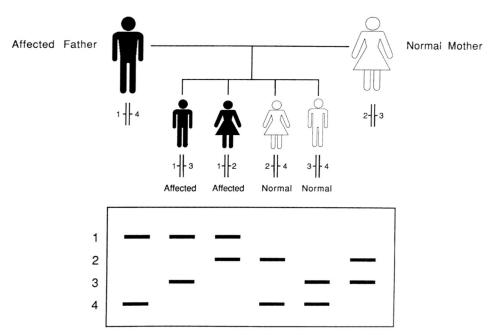

Figure 15–6. DNA analysis of autosomal dominant disorders. Example: Polycystic kidney disorder. (From Taylor HA, Schroer RJ, Phelan MC, Schwartz CE: Counseling Aids for Geneticists, ed 2. Greenwood, SC, Greenwood Genetic Center, 1989.)

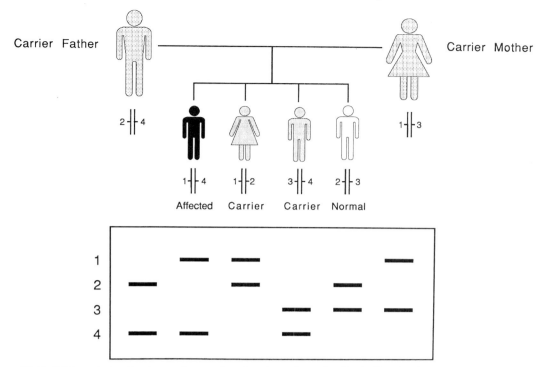

Figure 15–7. DNA analysis of autosomal recessive disorders. Example: Cystic fibrosis. (From Taylor HA, Schroer RJ, Phelan MC, Schwartz CE: Counseling Aids for Geneticists, ed 2. Greenwood, SC, Greenwood Genetic Center, 1989.)

Twin Studies

Studies of twins have been of great value in enriching our understanding of the relative contributions of genetic and environmental factors to the causation of human disease. There are two types of twins: monozygotic (identical) and dizygotic (fraternal). Monozygotic twins arise from the same fertilized ovum and are said to share 100% of their genetic material. Dizygotic twins, however, are like ordinary siblings who just happened to develop in the uterus at the same time. Like ordinary siblings, they share, on the average, 50% of their genetic material.

If we look at occurrence of a disease in identical twins who, in effect, have identical genetic material, what are the possible findings? Both twins may have the disease, or both twins may not have the disease—that is, the members of the pair may be *concordant* for the disease. It is also possible that we find one of the twins has the disease and the other does not; in this case the twin pairs are *discordant* for the disease.

If monozygotic twins are concordant for a disease, what does it tell us about the role of genetic factors? Could the disease be genetic? Yes, because the twins have identical genetic material. Could it be environmental? Yes, because it is well recognized that parents often raise identical twins in a similar fashion, so that they are exposed to many of the same environmental factors. So an observed concordance in monozygotic twins does not clearly indicate whether a disease is genetic or environmental in origin.

What if monozygotic twins are discordant for a certain disease—that is, one has the disease and the other does not? Is this observation consistent with a genetic hypothesis? No—because the discordant twins share the same genetic material but have a different disease experience, the disease would have to be mainly environmental in origin.

In dizygotic twins, both environmental and genetic factors are operant. If a disease is genetic, we would expect less concordance in dizygotic twins than in monozygotic twins.

How do we calculate the rates of concordance and of disconcordance in twins? Figure 15–8 shows a cross-tabulation of twins 1 and 2. The numbers in each cell are therefore numbers of *twin pairs*: thus, there are a pairs (in which both twin 1 and 2 have the disease); d pairs (in which neither twin 1 nor 2 has the disease); b pairs (in which twin 1 does not have the disease but twin 2 does); and c pairs (in which twin 1 has the disease but twin 2 does not).

		TWIN 1	
		Has Disease	Does Not Have Disease
TWIN 2	Has Disease	a	b
	Does Not Have Disease	c	d

Figure 15–8. Concordance in twins for a dichotomous variable such as leukemia.

If we want to calculate the concordance rate in twins, most twins will fall into the *d* category—that is, neither will have the disease. We therefore usually look at the other three cells—those twin pairs in which at least one of the twins has the disease. We can calculate the concordance rate in twin pairs in which at least one twin has the disease as follows:

$$\frac{a}{a+b+c}$$

We can also calculate the discordance rate in all twin pairs in which at least one twin has the disease as:

$$\frac{b+c}{a+b+c}$$

Table 15–3 shows concordance rates for leukemia in monozygotic and dizygotic twin pairs. Here we see that the percentage of concordant pairs is notably high for congenital leukemia, which is strongly suggestive of a major genetic component in causation when the disease occurs near the time of birth.

How are concordance data used? Let us look at a few examples. Table 15–4 shows reported concordance rates for alcoholism in monozygotic and dizygotic twins reported in several studies.[11–14] Almost all of the reported studies show higher concordance rates for monozygotic than for dizygotic twins; the findings from only one study with a relatively small number of twins were not consistent with those of the others. Thus, in general, the data reported in the literature strongly suggest a genetic component in the etiology of alcoholism.

Table 15–5 shows concordance rates in New York State for neural tube defects (anencephaly and spina bifida). Notice that the table refers only to cotwins and does not distinguish between monozygotic and dizygotic twins. The reason for this is that the data were obtained from birth certificates in which zygosity data are generally not available. No contacts were made with individuals and families. As seen in this study, routinely available data may be useful for certain studies, but because they are not gathered for study purposes, such data often are limited in the detail needed to answer specific questions. It should be pointed out that good evidence of zygosity is often not obtained in many twin studies, and when examining data such as those shown in Tables 15–3 and 15–4, we must ask on what basis the twin pairs were labeled monozygotic or dizygotic. (Remember the caveat discussed earlier: If you are shown differences between groups or changes over time, the first question to ask is, Are they real? If you are convinced that a difference or change is real and not artifactual, then and only then should you proceed to interpret the findings.)

One problem in interpreting concordance data is

Table 15–3. Age Distribution in Published Clinical Reports of Childhood Leukemia in Twins, 1928–1974

	Monozygotic Pairs		Dizygotic Pairs	
	Concordant	*Discordant*	*Concordant*	*Discordant*
Perinatal–congenital	14	1	1	1
Age 2–7 yr	6	13	3	5
Age 7–12 yr	1	8	—	1
Age 12 yr and older	5	14	0	3
Total	26	36	4	10

From Keith L, Brown ER, Ames B, et al: Leukemia in twins: Antenatal and postnatal factors. Acta Genet Med Gemellol 25:336–341, 1976.

Table 15–4. Concordance for Alcoholism in Monozygotic (MZ) and Dizygotic (DZ) Twin Pairs Identified Through an Alcoholic Member*

Author (Year)	No. of Twin Pairs	MZ (%)	DZ (%)	Ratio of MZ:DZ Concordance
Kaij (1960)	174	71	32	2.2
Hrubec et al. (1981)	15,924	26	13	2.0
Murray et al. (1983)	56	21	25	0.8
Pickens et al. (1991)	86 (M)	59	36	1.6
	44 (F)	25	5	5.0

Adapted from Lumeng L, Crabb DW: Genetic aspects and risk factors in alcoholism and alcoholic liver disease. Gastroenterology 107:572–578, 1994.

publication bias—that is, a selection bias related to which cases are reported and which are ultimately accepted for publication by a journal. An observation of an infrequent or unusual disease in both members of a pair of twins is often clinically striking. A clinician is therefore much more likely to report such a concordant pair than to report a discordant pair. Journals may also be more likely to accept reports of concordant twin pairs for publication than they are to accept reports of discordant twin pairs. Therefore, many discordant pairs that are never reported are probably missing in tables that summarize data from the literature.

So far we have discussed concordance for a discrete variable, such as leukemia or schizophrenia, either present or absent. But often we are interested in concordance for a continuous variable, such as blood pressure. In this case we would plot the data for twin 1 against the data for twin 2 and calculate the correlation coefficient (*r*) as seen in Figure 15–9: The correlation coefficient can range from −1 to +1.

A correlation coefficient of +1 indicates a full positive correlation, 0 indicates no correlation, and −1 indicates a full inverse correlation. If we plot

such data for monozygotic twin pairs and for dizygotic twin pairs, as shown in Figure 15–10, we would expect to find a stronger correlation for monozygotic than for dizygotic twins if the disease or characteristic is genetically determined.

Table 15–6 shows correlation coefficients for systolic blood pressure among relatives. The highest coefficient is seen in monozygotic twins; the values for dizygotic twins and ordinary siblings are close. Also of interest is that virtually no correlation exists between spouses. A strong correlation between spouses (who are not biologically related) would suggest a role for environmental factors. (An alternate suggestion, however, could be that people seek out individuals like themselves for marriage. Thus, individuals with type A personalities, for example, may seek out other individuals with type A personalities for marriage. In such a situation we might arrive at a high spousal correlation even for conditions that are not environmentally determined.)

Another example of the value of family studies and twin studies in assessing the relative contribu-

Table 15–5. Concordance Rates of Anencephaly and Spina Bifida (ASB) in New York State, 1955–1974

Incidence of ASB	1.3/1,000
Concordance rates	
Among co-twins	4/59 (6.8%)
Among full siblings	19/1,037 (1.8%)
Among half siblings	1/133 (0.8%)

From Janerich DT, Piper J: Shifting genetic patterns in anencephaly and spina bifida. J Med Genet 15:101–105, 1978.

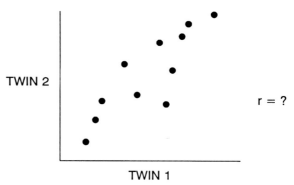

TWIN 2

r = ?

TWIN 1

Figure 15–9. Concordance in twins for a continuous variable such as systolic blood pressure.

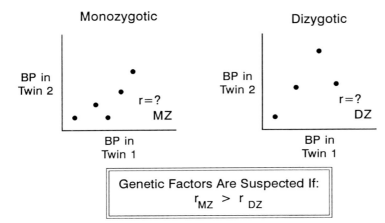

Genetic Factors Are Suspected If:

$$r_{MZ} > r_{DZ}$$

Figure 15–10. Use of concordance rates for continuous variables such as blood pressure [BP] to explore the etiologic role of genetic factors.

tions of genetic and environmental factors to disease causation is seen in the case of Hodgkin's disease. Years ago the incidence of Hodgkin's disease was shown to be bimodal when plotted against age: one peak occurred in the 20s and a second occurred at about age 70 years[15] (Fig. 15–11). Recent data suggest that the histologic type of disease varies by age: the young adult form of the disease is mainly the nodular sclerosing form, and the mixed cell type increases with increasing age.[16]

Over the years a large number of studies have implicated both environmental and genetic factors. Environmentally, small sibship size and higher socioeconomic status have been associated with increased risk of Hodgkin's disease, suggesting that Hodgkin's disease may be a rare sequel to a common childhood infection.[17] Epstein-Barr virus infection has been implicated. At the same time, familial clusters and increased risk of the disease among siblings of Hodgkin's disease patients have suggested a strong genetic component. In 1995, Mack and co-workers[18] reported a study of concordance for Hodgkin's disease in monozygotic and dizygotic

twin pairs that had been identified by Hodgkin's disease in one of its members. As indicated in Table 15–7, 6% of the monozygotic twin pairs were concordant for Hodgkin's disease compared with 0% of the dizygotic pairs.

The median age at diagnosis of the concordant twins was 25.5 years, and most of the cases in the concordant pairs for whom information was available were of the nodular sclerosing histologic subtype. Most of the previously reported sibships with multiple cases were also of this subtype. Although these data suggest a genetic susceptibility to Hodgkin's disease, such a susceptibility does not itself appear to account fully for all cases of the disease. The findings are therefore also consistent with a role for, and possibly an interaction with, environmental factors such as infection.

Adoption Studies

We have said that one problem in interpreting the findings from twin studies is that even monozygotic twins who share the same genetic constitution also

Table 15–6. Correlation Between Relatives for Systolic Blood Pressure

Relatives Compared	Correlation Coefficients
Monozygotic twins	.55
Dizygotic twins	.25
Siblings	.18
Parents-offspring	.34
Spouses	.07

Adapted from Feinleib M, Garrison MS, Borhani N, et al: Studies of hypertension in twins. *In* Paul O (ed): Epidemiology and Control of Hypertension. New York, Grune & Stratton, 1975, pp 3–20.

Table 15–7. Concordance Rates for Hodgkin's Disease in Twin Pairs with an Affected Member

Types of Pair	No. of Pairs	Concordant Pairs	
		No.	%
Monozygotic	179	10	6
Dizygotic	187	0	0

Adapted from Mack TM, Cozen W, Shibata DK, et al: Concordance for Hodgkin's disease in identical twins suggesting genetic susceptibility to the young-adult form of the disease. N Engl J Med 332:413–418, 1995.

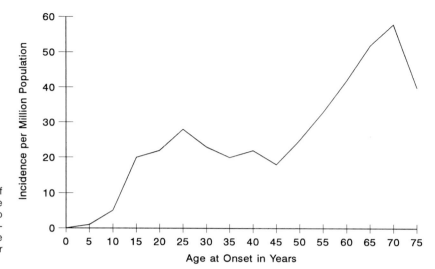

Figure 15–11. Incidence of Hodgkin's disease in the white population of Brooklyn, 1943 to 1957. (From MacMahon B: Epidemiologic evidence on the nature of Hodgkin's disease. Cancer 10:1045, 1957.)

share much of the same environment. In such studies it is therefore difficult to tease out the relative contributions of genetic and environmental factors to the cause of disease. One approach to addressing this problem would be to identify twin pairs in which one twin was adopted by another family and the other was not, so that they do not share a common environment. This is the basis for adoption studies. However, because such twins are difficult to find, the usual approach is to compare adopted children in the following way. Suppose we are interested in whether schizophrenia is primarily genetic or environmental in origin, and we are considering conducting a study using adopted children (Table 15–8).

We can examine offspring of normal biologic parents who are adopted and reared by schizophrenic parents. If the disease is genetic in origin, what would we expect the risk of schizophrenia to be in these children? It should approximate what is seen in the rest of the population because the environment would not have an effect in increasing the risk. If the disease is largely environmental, we would expect that being reared in an environment

with schizophrenic adoptive parents would increase the risk of schizophrenia in these children. We could also examine offspring of normal biologic parents reared by normal adoptive parents and we would expect them to have the usual rate of schizophrenia.

We could also examine offspring of schizophrenic biologic parents who have been adopted and reared by normal parents. In this case, if the disease is genetic, we would expect the children to have an increased risk. If the disease is environmental, we would expect them to have the usual rate of schizophrenia.

In interpreting data from adoption studies, certain factors need to be kept in mind. The first is the age at which the adoption took place. If the adoption occurred in late childhood, for example, part of the child's environment was that of the biologic parents. We would ideally like to study children who are adopted at birth. Another complicating issue is that after adoption some children maintain relationships with their biologic parents, including visits and other exposures to the environment of the biologic parents, so that the separation between environments of biologic parents and adoptive parents is not complete.

Many fine adoption studies have been conducted in Scandinavian countries, which have excellent disease registries and record linkage systems. They also have adoption registries and psychiatric registries. As an example, Table 15–9 shows data from a study of schizophrenia carried out by Kety and Ingraham in which they studied rates of schizophrenia in biologic relatives and in adoptive relatives of

Table 15–8. Types of Subjects Compared in Studies of Schizophrenia in Adopted Offspring

1. Offspring of normal biologic parents reared by schizophrenic adopting parents
2. Offspring of normal biologic parents reared by normal adopting parents
3. Offspring of schizophrenic biologic parents reared by normal adopting parents

Table 15–9. Schizophrenia in Biologic and Adoptive Relatives of Adoptees Who Became Schizophrenic (National Study of Adoptees in Denmark)

	Biologic Relatives			Adoptive Relatives		
	Total No.	Schizophrenic		**Total No.**	Schizophrenic	
		No.	*%*		*No.*	*%*
Adoptees who became schizophrenic (N = 34)	275	14	5	111	0	0
Control adoptees (no serious mental disease) (N = 34)	253	1	0.4	124	0	0

From Kety SS, Ingraham LJ: Genetic transmission and improved diagnosis of schizophrenia from pedigrees of adoptees. J Psychiatr Res 26:247–255, 1992.

adopted children.[19] Using the adoption registry and the psychiatric registry, they identified 34 adoptees who later became schizophrenic and also identified 34 adoptees without serious mental disease. They then examined the rates of schizophrenia in the biologic and in the adoptive relatives of the schizophrenic adoptees and in the control adoptees. The rate of schizophrenia in the biologic relatives of the schizophrenic adoptees was 5.1%, compared with 0.4% in the biologic relatives of control adoptees without serious mental disease. The findings strongly suggest that there is a significant genetic component in the cause of schizophrenia.

Table 15–10 shows correlation coefficients for parent-child aggregation of blood pressure, comparing biologic children with adopted children. Clearly, the correlations are much weaker (and approach 0) for correlations between parents and adopted children than between parents and biologic children. The findings strongly suggest a significant genetic component in determination of blood pressure.

TIME TRENDS IN DISEASE INCIDENCE

If we observe time trends in disease, with incidence either increasing or decreasing over a period of time, and if we are convinced that the trend is

Table 15–10. Correlation Coefficients for Parent-Child Aggregation of Blood Pressure

	Between Parents and	
	Biologic Child	**Adopted Child**
Systolic	.32 (P<.001)	.09 (NS)
Diastolic	.37 (P<.001)	.10 (NS)

Abbreviation: NS, not significant.
Adapted from Biron P, Mongeau JG, Bertrand D: Familial aggregation of blood pressure in 558 adopted children. CMAJ 115:773–774, 1975.

real, the observation implicates environmental factors in the causation of the disease. Clearly, genetic characteristics of human populations generally do not change over relatively short periods.

INTERNATIONAL STUDIES

Figure 15–12 shows age-adjusted death rates for stomach cancer in a number of countries. Note that the highest rate is seen in Japan, and the rates in the United States are quite low. Are the differences real? Could they be due to differences in quality of medical care or in access to medical care in different countries? Could they be due to international differences in how death certificates are completed? The differences seen in Figure 15–12 appear to be real.

Figure 15–13 shows comparable data for breast cancer in women. Here we see that one of the lowest rates in the world is in Japan. Are differences between countries due to environmental or to genetic factors? The answer is probably both. How can we tease apart the relative contributions of genetic and environmental factors to international differences in risk of disease? We can do so by studying migrants in a manner analogous to that just described for adoption studies.

Migrant Studies

Let us assume that a Japanese individual living in Japan, a country with a high risk for stomach cancer, moves to the United States, a country with a low incidence of stomach cancer. What would we expect to happen to this person's risk of stomach cancer? If the disease is primarily genetic in origin, we would expect the high risk of stomach cancer to be retained even when people move from a high-risk to a low-risk area. However, if the disease is

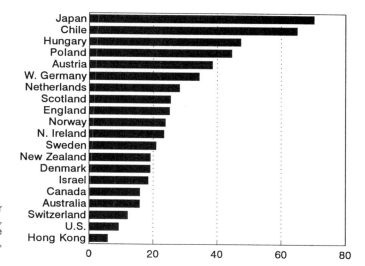

Figure 15–12. Age-adjusted death rates per 100,000 for stomach cancer in 20 countries, males, 1976–1977. (Data from Page HS, Asire AJ: Cancer Rates and Risks, ed 3. Washington, DC, NIH publication no. 85–691, 1985.)

environmental in origin, we would expect that over time the risk for such a migrant group would shift toward the lower risk of the adoptive country.

Table 15–11 shows standardized mortality ratios (SMRs) for stomach cancer in Japanese men living in Japan, Japanese men who migrated to the United States (Issei), and the children of the Japanese migrants (Nisei) born in the United States, compared with SMRs of U.S. white males. We see that the SMRs progressively shift toward the lower SMR of U.S. whites. These data strongly suggest that a significant environmental component is involved.

We should bear in mind that when a person migrates to his country of adoption, he and his family do not immediately shed the environment of their country of origin. Many aspects of their origi-

nal culture are retained, including certain dietary preferences. Thus, the microenvironment of the migrant, particularly environmental characteristics related to lifestyle, are generally a combination of those of the country of origin and those of the country of adoption. Another important consideration is the age at which the person migrated; in interpreting the findings from migrant studies it is important to know how much of the person's life was spent in the country of origin and how much in the country of adoption.

Let us turn to another example. Risk of multiple sclerosis has been demonstrated to be related to latitude: the greater the distance from the equator, the greater the risk. This observation is very intriguing and has stimulated much research, but ques-

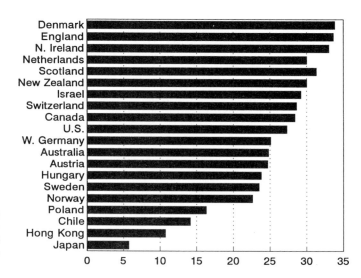

Figure 15–13. Age-adjusted death rates per 100,000 for breast cancer in 20 countries, females, 1976–1977. (Data from Page HS, Asire AJ: Cancer Rates and Risks, ed 3. Washington, DC, NIH publication no. 85–691, 1985.)

Table 15–11. Standardized Mortality Ratios (SMRs) for Cancer of the Stomach in Japanese Men, Issei, Nisei, and U.S. White Males

	SMRs
Japanese men	100
Issei*	72
Nisei*	38
U.S. white males	17

*Issei and nisei are first- and second-generation Japanese migrants, respectively.

From Haenzel W, Kurihara M: Studies of Japanese migrants: I. Mortality from cancer and other disease among Japanese in the United States. J Nat Cancer Inst 40:43–68, 1968.

tions remain about the extent to which the relationship to latitude is a result of environmental factors and about how we can ascertain which environmental factors might be involved.

This observation provides an excellent opportunity to conduct migrant studies to look, for example, at people who have migrated from high-risk to low-risk areas. One country that lent itself very nicely to such a study is Israel, which by latitude is a low-risk country for multiple sclerosis. Israel has had successive waves of immigration during the 20th century. Some of the migrants have come from high-risk areas, such as the relatively northerly latitudes of the United States, Canada, and Northern Europe, whereas others have come from low-risk latitudes closer to the equator, including areas of North Africa and the Arabian peninsula.

Table 15–12 shows data for incidence of multiple sclerosis in European and African-Asian migrants to Israel. (The disease is not common and the sample sizes are therefore small.)

First let us look at the rates for African-Asian migrants who have moved from one low-risk area

Table 15–12. Incidence of Multiple Sclerosis (MS) Per 100,000 Among European, African, and Asian Immigrants to Israel by Age at Immigration

Age at Immigration	Incidence of MS in Migrants	
	European	African and Asian
<15	0.76	0.65
15–29	3.54	0.40
30–34	1.35	0.26

Adapted from Alter M, Leibowitz V, Speer J: Risk of multiple sclerosis related to age at immigration to Israel. Arch Neurol 15:234–237, 1966.

to another. Their risk remains low. Now examine the data for European migrants who have migrated from a high-risk area (Europe) to a low-risk area (Israel). Europeans who migrated before age 15 years (top row) have a low rate, similar to that of African-Asian migrants. However, Europeans who migrated after age 15 years tend to retain the high rate of their country of origin. These findings have suggested that the risk of multiple sclerosis is determined in childhood and that the critical factor is whether childhood years are spent in a high-risk or a low-risk area. A person who has spent childhood years in a low-risk area retains a low risk; one who has spent childhood years in a high-risk area retains a high risk, even after later migration to a low-risk area. This has suggested that some event in childhood, possibly infectious in origin, may be of importance in the causation of multiple sclerosis; this has led to research on slow virus infections as a possible etiologic agent in this disease.

What are the problems with migrant studies? First, migrants are not representative of the populations of their countries of origin. We must therefore ask what factors led these people to migrate (selection factors)? For example, people who are seriously ill or disabled generally do not migrate. Other factors, including socioeconomic and cultural characteristics, are also related to which persons are likely to migrate and which are not. Consequently, we must ask whether we can legitimately compare the rates in Issei and Nisei with rates in native Japanese, given this problem of selection. Second, what was the age at migration? How many years did the migrants spend in their country of origin and how many in their country of adoption? Third, migrants do not completely shed the environment of their country of origin after they migrate.

All these factors must be considered in interpreting the results of migrant studies. There is an obvious parallel with adoption studies, and as seen in Table 15–13, many of the issues that arise in interpreting the findings are similar for the two types of studies.

INTERACTION OF GENETIC AND ENVIRONMENTAL FACTORS

When both genetic and environmental factors are found to have roles in the development of human disease, the nature of the relationship of the two types of factors needs to be elucidated. Certain diseases are largely environmental, whereas others

Table 15–13. Issues in Interpreting the Results of Adoption and Migrant Studies

Adoption Studies	Migrant Studies
• Adoptees are highly selected.	• Migrants are highly selected.
• Age at adoption varies.	• Age at migration varies.
• Adoptees may retain various degrees of contact with their biologic parent(s).	• Migrants may retain many elements of their original environment, particularly those related to culture and lifestyle.

are largely genetic in origin. However, the question of genetic susceptibility to environmental factors and the possibility of interaction between them need to be addressed. Advances in molecular biology have facilitated the integration of epidemiology and laboratory genetics. For example, oral contraceptive (OC) use has long been known to increase a woman's risk of venous thrombosis. Vandenbroucke and colleagues[20] studied the question of whether the factor V Leiden mutation, which is known to enhance susceptibility to thrombosis, may play a role in the increased thrombosis risk in women taking OCs. They conducted a case-control study of 155 premenopausal women who had developed deep venous thrombosis and 169 population controls.

As seen in Table 15–14, the risk of thrombosis among carriers of the mutation was increased about seven- to nine-fold compared to those without the mutation. Compared with women who were noncarriers of the factor V Leiden mutation and did not use OCs, women who were both carriers and users of OCs had more than a 30-fold increase in risk. The findings shown here slightly exceed what

Table 15–14. Estimated Population Incidence per 10,000 Person-Years of First Venous Thrombosis in Women Aged 15 to 49 Years According to Presence of Factor V Leiden Mutation and Use of Oral Contraceptives

	Factor V Leiden Mutation	
	Absent	*Present*
Did not use oral contraceptives	0.8	5.7
Used oral contraceptives	3.0	28.5

Adapted from Vandenbroucke JP, Koster T, Briët E, et al: Increased risk of venous thrombosis in oral contraceptive users who are carriers of factor V Leiden mutation. Lancet 344:1453–1457, 1994.

would be expected in a multiplicative model and therefore suggest interaction.

In 1995, Brennan and colleagues working in Sidransky's laboratory reported a study of cigarette smoking and squamous cell cancer of the head and neck.[21] They found that in patients with invasive cancer of the head and neck, smoking was associated with a marked increase in mutations in the p53 gene, normally a tumor suppressor. Such mutations are likely to contribute to both the inception and growth of cancers. The investigators studied tumor samples from 129 patients with head and neck cancer and found p53 mutations in 42% of the patients (54 of 129). Patients who smoked at least 1 pack/day for at least 20 years were more than twice as likely to have mutations in p53 as patients who were non-smokers. Patients who smoked and drank more than 1 oz of hard alcohol per day were 3.5 times as likely to have mutations in p53 than patients who neither smoked nor drank. As seen in Figure 15–14, p53 mutations were found in 58% of patients who both smoked and drank, in 33% of patients who smoked but did not drink, and in 17% of patients who neither smoked nor drank. Furthermore, the type of mutation found in patients who neither smoked nor drank seemed likely to be endogenous rather than exogenous, i.e., caused by environmental mutagens. The findings suggest that cigarette smoking may tend to inactivate the p53 tumor suppressor gene and thus provide a molecular basis for the well-recognized relationship of cigarette smoking and head and neck cancer.

A further step in this approach is to identify a specific gene defect that is associated with a certain environmental exposure. An example is seen in findings linking a specific defect in the p53 gene to aflatoxin exposure in patients with hepatocellular carcinoma (HCC). In Chapter 14, the positive synergism of hepatitis B virus (HBV) and aflatoxin B_1 exposure in increasing the risk of HCC is discussed. In order to determine whether the frequency of a specific mutation in the p53 tumor suppressor gene (a "hot spot" mutation at codon 249) was related to the risk of aflatoxin exposure, Ozturk and co-workers screened HCC samples from 14 countries.[22] The mutation was found in 17% of tumor samples (12/72) from four countries in southern Africa and the southeast coast of Asia but in none of 95 samples from other geographic locations including North America, Europe, the Middle East, and Japan. The four countries in which the mutation was found, China, Vietnam, South Africa, and Mozambique, have most of the cases of HCC in the world

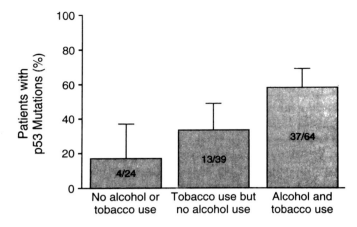

Figure 15–14. Association of p53 gene mutations with cigarette smoking and alcohol consumption in 129 patients with squamous cell carcinoma of the head and neck. (From Brennan JA, Boyle JO, Koch WM, et al: Association between cigarette smoking and mutation of the p53 gene in squamous cell carcinoma of the head and neck. N Engl J Med 332:712–717, 1995.)

and share a similar warm and humid climate, which favors the growth of aflatoxin-producing molds. The rate of HBV carriage was high but did not vary significantly among the countries studied. However, the risk of aflatoxin exposure did vary among these countries and presence of the mutation was found to correlate with the risk of exposure to aflatoxins.

Further support for these findings was provided by Aguilar and colleagues who studied samples of normal liver from three geographic areas that varied in their risk of aflatoxin exposure: negligible levels (United States), low levels (Thailand), and high levels (Qidong, China).[23] The frequency of the mutation paralleled the level of aflatoxin B_1 exposure, suggesting that aflatoxin has a causative and probably early role in the development of liver tumors.

Thus, studies combining epidemiologic and molecular methods may prove invaluable in confirming an etiologic role for certain environmental agents by demonstrating their specific gene effects. Moreover, such studies may also suggest biologic pathways and mechanisms that may be involved in the development of certain cancers and other diseases. However, combined epidemiologic and molecular studies may also help reduce the likelihood that a disease is primarily caused by environmental factors. For example, Harris (1993)[24] pointed out that the exact nature of the p53 mutation can be valuable in indicating that a certain cancer did not result from an environmental carcinogen but instead was caused by endogenous mutagenesis, such as was seen in the study just described of patients with head and neck cancers who were nondrinkers and nonsmokers. Germline mutations in p53 can also indicate that a person has an increased susceptibility to cancer as originally proposed by Knudson in 1971 (and discussed earlier in this chapter).[6]

However, despite the excitement of the results of such studies, in most situations in which both ge-

netic and environmental factors have been implicated, available information is not yet sufficient to delineate the specific nature of their relationship in disease causation.

SUMMARY

This chapter has described some of the epidemiologic approaches used to assess the relative contributions of genetic and environmental factors to the cause of human disease. The link of epidemiology and genetics has become increasingly recognized, and a field called *genetic epidemiology* has emerged.[10] Most epidemiologic studies are directed at the identification of environmental factors in disease, but when designing and conducting studies and interpreting their results, it is important to bear in mind that individuals who are subjects in epidemiologic studies differ not only in environmental exposures but also in their genetic susceptibilities. Therefore, family-based designs should increasingly be considered in epidemiologic studies of risk factors, including case-control as well as other types of studies. Finally, genetic markers of susceptibility that are developed in the laboratory are proving increasingly valuable in epidemiologic studies that address the etiology of human disease.

References

1. Hogben L: Nature and Nurture. New York, WW Norton, 1939.
2. Miki Y, Swensen J, Shattuck-Eidens D, et al: A strong candidate for the breast and ovarian cancer susceptibility gene *BRCA1*. Science 266:66–71, 1994.
3. Struewing JP, Abeliovich D, Peretz T, et al: The carrier frequency of the *BRCA1* 185delAG mutation is approximately 1 percent in Ashkenazi Jewish individuals. Nature Genet 11:198–200, 1995.
4. Savitsky K, Bar-Shira A, Gilad S: A single ataxia telangiectasia gene with a product similar to PI-3 kinase. Science 268:1749–1753, 1995.

5. Nowak R: Discovery of AT gene sparks biomedical research bonanza. Science 268:1700–1701, 1995.
6. Knudson AG Jr: Mutation and cancer: Statistical study of retinoblastoma. Proc Natl Acad Sci USA 68:820–823, 1971.
7. Cavenee WK, Dryja TP, Phillips RA, et al: Expression of recessive alleles by chromosomal mechanisms in retinoblastoma. Nature 305:779–784, 1983.
8. Benedict WF, Fung WT, Murphree L: The gene responsible for the development of retinoblastoma and osteosarcoma. Cancer 62:1691–1694, 1988.
9. Childs B, Scriver CR: Age at onset and causes of disease. Perspect Biol Med 29:437, 1986.
10. Khoury MJ, Beaty TH, Cohen BH, Fundamentals of Genetic Epidemiology. New York, Oxford University Press, 1993.
11. Kaij L: Studies on the Etiology and Sequels of Abuse of Alcohol. Lund, Hakan Ohlssons Boktryckeri, 1960.
12. Hrubec Z, Omenn GS: Evidence of genetic predisposition to alcoholic cirrhosis and psychosis: Twin concordance for alcoholism and its end points by zygosity among male veterans. Alcohol Clin Exp Res 5:207–215, 1981.
13. Murray RM, Clifford C, Gurlin HM: Twin and alcoholism studies. In Galanter M (ed): Recent Developments in Alcoholism, vol 1. New York, Plenum, 1983, pp 25–47.
14. Pickens RW, Svikis DS, McGue M, et al: Heterogeneity in the inheritance of alcoholism: A study of male and female twins. Arch Gen Psychiatry 48:19–28, 1991.
15. MacMahon B: Epidemiology of Hodgkin's disease. Cancer Res 26:1189–1200, 1966.
16. Diehl V, Tesch H: Hodgkin's disease: Environmental or genetic? N Engl J Med 332:461–462, 1995.
17. Gutensohn N, Cole P: Childhood social environment and Hodgkin's disease. N Engl J Med 304:135-140, 1980.
18. Mack TM, Cozen W, Shibata DK, et al: Concordance for Hodgkin's disease in identical twins suggesting genetic susceptibility to the young-adult form of the disease. N Engl J Med 332:413–418, 1995.
19. Kety SS, Ingraham LJ: Genetic transmission and improved diagnosis of schizophrenia from pedigrees of adoptees. J Psychiatr Res 26:247–255, 1992.
20. Vandenbroucke JP, Koster T, Bríët E, et al: Increased risk of venous thrombosis in oral-contraceptive users who are carriers of factor V Leiden mutation. Lancet 344:1453–1457, 1994.
21. Brennan JA, Boyle JO, Koch WM, et al: Association between cigarette smoking and mutation of the p53 gene in squamous-cell carcinoma of the head and neck. N Engl J Med 332:712–717, 1995.
22. Ozturk M, Bressac B, Puisieux A, et al: p53 mutation in hepatocellular carcinoma after aflatoxin exposure. Lancet 338:1356–1359, 1991.
23. Aguilar F, Harris CC, Sun T, et al: Geographic variation of p53 mutational profile in non-malignant human liver. Science 264:1317–1319, 1994.
24. Harris C: p53: At the crossroads of molecular carcinogenesis and risk assessment. Science 262:1080–1081, 1993.

Review Questions

1. If a greater proportion of monozygotic twin pairs are found to be concordant for a certain disease than are dizygotic twin pairs, the observation suggests that the disease is most likely due to:
   a. Exclusively environmental factors
   b. Exclusively hereditary factors
   c. Hereditary factors almost exclusively, with some non-hereditary factors possibly playing a role
   d. Environmental and genetic factors almost equally
   e. Gender differences in monozygotic twins

Question 2 is based on the information given below:

In a familial study of schizophrenia, the following concordance rates were observed within various pairs of relatives:

Pair	Concordance Rate (%)
Husband-wife	5
Parent-child	40
Monozygotic twins	65
Dizygotic twins	42
Ordinary siblings	40

2. A reasonable conclusion to be drawn from these data is:
   a. Genetic factors are unimportant in the etiology of schizophrenia
   b. The data suggest a potentially important genetic component
   c. The incidence of schizophrenia within relative pairs is highest in monozygotic twins
   d. The prevalence of schizophrenia within relative pairs is highest in monozygotic twins
   e. Twins are less likely to develop schizophrenia than are ordinary siblings

Question 3 is based on the information given below:

In a study of Japanese migrants to the United States, the following standardized mortality ratios (SMRs) were found for disease X:

Group	SMR (%)
Native Japanese living in Japan	100
Japanese migrants	105
Children of Japanese ancestry	108
United States whites	591

3. These findings suggest that:
   a. Environmental factors are the major determinants of these SMRs
   b. Genetic factors are the major determinants of these SMRs
   c. Environmental factors associated with the migrant culture are probably involved
   d. Migrants are highly selected and are non-representative of the population in their native country
   e. International differences in coding death certificates for disease X are an important determinant of these SMRs

4. When the incidence of a disease is studied in adopted children and compared to its incidence in biologic relatives and in adoptive relatives, all of the following are relevant concerns *except*:
   a. Age at onset
   b. Amount of contact maintained by the adoptee with his(her) biologic parents
   c. Marital status of the biologic parents
   d. Selection factors relating to who is adopted and who is not
   e. *c* and *d*

5. If an association is found between the incidence of a disease and a certain genetically determined characteristic:
   a. The disease is clearly genetic in origin
   b. Genetic factors are at least implicated in all cases of the disease
   c. Genetic factors are implicated in at least some cases of the disease
   d. A role for environmental factors is excluded
   e. Expression of the disease is likely to be unavoidable

Applying Epidemiology to Evaluation and Policy

In Section II, we reviewed the major types of study design used in epidemiology and examined how the results of epidemiologic studies are used for demonstrating associations and deriving causal inferences. Although the methodologic issues discussed are interesting and intriguing, much of the excitement in epidemiology stems from the fact that its results have direct application to problems involving human health. The challenges that are therefore involved include deriving valid inferences from the data generated by epidemiologic studies, ensuring appropriate communication of the findings and their interpretations to policy-makers and the general public, and dealing with the ethical problems that arise because of the close link of epidemiology to human health and to clinical and public health policy.

This section discusses the uses of epidemiology in evaluating both health services (Chapter 16) and screening programs (Chapter 17). We then turn to some of the specific issues involved in the application of epidemiology to issues of policy (Chapter 18), and finally address some of the major ethical and professional considerations that arise in the context both of conducting epidemiologic investigations and of utilizing the results of epidemiologic studies for improving the health of the community and enhancing the effectiveness of clinical care (Chapter 19).

CHAPTER 16

Using Epidemiology to Evaluate Health Services

Perhaps the earliest example of an evaluation is the description of the creation given in the book of Genesis, 1:1–4, which is shown in the original Hebrew in Figure 16–1. Translated, with the addition of a few subheadings, it reads as follows:

BASELINE DATA
In the beginning God created the heaven and the earth. And the earth was unformed and void and darkness was on the face of the deep.

IMPLEMENTATION OF THE PROGRAM
And God said, "Let there be light." And there was light.

EVALUATION OF THE PROGRAM
And God saw the light, that it was good.

FURTHER PROGRAM ACTIVITIES
And God divided the light from the darkness.

This excerpt includes all of the basic components of the process of evaluation: baseline data, implementation of the program, evaluation of the program, and implementation of new program activities on the basis of the results of the evaluation. However, two problems arise in this description. First, we are not given the precise criteria that were used to determine whether the program was "good"; we are only told that God saw that it was good. Second, this evaluation exemplifies a frequently observed problem: the program director is assessing his own program. Both conscious and subconscious biases can arise in evaluation. Furthermore, even if the program director administers the program superbly, he may not necessarily have the specific skills that are needed for conducting a rigorous evaluation of the program.

Dr. Wade Hampton Frost, a leader in epidemiology in the early part of the 20th century, addressed the use of epidemiology in the evaluation of public health programs in a talk presented to the American Public Health Association in 1925.[1] He wrote, in part, as follows:

The health officer occupies the position of an agent to whom the public entrusts certain of its resources in public money and cooperation, to be so invested that they may yield the best returns in health; and in discharging the responsibilities of this position he is expected to follow the same general principles of procedure

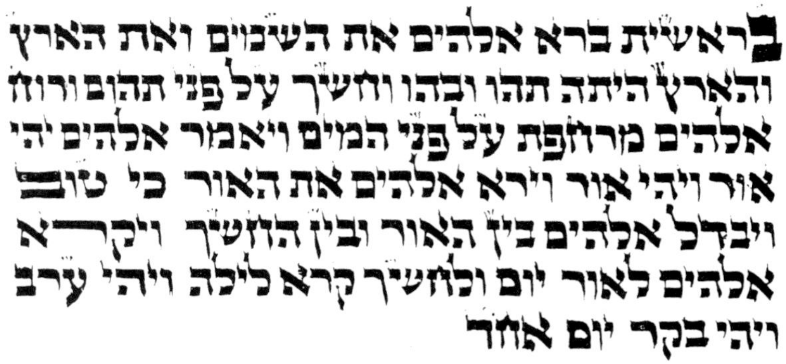

בְּרֵאשִׁית בָּרָא אֱלֹהִים אֵת הַשָּׁמַיִם וְאֵת הָאָרֶץ
וְהָאָרֶץ הָיְתָה תֹהוּ וָבֹהוּ וְחֹשֶׁךְ עַל פְּנֵי תְהוֹם וְרוּחַ
אֱלֹהִים מְרַחֶפֶת עַל פְּנֵי הַמָּיִם וַיֹּאמֶר אֱלֹהִים יְהִי
אוֹר וַיְהִי אוֹר וַיַּרְא אֱלֹהִים אֶת הָאוֹר כִּי טוֹב
וַיַּבְדֵּל אֱלֹהִים בֵּין הָאוֹר וּבֵין הַחֹשֶׁךְ וַיִּקְרָא
אֱלֹהִים לָאוֹר יוֹם וְלַחֹשֶׁךְ קָרָא לַיְלָה וַיְהִי עֶרֶב
וַיְהִי בֹקֶר יוֹם אֶחָד

Figure 16–1. The earliest known evaluation. (Genesis 1:1–4.)

217

as would be a fiscal agent under like circumstances. . . .

Since his capital comes entirely from the public, it is reasonable to expect that he will be prepared to explain to the public his reasons for making each investment, and to give them some estimate of the returns which he expects. Nor can he consider it unreasonable if the public should wish to have an accounting from time to time, to know what returns are actually being received and how they check with the advance estimates which he has given them. Certainly any fiscal agent would expect to have his judgment thus checked and to gain or lose his clients' confidence in proportion as his estimates were verified or not. . . .

However, as to such accounting, the health officer finds himself in a difficult and possibly embarrassing position, for while he may give a fairly exact statement of how much money and effort he has put into each of his several activities, he can rarely if ever give an equally exact or simple accounting of the returns from these investments considered separately and individually. This, to be sure, is not altogether his fault. It is due primarily to the character of the dividends from public health endeavor, and the manner in which they are distributed. They are not received in separate installments of a uniform currency, each docketed as to its source and recorded as received; but come irregularly from day to day, distributed to unidentified individuals throughout the community, who are not individually conscious of having received them. They are positive benefits in added life and improved health, but the only record ordinarily kept in morbidity and mortality statistics is the partial and negative record of death and of illness from certain clearly defined types of disease, chiefly the more acute communicable diseases, which constitute only a fraction of the total morbidity.

Dr. Charles V. Chapin commented on Frost's presentation:

Dr. Frost's earnest demand that the procedures of preventive medicine be placed on a firm scientific basis is well timed. Indeed, it would have been opportune at any time during the past 40 years and, it is to be feared, will be equally needed for 40 years to come.

Chapin clearly underestimated the number of years; the need remains as critical today, more than 70 years later, as it was in 1925.

STUDIES OF PROCESS AND OUTCOME

Studies of Process

At the outset we should distinguish between process and outcome studies. *Process* means that we decide what constitutes the components of good care. Such a decision is often made by an expert panel. We can then assess a clinic or health care provider, review relevant records, and determine to what extent the care provided meets the established criteria. For example, we can determine what percentage of patients have had blood pressure measured. The problem with such process measures is that they do not indicate whether the patient is better off; monitoring blood pressure, for example, does not ensure that the patient's blood pressure is under control. Second, because process assessments are based on expert opinion, the criteria used in process evaluations may change over time as expert opinion changes. For example, in the 1940s, the accepted standard of care of premature babies required that such infants be placed in 100% oxygen, and incubators were monitored to be sure that such levels were maintained. However, with recognition of the role of high oxygen concentration in producing retrolental fibroplasia—a blindness of premature newborns—such a concentration was deemed unacceptable.

Studies of Outcomes

Given the limitations of process studies, the remainder of this chapter focuses on outcome measures. *Outcome* denotes whether or not a patient benefits from the medical care provided. Health outcomes are the domain of epidemiology. Although such measures have traditionally been mortality and morbidity, interest in outcome research in recent years has expanded the measures of interest to include patient satisfaction, quality of life, degree of dependence and disability, and similar measures.

EFFICACY, EFFECTIVENESS, AND EFFICIENCY

Three terms often encountered in the literature dealing with evaluation of health services are *efficacy*, *effectiveness*, and *efficiency*.

Efficacy

Does the agent or intervention "work" under ideal, "laboratory" conditions? We test a new drug in a group of patients who have agreed to be hospitalized and who are observed as they take their therapy. Or a vaccine is tested in a group of consenting subjects. Thus, efficacy is a measure in a situation in which all conditions are controlled to maximize the effect of the agent.

Effectiveness

If we administer the agent in a "real-life" situation, is it effective? For example, when the vaccine just referred to is tested in a community, many individuals may not come in to be vaccinated. Or, an oral medication may have such an undesirable taste that no one will take it (so that it will prove ineffective), despite the fact that under controlled conditions, when compliance was ensured, the drug was shown to be efficacious.

Efficiency

If an agent is shown to be effective, what is the cost-benefit ratio? Is it possible to achieve our goals in a cheaper and better way? Cost includes not only money, but also discomfort, pain, absenteeism, disability, and social stigma.

If a health care measure has not been demonstrated to be effective, there is little point looking at efficiency, for if it is not effective, the cheapest alternative is not to use it at all. At times, of course, political and societal pressures may drive a program even if it is not effective. However, this chapter will focus only on the science of evaluation and specifically on the issue of effectiveness in evaluating health services.

MEASURES OF OUTCOME

If efficacy of a measure has been demonstrated—that is, if the methods of prevention and intervention that are of interest have been shown to work, we can then turn to evaluating effectiveness. What guidelines should we use in selecting an appropriate outcome measure to serve as an index of effectiveness? First, the measure must be clearly quantifiable—that is, we must be able to express it in quantitative terms. Second, the measure of outcome should be relatively easy to define and diagnose. If it is to be used in a population study, we

Table 16–1. Some Possible Endpoints for Measuring Success of a Vaccine Program

1. No. (or proportion) of people immunized
2. No. (or proportion) of people at (high) risk who are immunized
3. No. (or proportion) of people immunized who show serologic response
4. No. (or proportion) of people immunized and later exposed in whom clinical disease does not develop
5. No. (or proportion) of people immunized and later exposed in whom clinical or subclinical disease does not develop

would certainly not want to depend on an invasive procedure for assessing any benefits. Third, it should lend itself to standardization for study purposes. Fourth, the population served (and the comparison population) must be at risk for the same condition for which an intervention is being evaluated. For example, it would obviously make no sense to test the effectiveness of a sickle cell screening program in a white population.

The type of outcome endpoint that we select should depend on the question that we are asking. Although this may seem self-evident, it is not always immediately apparent. Table 16–1 shows possible endpoints in evaluating the effectiveness of a vaccine program. Whatever outcome we select should be explicitly stated so that others reading our report will be able to make their own judgments regarding the appropriateness of the measure selected and the quality of the data. Whether the measure we have selected is indeed an appropriate one depends on clinical and public health aspects of the disease in question.

Table 16–2 shows possible choices of measures for assessing the effectiveness of a throat culture program in children. Measures of volume of ser-

Table 16–2. Some Possible Endpoints for Measuring Success of a Throat Culture Program

1. No. of cultures taken (symptomatic or asymptomatic)
2. No. (or proportion) of cultures positive for streptococcal infection
3. No. (or proportion) of persons with positive cultures for whom medical care is obtained
4. No. (or proportion) of persons with positive cultures for whom proper treatment is prescribed *and* taken
5. No. (or proportion) of positive cultures followed by a relapse
6. No. (or proportion) of positive cultures followed by rheumatic fever

vices provided, numbers of cultures taken, and number of clinic visits have been traditional favorites because they are relatively easy to count and are helpful in justifying requests for budgetary increases for the program in the following year. However, such measures tell us nothing about effectiveness. We therefore move to other possibilities listed in this table. Again, the most appropriate measures should depend on the question being asked. The question must be specific. It is not enough to just ask, How good is the program?

EVALUATION USING GROUP DATA

Regularly available data such as mortality data and hospitalization data are often employed in evaluation studies. Such data can be obtained from different sources, and such sources may differ in important ways. For example, Figure 16–2 shows discharge rates for short-term hospital stays in the United States from two sources: the National Hospital Discharge Survey (NHDS) and the National Health Interview Survey (NHIS).

Although the trends are similar, the magnitude of the rates differs. The NHDS uses hospital records of inpatients discharged from short-stay non-federal

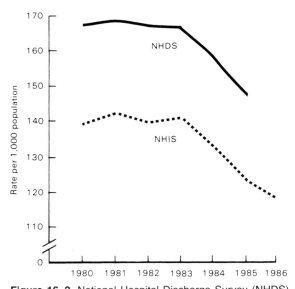

Figure 16–2. National Hospital Discharge Survey (NHDS) and National Health Interview Survey (NHIS) short-stay hospital discharge rates: United States, 1980–1986. (From Moss AJ, Moien MA: Recent declines in hospitalization: United States, 1982–1986. Data from the National Health Interview Survey and the National Hospital Discharge Survey. NCHS Advance Data, Vital and Health Statistics of the National Center for Health Statistics, no. 140, p. 2, 1987.)

hospitals. The NHIS uses personal interviews, and people tend to forget many of their past hospitalizations. The NHIS also includes discharges from federal hospitals, most of which are Veterans Administration hospitals. The NHDS includes patients who die in the hospital as well as those admitted from nursing homes, two groups not included by the NHIS. The NHDS—but not the NHIS—counts as discharges persons who are hospitalized for less than 1 day. The point is that in evaluating any modality of health care, we must identify and understand the sources of data that will be used, such as who or what is included or excluded and how data are categorized. We then assess the impact of these characteristics and the validity of the data obtained, as well as examine possible biases that may be introduced. If we are only interested in changes over time—*trends*—the issues may not be critical, but if we are interested in absolute values, the issues may be very important.

One area in which existing sources of data are often used in evaluation studies is prenatal care. Birth certificates are often used because they are easily accessible and provide certain medical care data, such as the trimester in which prenatal care was begun. However, birth certificates for women with high-risk pregnancies more often have missing data than those for women with low-risk pregnancies. The quality of the data used in birth certificates may also differ regionally and internationally, and may complicate any comparisons made.

A number of other interesting issues arise in examining the question of the effectiveness of prenatal care, specifically the number of prenatal visits, and an outcome such as prematurity. Several potential biases may be introduced into this type of analysis. For example, other things being equal, a woman who delivers prematurely will have fewer prenatal visits (i.e., the pregnancy was shorter so that there was less time in which it was possible for her to ''be at risk'' for prenatal visits). The result would be an artifactual relationship between fewer prenatal visits and prematurity, only because the period of gestation was shorter. However, the bias can also operate in the other direction: A woman who begins prenatal care in the last trimester of pregnancy is not going to have an early premature delivery, as she has already carried the pregnancy to the last trimester. This would lead to an observed association of fewer prenatal visits with a smaller likelihood of early premature delivery. Finally, women who have had medical complications in the past may come for more prenatal visits, but they may also be at greater risk for a bad outcome. Thus, the potential biases can run in either direction.

Two approaches to evaluating health services using ecologic studies are those of avoidable mortality and the use of health indicators. *Avoidable mortality* analyses assume that the rate of "avoidable deaths" should vary inversely to the availability, accessibility, and quality of medical care in different geographic regions. Thus, ideally, avoidable mortality would serve as a measure of the adequacy and effectiveness of care in an area. Changes over time could be plotted and comparisons made with other areas. Unfortunately, the necessary data are lacking for many of the conditions suggested for avoidable mortality analyses. Moreover, data on confounders may not be available and the resulting inferences may therefore be open to question.

Another approach has been to use *health indicators*. In this approach, certain sentinel conditions are assumed to reflect the general level of health care, and changes in the incidence of such conditions are plotted over time and compared with data for other populations. The changes and differences found are then related to changes in the health service sector and inferences regarding causation are derived. It is difficult to know, however, what criteria need be met in order for a given condition to be acceptable as a valid health indicator.

EVALUATION USING INDIVIDUAL DATA

Because of the limitations inherent in studies using group data, that is, studies in which we do not have data on both health care (exposure) and outcome for each individual, studies using individual data are generally preferable. If we wish to compare two populations, one receiving the care being evaluated and one not receiving it, we must ask the following two questions to be able to derive inferences about the effectiveness of care:

1. Are the characteristics of those two populations comparable, demographically, medically, and in terms of factors relating to prognosis?
2. Are the measurement methods comparable (e.g., diagnostic methods and the way disease is classified) in both groups?

Both issues have been discussed in earlier chapters because they also apply to questions of etiology, prevention, and therapy, and they must therefore be considered in any type of study design.

An important issue in using epidemiology to study outcomes for the evaluation of health services is the need to address prognostic stratification. If a change in health outcome is observed after a certain type of care has been delivered, can we necessarily conclude that the change is due to the health care provided, or could it be a result of differences in prognosis based on pre-existing disease, in severity, or in other associated conditions that bear on prognosis? To address these issues, such outcome studies must carry out a prognostic stratification by studying case mix and by carefully characterizing the individuals studied on the basis of disease severity.

Let us first turn to some *cohort designs* used in evaluation.

Randomized Designs

Randomization eliminates the problem of selection bias resulting either from self-selection by the patient or selection of the patient by the health care provider. Usually, the assignments are to one type of care or to the other rather than to care and no care (Fig. 16–3). For many reasons, both ethical and practical, randomizing to no care is usually not considered.

The randomized design can be applied to many types of health care questions. As an example, Figure 16–4 shows the results of a randomized trial of physician education. The program evaluated was designed to reduce the use of unindicated pelvimetry studies in pregnant women. A group of hospitals were randomized, and in one of the hospital groups,

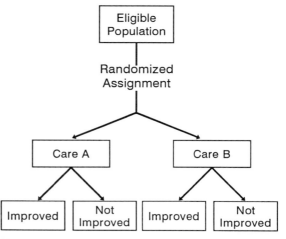

Figure 16–3. Design of randomized study comparing care A and care B.

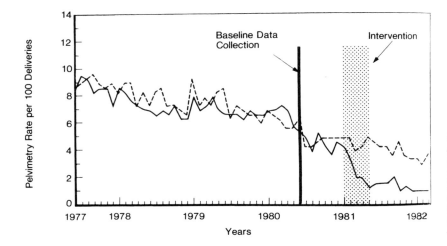

Figure 16–4. Rates of pelvimetry over time in study and control groups. *Symbols: solid line,* study group; *dashed line,* control group. (From Chassin MR, McCue SM: A randomized trial of medical quality assurance. Improving physicians' use of pelvimetry. JAMA 256:1012–1016, 1986.)

physicians received intensive education in the appropriate use of pelvimetry; in the other they did not. A clear difference in pelvimetry usage resulted.

Non-randomized Designs

Everything we do in health care cannot be subjected to randomized trials for several reasons. First, such trials are often logistically complex and extremely expensive. Because so many different health care measures are in use at any time, it is not feasible to subject all of them to randomized evaluations. Second, ethical problems are often perceived to occur in randomizing in health services evaluation studies so that randomizing may be viewed as an unacceptable process both by many patients and by health care providers. Third, randomized trials often take a long time to complete, and because programs and health problems change over time, when the results of the study are finally obtained and analyzed they may no longer be entirely relevant. For these reasons, many health care researchers are looking for alternative approaches that may at least yield some information. A term in current use—*outcomes research*—generally refers to the obtaining of data from non-randomized studies, which often employ large existing data sets.

Before-After Design (Historical Controls)

If randomization is not possible or will not be used for any reason, one possible study design to evaluate a program is to compare people who received care before a program was established (or before the health care measure became available) with those who received care from the program

after it was established or after the measure became available. What are the problems with this before-after design? First, the data obtained in each of the two periods are frequently not comparable in terms of either quality or completeness. Often, when a new form of health service delivery is developed, a decision is made to evaluate the program by studying people who were treated in the past, before the program began, as a comparison group. As a result, the data available for people after the program was started may be collected using a well-designed research instrument, whereas data for past patients may be available only from health care records that had been designed and used only for clinical or administrative purposes at that time. Hence, if we observe a difference in outcome, we may not know if the observed difference is a result of the effect of the program or of differences in the quality of data from the two time periods.

Second, if we see a difference—for example, mortality is lower after a program was initiated than before the program was initiated—we do not know whether the difference is due to the program itself or to other factors that may have changed over time, such as housing, nutrition, other aspects of lifestyle, or other health services.

Third, a problem of selection exists. Often, it is difficult to know whether the population studied after a program was established is actually similar to that seen before the program was established in terms of other factors that might affect outcome.

Does this mean that before-after studies have no value? No, it does not. But it does mean that such studies only provide a suggestion—and are rarely conclusive—in demonstrating the effectiveness of a health service.

A before-after design was used in a study to assess the impact of the Medicare prospective payment system (PPS) in the United States on quality of care.[2] The study was stimulated by concern that the PPS, with its closely regulated length of hospital stays and incentives for cost-cutting, might have adversely affected the quality of care. The before-after design was selected because the PPS was instituted nationwide, so a prospective cohort design could not be used. Data for almost 17,000 Medicare patients who were hospitalized in 1981–1982 prior to when the PPS was instituted were compared with data for patients hospitalized in 1985–1986 after the PPS was in place. Quality of care was evaluated for five diseases: (1) congestive heart failure, (2) myocardial infarction, (3) pneumonia, (4) cerebrovascular accident, and (5) hip fractures. Outcome findings were adjusted for level of patient sickness on admission to the hospital. Although PPS was not found to be associated with an increase in either 30-day mortality or 6-month mortality, an increase was observed in instability at discharge (defined as the presence of conditions at discharge that clinicians agree should be corrected prior to discharge or monitored after discharge, and that may result in poor outcomes if not corrected).[3] The authors point out that other factors may also have changed during the time before and after institution of the PPS. Although the before-after design was probably the only design possible for the issue addressed in this study, the study is nevertheless susceptible to some of the problems of this type of design that were discussed earlier.

Simultaneous Non-randomized Design (Program–No Program)

One option for avoiding the problem of changes over calendar time is to conduct a simultaneous comparison of two populations that are not randomized, in which one population is served by the program and the other is not. This type of design is in effect a cohort study in which the type of health care being studied represents the "exposure." As in any cohort study, the problem arises of how to select exposed and non-exposed groups for study.

An example of a simultaneous, non-randomized study is one reported by Jollis and co-workers[4] who examined the relationship of in-hospital mortality and need for bypass surgery during the index hospitalization in patients who underwent percutaneous transluminal coronary angioplasty with the volume of angioplasties carried out by the hospital. As seen in Table 16–3, a dose-response relationship was found, with the highest in-hospital mortality and the highest rate of unplanned bypass surgery occurring in hospitals that had the smallest volume of angioplasties per year.

The finding that hospitals that perform more angioplasties have lower short-term mortality has important potential policy implications and argues for the regionalization of angioplasty services.

Comparison of Utilizers and Non-utilizers

One approach for a simultaneous non-randomized study is to compare a group of people who utilize a health service with a group of people who do not (Fig. 16–5).

The problems of self-selection inherent in this type of design have long been recognized. Many years ago, Stine and colleagues[5] reported the results of a study of prenatal care to young women under age 17 years who were delivered of children in Baltimore from 1960 to 1961 (Table 16–4).

In this study, 1,397 young women received prenatal care and 315 did not. The neonatal death rate was 30.1 per 1,000 in those who received care and 88.9 in those who did not. The patients were not randomized, but decided themselves whether or not to seek care. As the authors pointed out, in the absence of randomization, we cannot conclude that the care reduced neonatal mortality. For we have the problem of selection: namely, those who came

Table 16–3. In-Hospital Mortality and Rates of Bypass Surgery During Index Hospitalization According to Hospital Volume of Angioplasty Procedures Each Year

	<50 Procedures/yr	50–100 Procedures/yr	>100 Procedures/yr
In-hospital mortality (%)	3.7	3.2	2.7
Bypass surgery during index hospitalization (%)	5.3	4.6	3.5

Adapted from Jollis JG, Peterson ED, DeLong ER, et al: The relation between the volume of coronary angioplasty procedures at hospitals treating Medicare beneficiaries and short-term mortality. N Engl J Med 331:1625–1629, 1994.

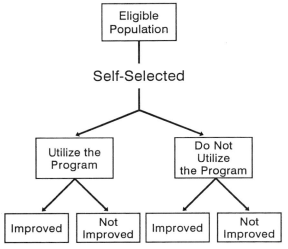

Figure 16–5. Design of a non-randomized cohort study comparing utilizers with non-utilizers of a program.

in for care were probably more motivated regarding a broad array of health and prevention issues compared with those who did not. Consequently, the neonatal mortality difference observed may be due as much to the characteristics of the two groups as to the care provided.

Although we can try to address the selection problem by characterizing the prognostic profile of those who utilize care and those who do not, so long as the groups are not randomized, we are left with a gnawing uncertainty as to whether some factors were not identified in the study that might have differentiated utilizers and non-utilizers and, therefore, affected the health outcome.

Comparison of Eligibles and Non-eligibles

Because of the problem of possible selection biases in comparing groups of utilizers with non-

Table 16–4. Relationship of Neonatal Mortality to History of Prenatal Care, Baltimore Residents, Younger Than 17 Years, 1960–1961

	Received Prenatal Care	Did Not Receive Prenatal Care
No. of births	1,397	315
No. of neonatal deaths	42	28
Neonatal deaths per 1,000 live births	30.1	88.9

Adapted from Stine OC, Rider RV, Sweeney E: School leaving due to pregnancy in an urban adolescent population. J Pub Health 54:1–6, 1964.

utilizers, another approach compares persons who are eligible for the care being evaluated with a group of persons who are not eligible (Fig. 16–6).

The assumption here is that eligibility or non-eligibility is not related to prognosis or outcome, and that no selection bias is therefore being introduced that might affect the inferences from the study. Eligibility criteria may include, for example, type of employer or census tract of residence. Even with this design, however, one must be on the alert for factors that may introduce selection bias. For example, census tract of residence may clearly relate to socioeconomic status, and the issue of finding an appropriate non-eligible population for comparison may be critical.

Combination Designs

As seen in Figure 16–7A, in all the non-randomized study designs that compare the morbidity level in persons who receive care with the morbidity level in those who do not, the assumption is that the original levels of morbidity in the two groups (A_1 and B_1) were comparable before the care was provided to group B. If so, we could interpret the finding of a lower level of morbidity in those receiving the care (B_2) than in those not receiving the care (A_2) as likely to have resulted from the care provided.

However, as seen in Figure 16–7B, it is possible that the groups might have been different originally and their prognoses may have differed at that time even without the care having been provided. If

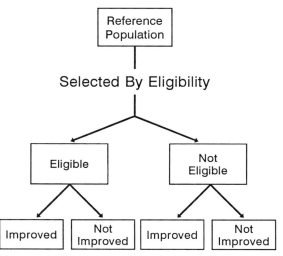

Figure 16–6. Design of a non-randomized cohort study comparing people eligible with people not eligible for a program.

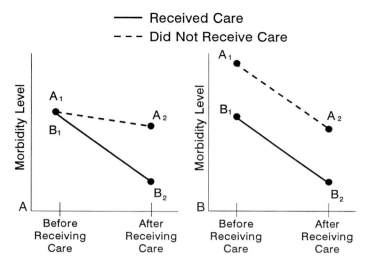

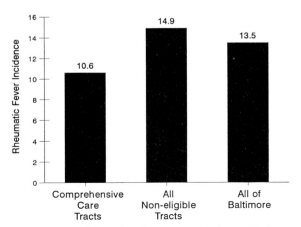

Figure 16–7. Two possible interpretations of an observed difference in morbidity between people receiving a health service and those not receiving the service.

such were the case, any differences in morbidity observed at time T_2 (B_2 lower than A_2) might only reflect the original differences at time T_1 and would not necessarily shed any light on the effectiveness of the care provided. Without having data on morbidity levels in the two groups at time T_1, the latter explanation of the observations could not be ruled out.

In view of this problem, another approach to program evaluation is to utilize a *combination design,* which involves both before-after and program–no program designs. This approach is demonstrated in the following example, in which outpatient care for sore throats in children was evaluated.

The study was designed to assess the effectiveness of outpatient care for sore throats in children by determining whether children who were eligible for such care had lower rates of rheumatic fever than did children who were not eligible.[6] The rationale was as follows: "Strep" throats are common in children. Untreated "strep" throats can lead to rheumatic fever. If "strep" throats are properly treated, rheumatic fever can be prevented. Therefore, if these programs are effective in treating "strep" throats, fewer cases of rheumatic fever should occur in the children who received the treatment.

In the mid-1960s, comprehensive care programs for children and youth were established in many inner cities, including in Baltimore. Eligibility for care in this program was determined by the census tract of tne child's residence. Rheumatic fever had already been shown to cluster in Baltimore's inner city.

It was possible to identify and compare several subgroups of Baltimore children and adolescents and to compare their rates of hospitalization for episodes of acute rheumatic fever with those for all of the city of Baltimore. The groups included residents of census tracts that met eligibility criteria for comprehensive care and residents of census tracts that did not meet eligibility criteria for comprehensive care. Both were compared with the city of Baltimore as a whole.

Figure 16–8 shows a program–no program comparison of rheumatic fever rates in black children. In children eligible for comprehensive care, the rheumatic fever rate was 10.6 per 100,000, compared with 14.9 in those who were not eligible.

Figure 16–8. Comprehensive care and rheumatic fever incidence, 1968–1970; Baltimore, black population, aged 5 to 14 years. (Adapted from Gordis L: Effectiveness of comprehensive-care programs in preventing rheumatic fever. N Engl J Med 289:331–335, 1973.)

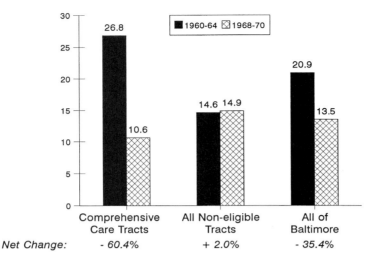

Figure 16–9. Comprehensive care and changes in rheumatic fever incidence, 1960–1964 and 1968–1970; Baltimore, black population, aged 5 to 14 years. (Adapted from Gordis L: Effectiveness of comprehensive-care programs in preventing rheumatic fever. N Engl J Med 289:331–335, 1973.)

Although the rate was lower in the eligible group in this simultaneous comparison, the difference was not dramatic.

The next analysis in this combination design examined changes in rheumatic fever rates over time in both eligible and non-eligible populations.

As seen in Figure 16–9, the rheumatic fever rate declined 60% in the eligible census tracts from 1960–1964 (before the programs were established) to 1968–1970 (after the programs were operating). In the non-eligible tracts, rheumatic fever incidence was essentially unchanged (+2%). Thus, both parts of the combination design are consistent with a decline related to the care available.

However, because many changes had occurred in the inner city during this time, it was not certain whether the care provided by the programs was indeed responsible for the decline in rheumatic fever. Another analysis was therefore carried out. In a child, a streptococcal throat infection can be either symptomatic or asymptomatic. Clearly, only a child with a symptomatic sore throat would have been brought to a clinic. If we hypothesize that the care in the clinic was responsible for the reduction in rheumatic fever incidence, we would expect the decline in incidence to be limited to children with symptomatic clinical sore throats who would have sought care, and not to have occurred in asymptomatic children who had no clinically apparent infections.

As seen in Figure 16–10, the entire decline was limited to children with prior clinically overt infection; no change in rheumatic fever incidence occurred in those whose sore throats were asymptomatic. These findings are therefore highly consistent with the suggestion that it was the medical care, or some factor closely associated with it, that was responsible for the decline in rheumatic fever incidence.

Case-Control Studies

The use of the case-control design for evaluating health services, including vaccines and other forms of prevention and screening programs, has elicited increasing interest. Although the case-control design has been primarily applied to etiologic studies, when appropriate data are obtainable, this design can serve as a useful, if limited, surrogate for randomized trials. Because this design requires definition and specification of cases, it is most applicable

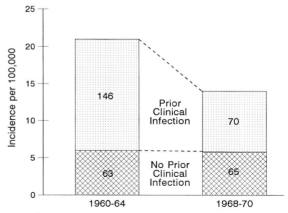

Figure 16–10. Changes in the annual incidence of first attacks of rheumatic fever in relation to preceding clinical respiratory infection. (Adapted from Gordis L: Effectiveness of comprehensive-care programs in preventing rheumatic fever. N Engl J Med 289:331–335, 1973.)

to studies of prevention of specific diseases. The "exposure" is then the specific preventive or other health measure being assessed. As in most health services research, stratification by severity and by other possible prognostic factors is essential for appropriate interpretation of findings. The methodologic problems associated with such studies (which are discussed extensively in Chapter 10) also arise when the case-control design is used for evaluation of effectiveness. In particular, selection of controls and issues of confounders need to be addressed in these studies.

CONCLUSION

This chapter has reviewed the application of basic epidemiologic study designs to the evaluation of health services. Many of the issues that arise are similar to those that arise in etiologic studies, although at times they present a different twist. In etiologic studies, we are primarily interested in the possible association of a potential causal factor and a specific disease, and factors such as health services often represent possible confounders that must be taken into account; in health care evaluation studies, we are primarily interested in possible associations of a health care or preventive measure and disease outcome, and factors such as pre-existing disease and other prognostic and risk factors become confounders that must be taken into consideration. Consequently, although many of the design issues remain, the focus in evaluation research is often on different issues of measurement and assessment. The randomized trial remains the optimal method for demonstrating the effectiveness of a health intervention. In initiating any evaluation study of health care, we should ask at the outset whether it is biologically and clinically plausible, given our current knowledge, to expect a specific benefit from the care being evaluated.

For practical reasons, non-randomized observations are also necessary and must be capitalized on in the attempt to expand efforts at evaluation. Critics of randomized trials have pointed out that such studies have included—and can only include—a small fraction of patients receiving care in the health care system. Although this is true, generalizability is a problem with any study, no matter how large the study population. Nevertheless, even as we further refine the methodology of clinical trials, we also need improved methods to enhance the information that can be obtained even from non-randomized evaluations of health services.

The study of specific components of care, rather than a care program per se, is essential. In this way, if an effective element can be identified in a mix of many modalities, the others can be eliminated and the quality of care can be enhanced in a cost-effective fashion.

In the next chapter, the discussion of evaluation is extended to a specific type of program: screening for disease in human populations.

References

1. Frost WH: Rendering account in public health. Am J Pub Health 15:394–398, 1925.
2. Kahn KL, Rubenstein LV, Draper D, et al: The effects of DRG-based prospective payment system on quality of care of hospitalized Medicare patients: An introduction to the series. JAMA 264:1953–1955, 1990.
3. Kosecroff J, Kahn KL, Rogers WH, et al: Prospective payment system and impairment at discharge: The "quicker and sicker" story revisited. JAMA 265:1980–1983, 1990.
4. Jollis JG, Peterson ED, DeLong ER, et al: The relation between the volume of coronary angioplasty procedures at hospitals treating Medicare beneficiaries and short-term mortality. N Engl J Med 331:1625–1629, 1994.
5. Stine OC, Rider RV, Sweeney I: School leaving due to pregnancy in an urban adolescent population. J Pub Health 54:1–6, 1964.
6. Gordis L: Effectiveness of comprehensive-care programs in preventing rheumatic fever. N Engl J Med 289:331–335, 1973.

Review Questions

1. All of the following are measures of *process* of health care in a clinic except:
   a. Proportion of patients in whom blood pressure was measured
   b. Proportion of patients who develop complications of a disease
   c. Proportion of patients advised to stop smoking
   d. Proportion of patients whose height and weight are determined
   e. Proportion of patients whose bill is reduced because of financial need

Question 2 is based on the informaion given below:

In-Hospital Case-Fatality Rates (CFRs) for 100 Male Patients Not Treated in a Coronary Care Unit (CCU) and for 100 Male Patients Treated in a CCU, According to Three Clinical Grades of Severity of Myocardial Infarction

Clinical Grade	Non-CCU (No. of Patients)			CCU (No. of Patients)		
	Total	*Died*	*CFR (%)*	*Total*	*Died*	*CFR(%)*
Mild	60	12	20	10	3	30
Severe	36	18	50	60	18	30
Shock	4	4	100	30	13	43

The results given above were based on a comparison of the last 100 patients treated before the CCU was installed and the first 100 patients treated within the CCU. All 200 patients were admitted during the same month.

You may assume that there is *only this one hospital* in the town, and that the natural history of MI was *unchanged* during this period.

2. The authors concluded that the CCU was very beneficial for male patients with severe myocardial infarction (MI) and for those in shock, because the in-hospital CFRs for these categories were much lower in the CCU. This conclusion:

   a. Is correct
   b. May be incorrect because CFRs were used rather than mortality rates
   c. May be incorrect because of a referral bias of cases to this hospital from hospitals in distant towns
   d. May be incorrect due to differences in the assignment of clinical severity grade before and after opening of the CCU
   e. May be incorrect because of failure to recognize a possible decrease in the annual *incidence rate* of MI in recent years

3. The extent to which a specific health care treatment, service, procedure, program, or other intervention does what it is intended to do when employed in a community-dwelling population is termed its:

   a. Efficacy
   b. Effectiveness
   c. Effect modification
   d. Efficiency
   e. None of the above

4. The extent to which a specific health care treatment, service, procedure, program, or other intervention produces a beneficial result under ideal controlled conditions is its:

   a. Efficacy
   b. Effectiveness
   c. Effect modification
   d. Efficiency
   e. None of the above

5. A major problem in using a historical control design for evaluating a health service using case-fatality rate (CFR) as an outcome is that if CFR is lower after provision of the health service was started, then:

   a. The lower CFR could be due to changing prevalence of the disease
   b. The lower CFR may be a result of decreasing incidence
   c. The lower CFR may be an indirect effect of the new health service
   d. CFR may have been affected by changes in factors that are not related to the new health service
   e. None of the above

CHAPTER 17

The Epidemiologic Approach to Evaluation of Screening Programs

In Section II, we discussed the design and interpretation of studies that aim to identify risk factors or etiologic factors for disease so that disease occurrence can be prevented—*primary prevention.* In this chapter, we address the early detection of disease that is carried out in the hope of improving prognosis—*secondary prevention.* The chapter focuses on the use of epidemiology for evaluating the effectiveness of screening programs. This subject is important both in clinical practice and in public health, for there is increasing acceptance of a physician's obligation to include prevention along with diagnosis and treatment as major responsibilities to patients.

In Chapter 4, the validity and reliability of screening tests were discussed. In this chapter, we discuss some of the methodologic issues that must be considered in deriving any inferences about the benefits that may accrue to persons who undergo screening with such tests.

The question of whether patients benefit from early detection of disease includes the many following components:

1. Can the disease be detected early?
2. What are the sensitivity and specificity of the test?
3. What is the predictive value of the test?
4. How serious is the problem of false-positive test results?
5. What is the cost of early detection in terms of funds, resources, and emotional impact?
6. Are the subjects harmed by screening tests?
7. Do the individuals in whom disease is detected early benefit from the early detection, and is there an overall benefit to those who are screened?

In this chapter we primarily address the last question. Several of the other questions in the preceding list are considered only in the context of the main issue.

The term *early detection of disease* means detecting a disease at an earlier stage than would usually occur in standard clinical practice. This denotes detecting disease at a presymptomatic stage, at which point the patient has no clinical complaint (no symptoms or signs) and, therefore, no reason to seek medical care for the condition. The assumption in screening is that an appropriate intervention is available for the disease that is detected and that the intervention can be more effectively applied if the disease is detected at an earlier stage.

At first glance, the question of whether people benefit from early detection of disease may seem somewhat surprising. Intuitively, it would seem obvious that early detection is beneficial and that intervention at an earlier stage of the disease process is more effective and/or easier to implement than later intervention. In effect, these assumptions represent a "surgical" view; for example, every malignant lesion is localized at some early stage, and at this stage it can be successfully excised before regional spread occurs, or certainly before widespread metastases develop. However, the intuitive attractiveness of such a concept should not blind us to the fact that throughout the history of medicine, deeply felt convictions have often turned out to be erroneous when they were not supported by data obtained from appropriately designed and rigorously conducted studies. Consequently, regardless of the attractiveness of the idea of the beneficial aspects of early disease detection, both to clinicians involved in prevention and therapy and to those involved in community-based prevention programs, the evidence to support the validity of this concept must be rigorously examined.

As in evaluating any type of health service, screening can be evaluated using process or outcome measures. Table 17–1 provides a list of operational measures that includes process measures as well as measurements of yield and information produced by the screening program.

We are particularly interested in the question of what benefit is gained by people who undergo screening in a screening program. However, just as is the case with evaluation of health services (discussed in Chapter 16), there is little advantage to improving the *process* of screening if persons who are screened derive no benefit. We will therefore examine some of the problems associated with determining whether early detection of disease confers benefits to the individual who undergoes screening (i.e., whether outcome is improved by screening).

What do we mean by *outcome*? To answer the question of whether patients benefit, we must precisely define what we mean by benefit, and what outcome or outcomes are considered to be evidence of patient benefit. Some of the possible outcome measures that might be used are shown in Table 17–2.

THE NATURAL HISTORY OF DISEASE

To discuss the methodologic issues involved in evaluating the benefit of screening, let us examine in further detail the natural history of disease (first discussed in Chapter 5).

Figure 17–1A is a schematic representation of the natural history of a disease in an individual. At

Table 17–1. Assessing the Effectiveness of Screening Programs Using Operational Measures

1. No. of people screened
2. Proportion of target populations screened and no. of times screened
3. Detected prevalence of preclinical disease
4. Total costs of the program
5. Costs per case found
6. Costs per previously unknown case found
7. Proportion of positive screenees brought to final diagnosis and treatment
8. Predictive value of a positive test in population screened

Adapted from Hulka BS: Degrees of proof and practical application. Cancer 62:1776–1780, 1988.

Table 17–2. Assessing the Effectiveness of Screening Programs Using Outcome Measures

1. Reduction of mortality in the population screened
2. Reduction of case-fatality in screened individuals
3. Increase in percent of cases detected at earlier stages
4. Reduction in complications
5. Prevention of/reduction in recurrences or metastases
6. Improvement of quality of life in screened individuals

some point, biologic onset of disease occurs. This may be a subcellular change, such as an alteration in DNA, and this point is generally undetectable. At some later point the disease becomes symptomatic, or clinical signs develop—that is, the disease moves into a clinical phase. The clinical signs prompt the patient to seek care, after which a diagnosis is made and appropriate therapy is instituted, the ultimate outcome of which may be cure, control of the disease, disability, or death.

As shown in Figure 17–1B, the onset of symptoms marks an important point in the natural history of a disease. The period after which the symptoms develop is the *clinical phase of the disease*. The period from biologic onset of the disease to the development of signs and symptoms is the *preclinical phase of the disease.*

If we want to detect disease earlier than usual through programs of health education, we could encourage symptomatic persons to seek medical care sooner. But a major challenge lies in identifying persons with disease who are asymptomatic. Our focus in this chapter is on identification of disease in persons who have not yet developed symptoms and who are in the preclinical phase of illness.

At some point during the preclinical phase it becomes possible to detect the disease by using available tests (Fig. 17–1C). The interval from this point to the development of signs and symptoms is the *detectable preclinical phase* of the disease. When disease is detected by screening, the time of diagnosis is advanced to an earlier point in the disease's natural history. The *lead time* is defined as the interval by which the time of diagnosis can be advanced by screening and early detection of disease compared with the usual time of diagnosis (Fig. 17–1D).

Another important concept in screening is the *critical point* in the natural history of a disease[1] (Fig. 17–2A). This is a point in the natural history before which treatment is more effective and/or less

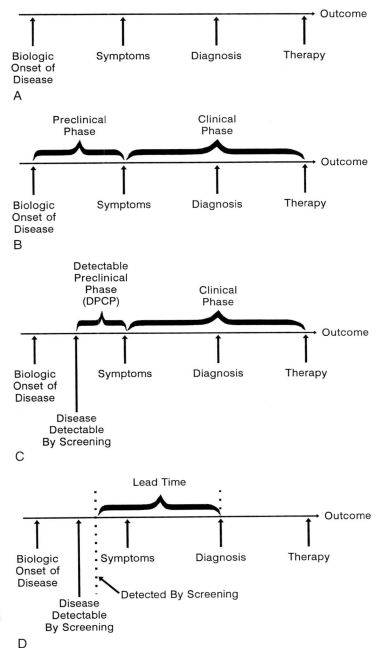

Figure 17–1. *A,* Natural history of disease. *B,* Natural history of disease with preclinical and clinical phases. *C,* Natural history of disease with detectable preclinical phase. *D,* Natural history of disease with lead time.

difficult to administer. If a disease is potentially curable, cure may be possible before this point, but not after. For example, in a woman with breast cancer, one critical point would be that at which the disease spreads from the breast to the axillary lymph nodes. If the disease is detected and treated before that point, prognosis is much better than after spread to the nodes has taken place.

As shown in Figure 17–2*B*, there may be multiple

critical points in the natural history of a disease. For example, in the patient with breast cancer, a second critical point may be that at which disease spreads from the axillary nodes to other parts of the body. Prognosis is still better when the disease is confined to the axillary lymph nodes than when systemic spread has occurred.

The critical point is a theoretical concept, and in a given disease we usually cannot identify when

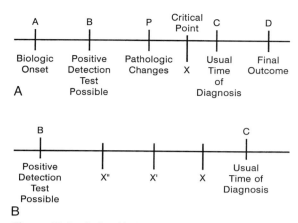

Figure 17–2. *A*, A critical point in the natural history of disease. *B*, Multiple critical points in the natural history of disease. (Adapted from Hutchison GB: Evaluation of preventive services. J Chron Dis 11:497–508, 1960.)

the critical point is reached. However, it is a very important idea in screening. For if we cannot envision one or more critical points in the natural history of a disease, there is clearly no rationale for screening and early detection. Early detection presumes that a biologic point exists in the natural history of a disease before which treatment will benefit a person more than if he or she is treated after that point.

THE PATTERN OF DISEASE PROGRESSION

We might expect to see a potential benefit from screening and early detection if the following two assumptions hold:

1. All or most clinical cases of a disease first go through a detectable preclinical phase.
2. In the absence of intervention, all or most cases in a preclinical phase progress to a clinical phase.

Both assumptions are reasonably self-evident. For example, if none of the preclinical cases progress to clinical cases, there is no reason to perform screening tests. Or, if none of the clinical cases passes through a preclinical phase, there is no reason to perform screening tests. Thus, both assumptions are important in assessing any potential benefit from screening. However, both assumptions are open to question. In certain situations, the preclinical phase may be so short that the disease is unlikely to be detected by any periodic screening program. Also, there is increasing evidence that

spontaneous regression may occur in some diseases, so not every preclinical case inexorably progresses to clinical disease.

For example, Figure 17–3A shows a schematic progression from normal cervix to cervical cancer. One would expect that detection of more cases at the in situ stage would be reflected in a commensurate reduction in the number of cases that progress to invasive disease.

However, evaluating the benefits of cervical cancer screening is complicated by the problem that some cases progress through the in situ stage so rapidly, and the preclinical stage is so brief, that for all practical purposes there is no preclinical stage during which disease can be detected by screening. In addition, nuclear DNA quantitation studies suggest that cervical intraepithelial abnormalities may exist either as a reversible state or as an irreversible precursor of invasive cancer. Data also suggest that some cases of cervical intraepithelial neoplasia detected by a Papanicolaou (Pap) smear regress spontaneously, particularly in the earlier stages, but also in the later stage (carcinoma in situ). In one study, 36% of women with abnormal Pap smears who refused any intervention were later found to have normal Pap smears. In addition, recent data suggest that in situ cervical neoplasia are associated with different types of papillomaviruses. Only neoplasia associated with certain types of papillomavirus progress to invasive cancer, so we may be dealing with heterogeneity of both causal agent and disease.

Thus, whereas the simple model of progression from normal cervix to invasive cervical cancer seen in Figure 17–3A would suggest that early detection followed by effective intervention would be reflected by a commensurate reduction in the number

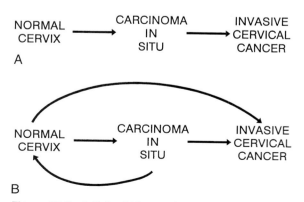

Figure 17–3. *A*, Natural history of cervical cancer: I. Progression from normal cervix to invasive cancer. *B*, Natural history of cervical cancer: II. Extremely rapid progression and spontaneous regression.

of invasive lesions that subsequently develop, a more accurate presentation of the natural history may be that seen in Figure 17–3*B*. The extent of both phenomena, spontaneous regression and extremely rapid progression, clearly influence the size of the decrease in invasive disease that might be expected to result from early detection and intervention and must therefore be taken into account in assessing the benefits of screening. Although these issues have been demonstrated for cervical cancer, they are clearly relevant to evaluating the benefits of screening for many diseases.

METHODOLOGIC ISSUES

To interpret the findings in a study designed to evaluate the benefits of screening, certain methodologic problems must be taken into account. Most studies of screening programs that have been carried out have not been randomized trials, because of the difficulties of randomizing a population for screening. The question is, therefore, why can't we just examine a group of people who have been screened and compare their mortality to that of a group of people who have not been screened?

Let us assume that we compare a population of people who have been screened for a disease with a population of people who have not been screened for the disease. Let us further assume that a treatment is available and will be used for those in whom disease is detected. If we find a lower mortality from the disease in those in whom disease was identified through screening than in those in whom disease was not detected in this manner, can we not conclude that screening and early detection of disease has been beneficial? Let us turn to some of the methodologic issues involved.

Selection Biases

Referral Bias (Volunteer Bias)

In deriving a conclusion about benefits of screening, the first question we might ask is whether there was a selection bias in terms of who was screened and who was not. We would like to be able to assume that those who were screened had the same characteristics as those who were not screened. However, there are many differences in the characteristics of those who participate in screening or other health programs and those who do not. Many studies have shown volunteers to be healthier than the general population and to be more likely to

comply with medical recommendations. If, for example, persons whose disease had a better prognosis from the outset were either referred for screening or were self-selected, we might observe lower mortality in the screened group even if early detection played no role in improving prognosis. Of course, it is also possible that volunteers may include many people who are at high risk and who volunteer for screening because they have anxieties based on a positive family history or lifestyle characteristics. The problem is that we do not know in which direction the selection bias might operate and how it might affect the study results.

The problem of selection bias that affects our interpretation of the findings is best addressed by carrying out the comparison using a randomized experimental study in which care is taken that the two groups are comparable in terms of their initial prognostic profiles (Fig. 17–4).

Length-Biased Sampling (Prognostic Selection)

The second type of selection problem that arises in interpreting the results of a comparison of a screened and an unscreened group is a possible selection bias; this does not relate to who comes for screening but rather to the type of disease that is detected by the screening. The question is: Does screening selectively identify cases of the disease for which there is a better prognosis, regardless of how early therapy is initiated in the natural history of the disease? Or, if the outcome of those in whom disease is detected by screening is better than the outcome of those who were not screened, and in whom disease was identified during the usual course of clinical care, could the better outcome among those who are screened result from selective

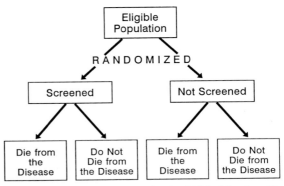

Figure 17– 4. Design of a randomized trial of the benefits of screening.

identification of persons with a better prognosis by screening, and be unrelated to the time of diagnostic and treatment interventions?

How could this come about? Recall the natural history of disease, with the clinical and preclinical phases, shown in Figure 17–1B. We know that the clinical phase of illness differs in different people. For example, some patients with colon cancer die soon after diagnosis, whereas others survive for many years. What appears to be the same disease may have a clinical phase of different length in different individuals.

What about the preclinical phase in these individuals? Actually, each patient has a single continuous natural history, which we divide into preclinical and clinical phases (Fig. 17–5) on the basis of the point in time at which signs and symptoms develop. In some, the natural history is brief and in others the natural history is protracted. This suggests that if a person has a slowly progressive natural history with a long clinical phase, the preclinical phase will also be long. In contrast, if a person has a rapidly progressive disease process and a short natural history, the clinical phase is likely to be short, and it seems reasonable to conclude that the preclinical phase will also be short. There are in fact data to support the notion that a long clinical phase is associated with a long preclinical phase and a short clinical phase with a short preclinical phase.

Remember that our purpose in screening is to detect the disease during the preclinical phase, because during the clinical phase the patient is aware of the problem and will seek medical care for symptoms. If we mount a one-time screening program in a community, which group of patients are we likely to identify: those with a short preclinical phase or those with a long preclinical phase?

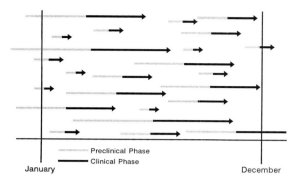

Preclinical Phase
Clinical Phase
January   December

Figure 17–6. Hypothetical population of individuals with long and short natural histories.

To answer this, let us consider a small population that is screened for a certain disease (Fig. 17–6). As shown here, each case has a preclinical and a clinical phase. The figure is drawn so that each preclinical phase is the same length as its associated clinical phase. Patients in the clinical phase will be identified in the usual course of medical care, so the purpose of the screening is to identify cases in the preclinical, presymptomatic state. Note that the lengths of the preclinical phases of cases represented here vary. The longer the preclinical phase, the more likely the screening program is to detect the case while it is still preclinical. For example, if we screen once a year for a disease for which the preclinical phase is only 24 hours long, we will clearly miss most of the cases during the preclinical phase. If, however, the preclinical phase is 1 year long, cases will be identified during the preclinical phase. Screening tends to selectively identify those cases that have longer preclinical phases of illness. Consequently, even if the subsequent therapy had no effect, screening would selectively identify persons with a long preclinical phase, and consequently a long clinical phase (i.e., those with a better prognosis). These people would have a better prognosis even without the screening program or even if there were no true benefits from screening.

This problem can be addressed in several ways. First is, again, to use an experimental randomized design in which care is taken to try and keep the groups comparable in terms of the lengths of the detectable preclinical phase of illness. However, this may not be easy. In addition, survival should be examined for all members of each group—that is, the screened and the non-screened. In the screened group, survival should be calculated for those in whom disease is detected by screening and for those in whom disease is detected between

A. <u>Short Natural History:</u>

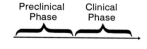

Preclinical   Clinical
Phase   Phase

B. <u>Long Natural History:</u>

Preclinical Phase   Clinical Phase

Figure 17–5. Short and long natural histories of disease: relationship of length of clinical phase to preclinical phase.

screening examinations, the so-called *interval cases*. We shall return to the importance of interval cases later in this chapter.

Lead Time Bias

Another problem that arises in examining survival in people who are screened and comparing it to survival in those who are not screened is a bias associated with the lead time—how much earlier can the diagnosis be made if the disease is detected by screening compared with the usual timing of the diagnosis if screening were not carried out?

Consider four individuals with a certain disease shown by the four timelines in Figure 17–7. The first shows usual time of diagnosis and usual time of death. The second timeline shows an earlier time of diagnosis but the same time of death. Survival seems better because the interval from diagnosis to death is longer, but the patient is not any better off, as death has not been delayed. The third timeline shows earlier diagnosis and a delay in death from the disease—clearly a benefit to the patient (assuming that quality of life is good). Finally, the fourth timeline shows earlier diagnosis with subsequent prevention of death from the disease.

The benefits we seek are delay or prevention of death. Although we have chosen to focus on mortality in this chapter, we could also have used morbidity, recurrences, quality of life, or patient satisfaction as valid measures of outcome.

Lead Time and Five-Year Survival

Five-year survival is a frequently used measure of therapeutic success, particularly in cancer therapy. Let us examine the possible effect of lead time on apparent 5-year survival.

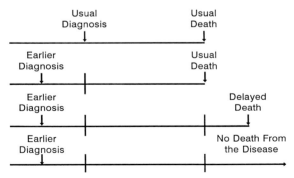

Figure 17–7. Possible outcomes of a screening program.

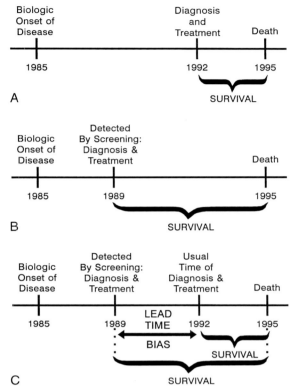

Figure 17–8. *A,* Lead time bias and 5-year survival: I. *B,* Lead time bias and 5-year survival: II. *C,* Lead time bias and 5-year survival: III.

Figure 17–8*A* shows the natural history of disease in a hypothetical patient with colon cancer, which was diagnosed in the usual clinical context without any screening. Biologic onset of the disease was in 1985. The patient became aware of symptoms in 1992, and had a diagnostic workup leading to a diagnosis of colon cancer. Surgery was performed in 1992 and the patient died of colon cancer in 1995. This patient has survived 3 years and clearly is not a 5-year survivor. If we use 5-year survival as an index of treatment success, this patient is a treatment failure.

Consider what might happen to this patient if he resides in a community in which a screening program is initiated (Fig. 17–8*B*). For this hypothetical example only, let us assume that there is actually no benefit from early detection—that is, the natural history of colon cancer is unaffected by early intervention. In this case, the patient is asymptomatic but undergoes a routine screening test in 1989, the result of which is positive. In 1989, surgery is performed and the patient dies in 1995. The patient

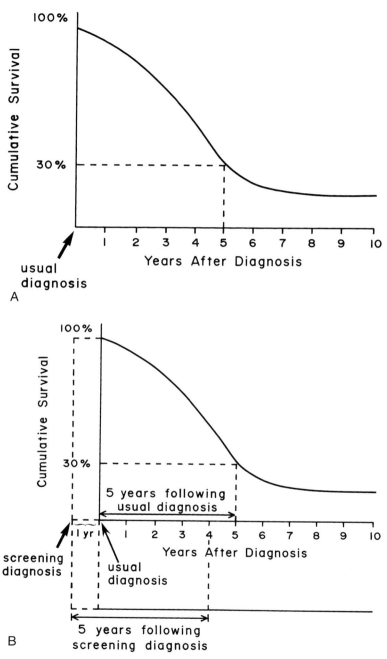

Figure 17–9. *A*, Lead time bias—I: 5-year survival when diagnosis is made without screening. *B*, Lead time bias—II: Shift of 5-year period by screening and early detection (lead time).

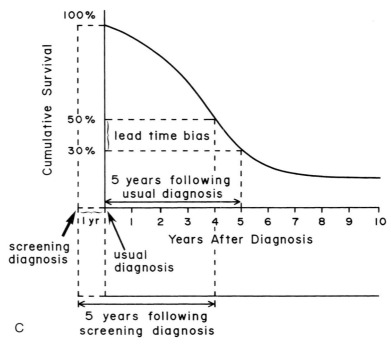

C

Figure 17–9 *Continued C*, Lead time bias—III: Bias in survival calculation resulting from early detection. (Modified from Frank JW: Occult-blood screening for colorectal carcinoma: The benefits. Am J Prev Med 1:3–9, 1985.)

has survived 6 years and is now clearly a 5-year survivor. However, he is a 5-year survivor not because death has been delayed, but because the diagnosis has been made earlier. When we compare this screening scenario with the scenario without screening (see Fig. 17–8A), it is apparent the patient has not derived any benefit from earlier detection in terms of having lived any longer; indeed the patient may have lost out in terms of quality of life, as the earlier detection of disease by screening gave him an additional 3 years of postoperative and other medical care, and may have deprived him of 3 years of normal life. This problem of an illusion of better survival only because of earlier detection is called the *lead time bias,* as shown in Figure 17–8C.

Thus, even in the absence of any true benefit from early disease detection, there will *appear* to be a benefit associated with screening, even if there is no delay in death, because of an earlier point of diagnosis from which survival is measured. This is not to say that early detection carries no benefit; rather, even without any benefit, the lead time associated with early detection suggests the appearance of a benefit in the form of enhanced survival. Lead time must therefore be taken into account in interpreting the results of non-randomized evaluations.

Figure 17–9A–C shows the effect of the bias resulting from lead time on quantitative estimates of survival.

Figure 17–9A shows the situation in which no screening activity is being carried out. Five years after diagnosis, survival is 30%. If we institute a screening program with a 1-year lead time, the entire frame is shifted to the left (Fig. 17–9B). If we now calculate survival at 5 years from the new time of diagnosis (Fig. 17–9C), survival appears to be 50%, but only as a result of lead time bias. The problem is that the apparently better survival is not a result of patients living longer, but it is rather a result of a diagnosis being made at an earlier point in the natural history of the disease.

Consequently, in any comparison of screened and unscreened populations we must make an allowance for an estimated lead time in an attempt to identify any prolongation of survival above and beyond that resulting from the artifact of lead time. If early detection is truly associated with improved survival, survival in the screened group should be greater than survival in the control group *plus the lead time.* We therefore have to generate some estimate of the lead time for the disease being studied.

Another strategy is to compare mortality from the disease in the entire group screened with that in the unscreened group, rather than just the case-fatality rate in those in whom disease has been detected by screening.

Overdiagnosis Bias

Another potential bias is that of overdiagnosis. At times, persons who initiate a screening program have almost limitless enthusiasm for the program. Even cytologists reading Pap smears may become so enthusiastic that they may tend to overread the smears (i.e., make false-positive readings). If they do overread, the result is that normal women are included in the group thought to have positive Pap smears. Consequently, the abnormal group will be diluted with women who are free of disease. If normal individuals in the screened group are more likely to be erroneously diagnosed as positive than are normal individuals in the unscreened group (e.g., identified as having cancer when in reality they do not), one could get a false impression of increased rates of detection and diagnosis of early-stage disease as a result of the screening. In addition, because many of the persons with a diagnosis of cancer would actually not have cancer, and would therefore have a good survival, the results would represent an inflated estimate of survival after screening in persons thought to have cancer. (In effect, this is a misclassification bias, as discussed in Chapter 14.) It is therefore essential that the diagnostic process be rigorously standardized in such studies.

STUDY DESIGNS FOR EVALUATION OF SCREENING

Non-randomized Studies

In discussing the methodologic issues involved in non-randomized studies of screening, we have in essence been discussing non-randomized observational studies of screened and unscreened persons—a cohort design (Fig. 17–10).

In recent years, the case-control design has gained increasing attention as a method of assessing the effectiveness of screening (Fig. 17–11).

In this design the "cases" are people with advanced disease—the type of disease we hope to prevent by screening. Several proposals have been made for appropriate controls for such a study. Clearly they should be "non-cases"—that is, people without advanced disease. Although the "controls" used in early case-control studies for evaluation of screening were people with disease in

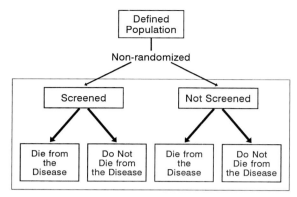

Figure 17–10. Design of a non-randomized cohort study of the benefits of screening.

an early stage, now many believe that people selected from the population from which the cases were derived are better controls. We then determine the prevalence of a history of screening among both the cases and the controls, so that screening is looked at as an "exposure." If screening is effective, we would expect to find a greater prevalence of screening history among the controls than among those with advanced disease, and an odds ratio can be calculated, which will be less than 1.0 if screening is effective.

Randomized Studies

In this type of study, a population is randomized, half to screening and half to no screening. Such a study is difficult to mount and carry out. Perhaps the best known randomized trial of screening is the trial of screening for breast cancer using mammography that was carried out at the Health Insurance Plan (HIP) of New York.[2] Shapiro and colleagues conducted a randomized trial in women enrolled in the prepaid HIP program. This study has become a classic in the literature in reporting evaluation of screening benefits through a randomized trial de-

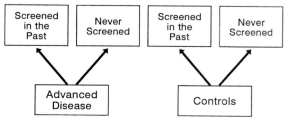

Figure 17–11. Design of a case-control study of the benefits of screening.

sign, and it serves as a model for future studies of this type.

The study was begun in 1963. It was designed to determine whether periodic screening using clinical examination and mammography reduced breast cancer mortality in women aged 40 to 64 years. Approximately 62,000 women were randomized into a study group and a control group of about 31,000 each (Fig. 17–12). The study group was offered screening examinations; 65% appeared for the first examination and were offered additional examinations at annual intervals. Most of these women had at least one of the three annual screening examinations that were offered. Screening consisted of physical examination, mammography, and interview. Control women received the usual medical care in the prepaid program. Many reports have been published from this outstanding study, and we will examine only a few of the results here.

Figure 17–13 shows the number of breast cancer deaths and the mortality rates in both the study group (women who were offered mammography) and the control group after 5 years of follow-up.

Note that the data for the study group include deaths among women screened and those who refused screening. Recall that in Chapter 6 we discussed the problem of unplanned crossover in randomized trials. In that context, it was pointed out that the standard procedure in data analysis was to analyze according to the original randomization—an approach known as "intention to treat." That is precisely what was done here. Once a woman was

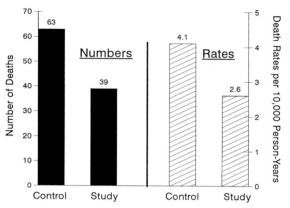

Figure 17–13. Numbers of deaths due to breast cancer, and mortality rates from breast cancer in control and study groups, 5 years of follow-up after entry into study. Data for study group include deaths among women screened and those who refused screening. (Data from Shapiro S, Venet W, Strax P, et al: Selection, follow-up, and analysis in the Health Insurance Plan Study: A randomized trial with breast cancer screening. Natl Cancer Inst Monogr 67:65–74, 1985.)

randomized to mammography, she was kept in that group for purposes of analysis even if she subsequently refused screening. We see that breast cancer deaths are much higher in the control group than in the study group.

Figure 17–14 shows 5-year case-fatality rates in the women who developed breast cancer in both groups.

Case-fatality in the control group was 41%. In the *total* study group—women who were randomized to mammography, regardless of whether or not they were actually screened—the case-fatality was 26%. Shapiro and co-workers then divided this group into those who were screened and those who refused screening. In those who refused screening, case-fatality was 34%. In those who were screened, case-fatality was 23%.

Shapiro and colleagues then compared survival in women whose breast cancer was detected at the screening examination with that in women whose breast cancer was identified between screening examinations—that is, no breast cancer was identified at screening, and before the next examination a year later, the woman had symptoms that led to the diagnosis of breast cancer. If the cancer had been detected through mammography, the case-fatality was only 13%. If, however, the breast cancer was an *interval cancer*, that is, diagnosed between examinations, the case-fatality was 38%. What could explain this difference in case-fatality? The likely explanation is that disease found between

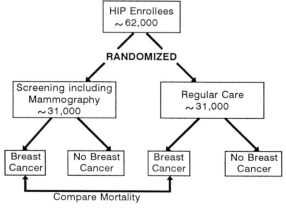

Figure 17–12. Design of the Health Insurance Plan (HIP) randomized controlled trial begun in 1963 to study the efficacy of mammography screening. (Data from Shapiro S, Venet W, Strax P, Venet L (eds): Periodic Screening for Breast Cancer: The Health Insurance Plan Project and Its Sequelae, 1963–1986. Baltimore, Johns Hopkins University Press, 1988.)

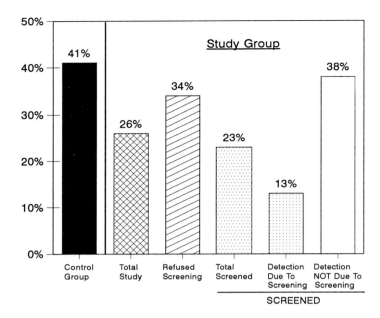

Figure 17–14. Five-year case-fatality rates among breast cancer patients. Rates for those in whom detection was due to screening allow for 1-year lead time. (Data from Shapiro S, Venet W, Strax P, et al: Ten- to 14-year effect of screening on breast cancer mortality. JNCI 69:349–355, 1982.)

regular mammographic examinations was rapidly progressive—not detectable at regular mammographic examination but identified before the next regularly scheduled examination a year later because it was so aggressive.

These observations also support the notion discussed earlier in this chapter that a long clinical phase is likely to be associated with a long preclinical phase: women in whom cancer findings were detected at screening had a long preclinical phase and had a case-fatality of only 13%, indicating a long clinical phase as well. The women who had normal mammograms and whose disease became clinically apparent before the next examination had a short preclinical phase and, given the group's high case-fatality, also had a short clinical phase.

Figure 17–15 shows deaths from causes *other than breast cancer* in both groups over 5 years. Mortality was much higher in those who did not come for screening than in those who did. Because the screening was only directed at breast cancer, why should those who came for screening and those who did not manifest different mortality rates for causes *other* than breast cancer? The answer is, clearly, volunteer bias—the well-documented observation that people who participate in health programs differ in many ways from those who do not: in their health status, attitudes, educational and socioeconomic levels, and other factors. This is another demonstration that for purposes of evaluating a health program, comparison of participants and non-participants is not a valid approach.

Before leaving our discussion of the HIP study, we might digress and mention an interesting application of these data that Shapiro and co-workers carried out.[3] Figure 17–16 shows that in the United States, 5-year relative survival rates from breast cancer are better in whites than in blacks.

The question has been raised whether this is due to a difference in the biology of the disease in blacks and in whites or to a difference between blacks and whites in accessing health care, which

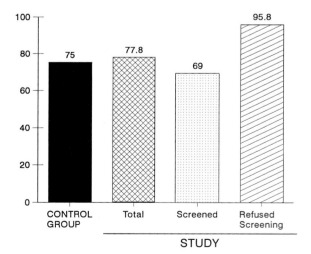

Figure 17–15. Mortality from all causes excluding breast cancer per 10,000 person-years, Health Insurance Plan (HIP). (Data from Shapiro S, Venet W, Strax P, et al: Selection, follow-up, and analysis in the Health Insurance Plan Study: A randomized trial with breast cancer screening. Natl Cancer Inst Monogr 67:65–74, 1985.)

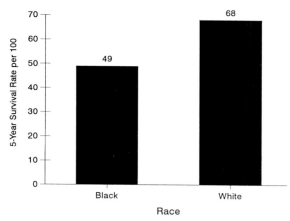

Figure 17–16. Five-year relative survival rates among breast cancer patients by race, women with breast cancer diagnosed 1964–1973 (SEER program). (Data from Shapiro S, Venet W, Strax P, et al: Prospects for eliminating racial differences in breast cancer survival rates. Am J Pub Health 72:1142–1145, 1982.)

may delay the diagnosis and treatment of the disease in black patients. Shapiro and colleagues recognized that the randomized trial of mammography offered an unusual opportunity to address this question. The findings are shown in Figure 17–17. Let us first look only at the survival curves for the control group, blacks and whites. The data are consistent with those in Figure 17–16: blacks and Hispanics had a worse prognosis than did whites. Now

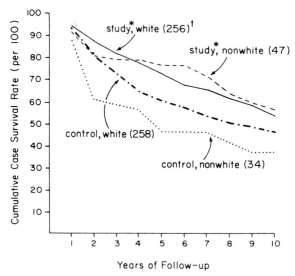

Figure 17–17. Cumulative case-survival rates, first 10 years after diagnosis by race, Health Insurance Plan (HIP) study and control groups. (From Shapiro S, Venet W, Strax P, et al: Prospects for eliminating racial differences in breast cancer survival rates. Am J Pub Health 72:1142–1145, 1982.)

let us look at the curves for whites and blacks in the study group of women who were screened and for whom there was therefore no difference in access to care or utilization of care, as screening was carried out on a regular schedule. We see considerable overlap of the two curves: essentially no difference. This strongly suggests that the screening had eliminated the racial difference in survivorship, and that the usually observed difference between the races in prognosis of breast cancer is in fact a result of poorer access to care or poorer utilization of care among blacks, with a consequent delay in diagnosis and treatment.

Screening for Cervical Cancer

Perhaps no screening test for cancer is employed more widely than the Pap smear. One would therefore assume that there has been overwhelming evidence of its effectiveness in reducing mortality from invasive cervical cancer. Unfortunately, there has never been a properly designed randomized, controlled trial of cervical cancer screening; and there probably never will be, because cervical cancer screening has been accepted as effective both by health authorities and by the public. This state of affairs is incredible, given the immense resources that have been invested worldwide in screening for cervical cancer.

At this point, one could not ethically do a randomized trial of Pap smears, despite the lack of conclusive evidence as to their effectiveness. In the absence of randomized trials, several alternative approaches have been used. Perhaps the most frequent evaluation design has been to compare incidence and mortality rates in populations with different rates of screening. A second approach has been to examine changes over time in rates of diagnosis of carcinoma in situ. A third approach has been that of case-control studies in which women with invasive cervical cancer are compared with control women, and the frequency of past Pap smears is examined in both groups. All of these studies are generally affected by the methodologic problems raised previously in this chapter.

Despite these reservations, the evidence indicates that many or most carcinomas in situ probably do progress to invasive cancer; consequently, early detection of cervical cancer in the in situ stage would result in a significant saving of life, even if it is lower than many optimistic estimates. Much of the uncertainty we face regarding screening for cervical cancer stems from the fact that no well-designed randomized trial was initially carried out. This observation points up that in the United States, a set of standards must be met before new pharmacologic agents are licensed for human use but another, less stringent, set of standards is used for new technology or new health programs. No drug would be licensed in the United States without evaluation through randomized, controlled trials, but no such evaluation is required before screening or other types of programs and procedures are introduced.

Screening for Neuroblastoma

Some of the issues just discussed are encountered in screening for neuroblastoma, which is a tumor that occurs in young children. The rationale for screening for neuroblastoma was outlined by Tuchman and colleagues[4]: (1) Outcome has improved little in the past several decades. (2) Prognosis is known to be better in children who manifest the disease before the age of 1 year. (3) At any age, children in advanced stages of disease have worse prognoses than those in early stages. (4) More than 90% of children presenting with clinical symptoms of neuroblastoma excrete higher than normal amounts of catecholamines in their urine. (5) These metabolites can easily be measured in urine samples obtained from diapers.

These facts constitute a strong rationale for neuroblastoma screening. Figure 17–18 shows data from Japan, where a major effort at neuroblastoma screening had been mounted. The percentages of children younger than 1 year in whom neuroblastoma was detected were compared before and

after initiation of screening in Sapporo, and these data were compared with birth data from Hokkaido, where no screening program was set up. After initiation of screening, a greater percentage of cases of neuroblastoma in children younger than 1 year was detected in Sapporo than in Hokkaido.

However, a number of serious problems arise in assessing the benefits of neuroblastoma screening. It is now clear that neuroblastoma is a biologically heterogeneous disease, and there is clearly a better prognosis from the start in some cases than in others. Many tumors have a good prognosis because they regress spontaneously, even without treatment. Furthermore, screening is most likely to detect slow-growing, less malignant tumors and is less likely to detect aggressive, fast-growing tumors. Thus, it is difficult to show that screening for neuroblastomas is, in fact, beneficial. These observations demonstrate the importance of an understanding of the biology and natural history of a disease when screening is being considered.

PROBLEMS IN ASSESSING THE SENSITIVITY AND SPECIFICITY OF TESTS

New screening programs are frequently initiated after a screening test becomes available for the first time. When such a test is developed, claims are often made—by manufacturers of test kits, investigators, or others—that the test has a high sensitivity and specificity. However, as we shall see, from a practical standpoint, this may often be difficult to demonstrate.

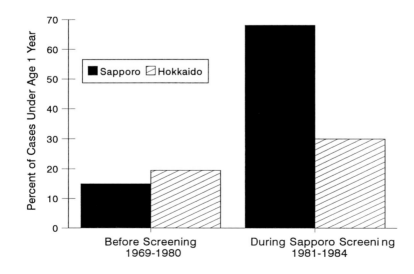

Figure 17–18. Percentage of neuroblastoma cases under 1 year of age in Sapporo and Hokkaido, Japan, before and after screening. (Adapted from Goodman SN: Neuroblastoma screening data. An epidemiologic analysis. AJDC 145:1415–1422, 1991, based on data from Nishi M, Miyake H, Takeda T, et al: Effects of the mass screening of neuroblastoma in Sapporo City. Cancer 60:433–436, 1987.)

Figure 17–19A shows a 2 × 2 table, as we have seen in earlier chapters, tabulating the reality (disease present or absent) against the test results (positive or negative).

To calculate sensitivity and specificity, data are needed in all four cells. However, often only those with positive test results ($a + b$) (seen in the *upper row* of the figure) are sent for further testing. Data for those who test negative ($c + d$) are frequently not available, because these patients do not receive further testing. For example, as shown in Figure 17–19B, the Western blot test serves as a gold standard for detecting human immunodeficiency virus (HIV) infection, and those with positive enzyme-linked immunosorbent assay (ELISA) results are sent for Western blot testing.

However, because those with negative ELISA results are generally not tested further, the data needed in the lower cells for calculating sensitivity and specificity are often not available from routine testing. To obtain such data, it is essential that some negative ELISA specimens also be sent for further testing, together with the ELISA-positive specimens.

The situation regarding the use of prostate-specific antigen (PSA) is even more difficult, as shown in Figure 17–19C. This test was originally used for monitoring response to treatment in patients with prostate cancer, but it has been used increasingly for detecting prostate cancer. But what are the sensitivity and specificity of the test in detecting prostate cancer?

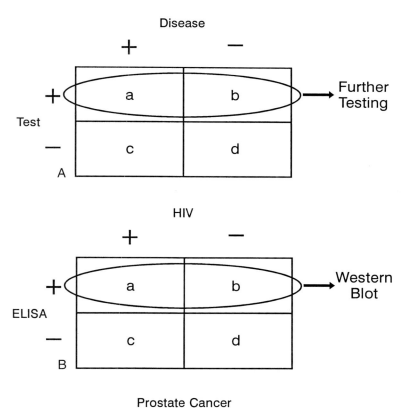

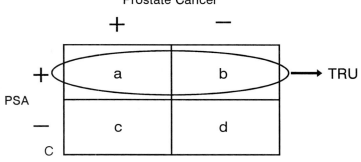

Figure 17–19. *A,* Problem of establishing sensitivity and specificity because of limited follow-up of those who test negative. *B,* Problem of establishing sensitivity and specificity because of limited follow-up of those who test negative for HIV using the ELISA test. *C,* Problem of establishing sensitivity and specificity because of limited follow-up of those who test negative using the prostate-specific antigen (PSA) test for prostatic cancer. TRU = transrectal ultrasound.

Men who have elevated PSA levels (positive test results) are often sent for further testing that includes transrectal ultrasound (TRU) and biopsy of the prostate. These procedures are expensive and are associated with pain and discomfort. Again, *only* those who have elevated PSA levels $(a + b)$ are sent for further testing, and data are missing for those with negative results $(c + d)$. In this case, however, in contrast to the situation for ELISA and Western blot tests, it is hard to conceive of a person with low PSA levels (normal results) being sent for TRU and biopsy solely to complete the data in the lower two cells. Hence, establishing the sensitivity and specificity of the PSA test is difficult at best.

INTERPRETING STUDY RESULTS THAT SHOW NO BENEFIT OF SCREENING

In this chapter thus far we have stressed the interpretation of results that show a difference between screened and unscreened groups. If, however, we are unable to demonstrate a benefit from early detection of disease, any of the following interpretations may be possible:

1. The apparent lack of benefit may be inherent in the natural history of the disease (e.g., the disease has no detectable preclinical phase or an extremely short detectable preclinical phase).
2. The therapeutic intervention currently available may not be any more effective when it is provided earlier than when it is provided at the time of usual diagnosis.
3. The natural history and currently available therapies may have the potential for enhanced benefit, but inadequacies of the care provided to those who screen positive may account for the observed lack of benefit (that is, there is efficacy, but poor effectiveness).

COST-BENEFIT ANALYSIS OF SCREENING

Some people respond to cost-benefit issues by concentrating only on cost, saying, If the test is cheap, why not perform it? However, although the test for blood in the stool, for example, in screening for colon cancer, costs only a few dollars for the filter paper kit and the necessary laboratory processing, to calculate the total cost of such a test we must include the cost of the colonoscopies that are done after the inital testing as well as the cost

of the complications that infrequently result from colonoscopy.

The balance of cost-effectiveness includes not only financial costs, but also non-financial costs to the patient, including anxiety, emotional distress, and inconvenience. Is the test itself invasive? Even if it is not, if the test result is positive, is invasive therapy warranted by the test result? What is the false-positive rate in such tests; that is, in what proportion of persons will invasive tests be carried out and/or anxiety be generated despite the reality that the individuals do not have the disease in question? Thus, the "cost" of a test is not just of the test procedure, but also the cost of the entire follow-up process that is set in motion by a positive result, even if it turns out to be a false-positive result. These considerations are reflected in the criteria used by the American Cancer Society for its 1980 recommendations on cancer-related check-ups (Table 17–3).

CONCLUSION

This chapter has reviewed some of the major sources of bias that must be taken into account in assessing study findings that compare screened and unscreened populations. The biases of selection for screening and prognostic selection can be addressed in large part by using a randomized, controlled trial as the study design. Reasonable estimates of the lead time can be made if appropriate information is available. Few of the methods currently employed for detecting disease early have been subjected to evaluation by randomized, controlled trials, and most are probably not destined to be. This is a result of several factors, including the difficulty and expense of conducting such studies and the ethical issues inherent in randomizing a population to receive or not receive modalities of care that are widely used and considered effective, even in the

Table 17–3. Criteria Used by the American Cancer Society for its 1980 Recommendations on Cancer-Related Check-up

1. There must be good evidence that each test or procedure recommended is medically effective in reducing morbidity or mortality.
2. The medical benefits must outweigh the risks.
3. The cost of each test or procedure must be reasonable compared with its expected benefits.
4. The recommended actions must be practical and feasible.

absence of strong supporting evidence. Consequently, we are obliged to maximize our use of evidence from non-randomized approaches, and to do so, the potential biases and problems discussed in this chapter must be taken into account.

In approaching programs of early disease detection, we need to be able to identify groups who are at high risk. This would include not only those at risk for developing the disease in question, but also those who are "at risk" of benefiting from the intervention. These are the groups for whom cost-benefit calculations will favor benefit. We must keep in mind that even if the screening test is not in itself invasive (e.g., Pap smear), the intervention mandated by a positive screening test result may be highly invasive (e.g., conization).

The overriding issue is how to make decisions when our data are inconclusive, inconsistent, or incomplete. We face this dilemma regularly, both in clinical practice and in the development of public health policy. These decisions must first take into consideration the existing body of relevant scientific evidence. In the last analysis, however, the decision of whether or not to screen for a disease is a value judgment that should take into account the incidence of the disease and its severity, the feasibility of detecting the disease early, the feasibility of intervening effectively in those with positive screening results, and the overall cost-benefit calculation for an early detection program.

To improve our ability to make appropriate decisions, additional research is needed regarding the natural history of disease and, specifically, regarding the definition of characteristics of individuals who are at risk for having a poor outcome. Before new screening programs are introduced, we should argue strongly for well-conducted randomized, controlled trials, so that we will not be operating in an atmosphere of uncertainty at the time in the future when such trials have become virtually impossible to conduct. Nevertheless, given the fact that most medical and public health practice—including early detection of disease—has not been subjected to randomized trials, and that decisions regarding early detection must be made on the basis of incomplete and equivocal data, it is essential that we as health professionals appreciate and understand the methodologic issues involved so that we can make the wisest use of the available knowledge on behalf of our patients. Even the best of intentions and passionate evangelism cannot substitute for rigorous evidence that supports the benefit of screening.

References

1. Hutchison GB: Evaluation of preventive services. J Chron Dis 11:497–508, 1960.
2. Shapiro S, Venet W, Strax P, Venet L (eds): Periodic Screening for Breast Cancer: The Health Insurance Plan Project and its Sequelae, 1963–86. Baltimore, Johns Hopkins University Press, 1988.
3. Shapiro S, Venet W, Strax P, et al: Prospects for eliminating racial differences in breast cancer survival rates. Am J Pub Health 72:1142–1145, 1982.
4. Tuchman M, Lemieus B, Woods WG: Screening for neuroblastoma in infants: Investigate or implement? Pediatrics 86:791–793, 1990.

Review Questions

Questions 1 through 4 are based on the information given below:

A new screening program was instituted in a certain country. The program used a screening test that is effective in detecting cancer Z at an early stage. Assume that there is no effective treatment for this type of cancer and, therefore, that the program results in no change in the usual course of the disease. Assume also that the rates noted are calculated from all known cases of cancer Z and that there were no changes in the quality of death certification of this disease.

1. What will happen to the apparent *incidence rate* of cancer Z in the country during the first year of this program?

   a. Incidence rate will increase
   b. Incidence rate will decrease
   c. Incidence rate will remain constant

2. What will happen to the apparent *prevalence rate* of cancer Z in the country during the first year of this program?
   a. Prevalence rate will increase
   b. Prevalence rate will decrease
   c. Prevalence rate will remain constant

3. What will happen to the apparent *case fatality rate* for cancer Z in the country during the first year of this program?
   a. Case fatality rate will increase
   b. Case fatality rate will decrease
   c. Case fatality rate will remain constant

4. What will happen to the apparent *mortality rate* from cancer Z in the country as a result of the program?

   a. Mortality rate will increase

   b. Mortality rate will decrease

   c. Mortality rate will remain constant

5. The best index (indices) for concluding that an early detection program for breast cancer truly improves the natural history of disease, 15 years after its initiation, would be:

   a. A smaller proportionate mortality for breast cancer 15 years after initiation of the early detection program compared to the proportionate mortality prior to its initiation

   b. Improved long-term survival rates for breast cancer patients (adjusted for lead time)

   c. A decrease in incidence of breast cancer

   d. A decrease in the prevalence of breast cancer

   e. None of the above

6. In general, screening should be undertaken for diseases with the following feature(s):

   a. Diseases with a low prevalence in identifiable subgroups of the population

   b. Diseases for which case fatality rates are low

   c. Diseases with a natural history that can be altered by medical intervention

   d. Diseases that are readily diagnosed and for which treatment efficacy has been shown to be equivocal in evidence from a number of clinical trials

   e. None of the above

7. Which of the following is *not* a possible outcome measure that could be used as an indicator of the benefit of screening programs aimed at early detection of disease?

   a. Reduction of case-fatality in screened individuals

   b. Reduction of mortality in the population screened

   c. Reduction of incidence in the population screened

   d. Reduction of complications

   e. Improvement in the quality of life in screened individuals

---

Question 8 is based on the information given below:

This diagram shows the natural history of disease X:

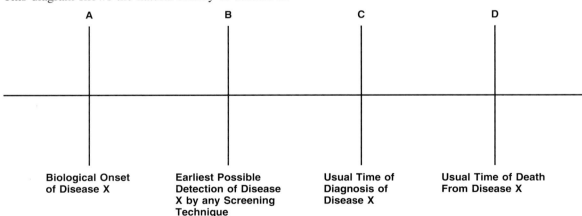

8. Assume that early detection of disease X through screening improves prognosis. In order for a screening program to be most effective, at which point in the natural history diagrammed above must the critical point be?

   a. Between A and B

   b. Between B and C

   c. Between C and D

   d. Anywhere between A and C

   e. Anywhere between A and D

CHAPTER 18

Epidemiology and Public Policy

A major role of epidemiology is to serve as a basis for developing policies that affect human health, including the prevention and control of disease. As seen in previous chapters, the findings from epidemiologic studies may be relevant both to issues in clinical practice and community health and to population approaches to disease prevention and health promotion. As discussed in Chapter 1, the practical applications of epidemiology are often viewed as being so integral to the discipline that they are incorporated into the very definition of epidemiology. Historically, epidemiologic investigations were initiated to address emerging challenges relating to human disease and the public health. Indeed, one of the major sources of excitement in epidemiology is the direct applicability of its findings to the alleviation of problems of human health. This chapter presents an overview of some issues and problems relating to epidemiology in its application to the formulation and evaluation of public policy.

EPIDEMIOLOGY AND PREVENTION

The importance of epidemiology in prevention has been emphasized in several of the preceding chapters. Identifying populations at increased risk, ascertaining the cause of their increased risk, and analyzing the costs and benefits of eliminating or reducing exposure to the causal factor or factors all require an understanding of basic epidemiologic concepts and of the possible interpretation of the findings of epidemiologic studies. In addition, assessing the strength of the evidence and identifying any limits on the inferences derived or on the generalizability of the findings is of critical importance. Thus, epidemiology can be considered to be the "basic science" of prevention.

How much epidemiologic data do we need to justify a prevention effort? Clearly, there is no easy answer to this question. Some of the issues involved are different depending on whether primary or secondary prevention is being considered. If we are discussing primary prevention, the answer depends on the seriousness of the condition, on the costs involved (in terms of dollars, human suffering, and loss of quality of life), on the strength of the evidence that implicates a certain causal factor or factors in the etiology of the disease in question, and on the difficulty of reducing or eliminating exposure to that factor.

With secondary prevention, the issues are somewhat different. We must still consider the severity of the disease in question. In addition, however, we must ask whether we can detect the disease earlier than usual, how invasive and expensive such detection would be, and whether a benefit accrues to a person who has the disease if treatment is initiated at an earlier-than-usual stage. Epidemiology is clearly an invaluable approach to resolving many of these issues.

In the final analysis, however, deciding how much data we need will be societally driven—dependent on a society's values and priorities. Epidemiology, together with other disciplines, can provide the necessary and relevant scientific data regarding a question of prevention. However, the final decision as to whether to initiate a prevention program will, it is hoped, use the scientific evidence, but it will be strongly influenced by economic and political considerations as well as by societal values.

POPULATION VS. HIGH-RISK APPROACHES TO PREVENTION

An important question in prevention is whether our approach should target groups that are known to be at high risk or whether it should extend primary prevention efforts to the general population as a whole. This issue was discussed by Rose in 1985[1] and later amplified by Whelton in 1994[2] in a discussion of hypertension prevention and prevention of deaths from coronary heart disease (CHD).

Epidemiologic studies have demonstrated that the risk of death from CHD steadily increases with increases in both systolic and diastolic blood pressure; there is no known threshold. Figure 18–1A shows the distribution of systolic blood pressures in 347,978 men who were screened for the Multiple Risk Factor Intervention Trial (MRFIT).

Figure 18–1B shows the risk of CHD mortality in relation to systolic blood pressure in this group; the risk increases steadily with higher blood pressure levels. Individuals with blood pressures of 180 mm Hg or higher had 5.65 times the risk of CHD death than those whose blood pressure was below 110 mm Hg. Figure 18–1C shows the numbers and percentages of excess CHD deaths due to hypertension at each blood pressure level. (Those with blood pressure below 110 mm Hg are defined as having no excess deaths.) Although fewer than one fourth of all individuals had hypertension, they accounted for more than two thirds of the excess CHD deaths. These observations argue for directing our preventive efforts to those at the highest extremes of systolic blood pressure, who have the highest relative risk.

However, almost 80% of the hypertensive persons had blood pressure in the 140 to 159 mm Hg range (stage 1). Stage 1 hypertension accounted for about 43% of the excess risk of dying from CHD in the total population and for almost 64% of the excess CHD death risk among hypertensive subjects. Thus, if we wish to address the overall burden of CHD deaths associated with elevated blood pressure, it is not enough to direct preventive efforts at those with the highest extremes of blood pressure. We also need to focus on those with less marked elevations in blood pressure if we are to prevent most of the excess deaths associated with increased blood pressure.

It therefore seems reasonable to combine a high-risk with a population approach: one set of preventive measures addressed to those at particularly high risk and another designed for primary prevention of hypertension and addressed to the population in general.

Such analyses can have significant implications for prevention programs. The types of preventive measures that might be used for high-risk individu-

als differ from those that are applicable to the general population. Those who are at high risk and know they are at high risk are more likely to tolerate more expensive, uncomfortable, and even more invasive procedures. However, in applying a preventive measure to a general population, the measure must have a low cost and be only minimally invasive; it needs to be associated with relatively little pain or discomfort if it is to be acceptable to the general population.

Figure 18–2 shows the goal of a population-based strategy, which is a downward shifting of the entire curve of blood pressure distribution when a blood pressure–lowering intervention is applied to an entire community. Because the blood pressure of most members of the population is above the very lowest levels that are considered optimal, even a small downward shift (shift to the left) in the curve is likely to have major public health benefits. In fact, such a shift would prevent more strokes in the population than would successful treatment limited to ''high-risk'' individuals. Furthermore, Rose[1] pointed out that the ''high-risk'' strategy is an interim expedient that is necessary for the protection of susceptible individuals. Ultimately, however, our hope is to understand the basic causes of the incidence of the disease—in this case, elevated blood pressure—and to develop and implement the necessary means for its (primary) prevention. Rose concluded that

> *Realistically, many diseases will long continue to call for both approaches, and fortunately competition between them is usually unnecessary. Nevertheless, the priority of concern should always be the discovery and control of the causes of incidence.*

EPIDEMIOLOGY, CLINICAL MEDICINE, AND OUTCOMES RESEARCH

Epidemiology can be considered the basic science of clinical investigation. Epidemiologic data are essential in clinical decision making in many situations. An understanding of epidemiology is crucial to designing meaningful studies of the natural history of disease, the quality of different diagnostic methods, and the effectiveness of clinical interventions.

Assessing the effectiveness of different modalities of therapy is ideally done through randomized clinical trials. However, for a variety of reasons, it is clear that randomized studies are not always

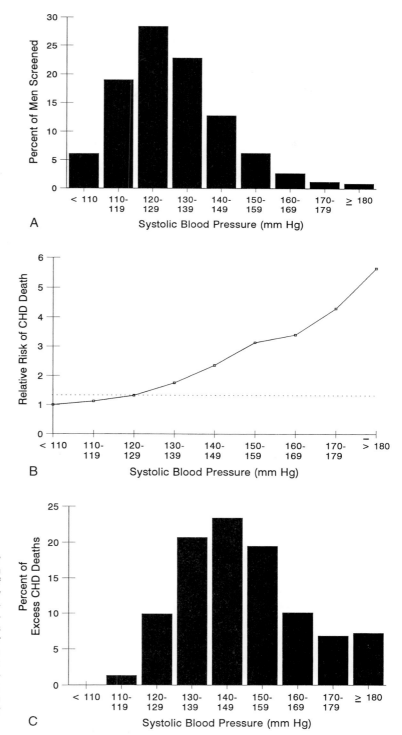

Figure 18–1. *A,* Percent distribution by baseline systolic blood pressure of men screened for MRFIT. *B,* Relative risk of coronary heart disease (CHD) mortality in relation to level of systolic blood pressure in men screened for MRFIT. *C,* Percent distribution of excess CHD deaths by level of systolic blood pressure for men screened for MRFIT. (Adapted from Stamler J, Dyer AR, Shekelle RB, et al: Relationship of baseline major risk factors to coronary and all-cause mortality, and to longevity: Findings from long-term follow-up of Chicago cohorts. Cardiology 82:191–222, 1993.)

possible. Moreover, there is often a long interval between the initiation of such trials and the availability of the results of such studies. Frequently, strong pressures are brought to bear for immediate answers to pressing questions regarding benefits and costs. As a result, in recent years there has been an increasing use of non-randomized observational studies for answering questions of effectiveness of

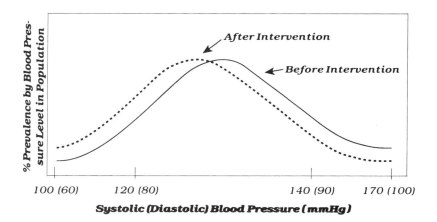

Figure 18–2. Representation of the effects of a population-based intervention strategy on the distribution of blood pressure. (From National Institutes of Health: Working Group Report on Primary Prevention of Hypertension, NIH publication No. 93–2669. Washington, DC, National Heart, Lung, and Blood Institute, 1993, p 8.)

care. These studies often use large existing data bases that are available from health insurers, health maintenance organizations, and drug manufacturers. The availability of such large data sets has made this approach attractive to many investigators. The term *outcomes research* has been applied to such studies.

Despite the popularity of this approach, however, outcomes research has elicited considerable controversy. The problems inherent in non-randomized epidemiologic studies, as discussed in detail previously, are particularly important when applied to assessing the effectiveness of medical care. In particular, in the absence of randomization, the potential for significant selection bias regarding who receives a certain drug or type of care generally cannot be eliminated and may be difficult or impossible to assess. Furthermore, the records that are utilized were often designed for billing or for other administrative purposes and not for research. As a result, they may lack critical relevant information that may be necessary for adequate analysis, including consideration of possible confounders. At this time, the potentials and limitations of outcomes research have not yet been adequately explored, so that conclusions based on such studies must be viewed with care.

RISK ASSESSMENT

A major use of epidemiology in relation to public policy is for risk assessment. Risk assessment has been defined as the characterization of the potential adverse health effects of human exposures to environmental hazards. Risk assessment is viewed as part of an overall process that flows from research to risk assessment and then to risk management, as shown in Figure 18–3.

The National Research Council (1983) listed four steps in the risk assessment process[3]:

1. *Hazard identification:* Determination of whether a particular chemical is or is not causally linked to particular health effects.
2. *Dose-response assessment:* Determination of the relationship between the magnitude of exposure and the probability of occurrence of the health effects in question.
3. *Exposure assessment:* Determination of the extent of human exposure before or after application of regulatory controls.
4. *Risk characterization:* Description of the nature, and often the magnitude, of human risk, including attendant uncertainty.

Clearly, epidemiologic data are essential in each of these steps, although epidemiology is not the only relevant scientific discipline in the risk-assessment process. In particular, toxicology plays a major role as well, and an important challenge remains to reconcile epidemiologic and toxicologic data when findings from the respective disciplines do not agree.

A number of important methodologic problems affect the use of epidemiology in risk assessment. Because epidemiologic studies generally address the relationship between an environmental exposure and the risk of a disease, rigorous assessment of each variable is critical. Perhaps the most significant problem is that of assessment of exposure.

Assessment of Exposure

It is important to distinguish between *macroenvironmental* and *microenvironmental* exposures.

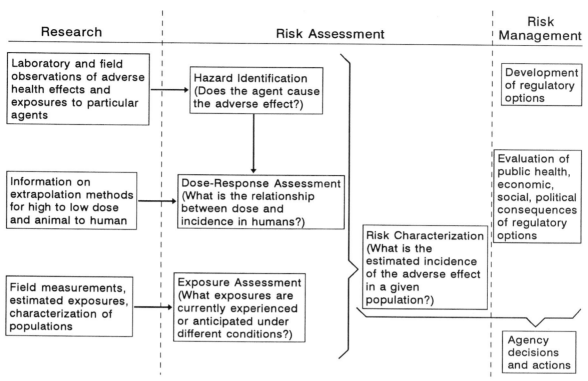

Figure 18–3. Relations among the four steps of risk assessment and between risk assessment and risk management. (Adapted from Committee on the Institutional Means for Assessment of Risks to Public Health, Commission on Life Sciences, National Research Council: Risk Assessment in the Federal Government: Managing the Process. Washington, DC, National Academy Press, 1983, p 21.)

Macroenvironmental exposures refer to exposures such as air pollution, which affect populations or entire communities. Microenvironmental exposures refer to environmental factors that affect a specific individual, such as diet, smoking, and alcohol consumption. From the prevention standpoint, macroenvironmental factors are in many ways easier to control and modify, as this can be accomplished by regulation (e.g., setting environmental standards for pollutants). In contrast, modification of microenvironmental factors depends on modifying individual habits and lifestyle, which is often a much greater challenge.

Data regarding exposure generally come from several types of sources (Table 18–1). Each type of source has advantages and disadvantages; the latter include lack of completeness and biases in reporting. Frequently, investigators utilize several sources of information regarding exposure, but a problem often results when different sources yield conflicting information.

Another problem in exposure assessment is that macroenvironmental factors generally affect many individuals simultaneously, so that individual expo-

sures may be difficult to measure. As a result, ecologic approaches are often used in which aggregate rather than individual measurements are used, and the aggregation is often carried out over large areas. The characteristics of the community are therefore ascribed to the individuals residing in that community, but the validity of characterizing an individual exposure by this process is often open to question. Furthermore, personal exposure histories are difficult to obtain either retrospectively or prospectively. In addition, the long latent or induction period between exposure and development of disease may make ascertainment of a long-past exposure particularly difficult.

Table 18–1. Sources of Exposure Data

1. Interviews
   a. Subject
   b. Surrogate
2. Employment or other records
3. Physician records
4. Hospital records
5. Disease registry records (e.g., cancer registries)
6. Death certificates

A somewhat parallel set of problems is seen when we try to characterize the occupational exposures of an individual worker and to link an exposure at work to an adverse health outcome. First, because a worker is likely to be exposed to many different agents in an industrial setting, it is often difficult to segregate the risk that can be ascribed to a single specific exposure. Second, because a long latent period often exists between the exposure and the subsequent development of disease, studies of the exposure-disease relationship may be difficult; for example, recall may be poor and records of exposure may have been lost. Third, increased disease risks may occur among those living near an industrial plant, so that it may be difficult to ascertain how much of a worker's risk results from living near the plant and how much is due to an occupational exposure in the work setting itself.

Perhaps the most fundamental problem in measuring exposures in epidemiologic studies is that all of the sources and measures discussed so far are indirect. For example, considerable interest has arisen in recent years over the possible health effects of electromagnetic fields (EMF). This interest followed the article of Wertheimer and Leeper in 1979,[4] which reported increased levels of leukemia in children living near high-voltage transmission lines. Subsequently, many methodologic questions have been raised, and the question of whether such fields are associated with adverse health effects remains unresolved.

In studying EMF, several approaches are used for measuring exposure, including the wiring configuration in the home, spot or 24-hour measurements of the fields, or self-reports of electrical appliance use. However, the results of different studies regarding risk of disease differ depending on the type of exposure measurement that was employed. In fact, actual magnetic field measurements, even 24-hour measurements, generate weaker associations with childhood leukemia than do those for wire configuration codes. This observation raises a question about any possible causal link between exposure to magnetic fields and occurrence of disease.

Even the best indirect measure of exposure often leaves critical questions unanswered. First, exposure is generally not dichotomous; data are therefore needed regarding the *dose* of exposure to explore a possible dose-response relationship. Second, it is important to know whether the exposure was continuous or periodic. For example, in the pathogenesis of cancer, a periodic exposure with alternat-ing exposure and non-exposure periods may allow for DNA repair during the non-exposure periods; in a continuous exposure, no such repair could take place. Finally, information about latency is critical: How long is the latent period and what is its range? This is essential so that we can focus efforts at ascertaining exposure on a time period that seems to be one in which a causal exposure might well have occurred.

Because of these problems in measuring exposure using indirect approaches, much interest has focused on the use of biologic markers of exposures. (Use of such biomarkers has been termed *biochemical epidemiology* or *molecular epidemiology*.) The advantage of using biomarkers is that such use can overcome the problem of limited recall or lack of awareness of an exposure. In addition, biomarkers can overcome errors resulting from variation in individual absorption or metabolism by focusing on a later step in the causal chain.

Biomarkers can be markers of exposure, markers of biologic changes resulting from exposures, or markers of risk or susceptibility. Figure 18–4 exemplifies schematically the different types of exposure we may choose to measure.

We might measure ambient levels of possibly toxic substances in a general environment, the levels to which a specific individual is exposed, the amount of substance absorbed, or the amount of substance or metabolite of the absorbed substance that reaches the target tissue. Biomarkers bring us closer to being able to measure an exposure at a specific stage in the process by which an exposure is linked to human disease. For example, we can measure not only environmental levels of a substance, but also DNA adducts that reflect bodily processes after absorption.

Nevertheless, despite these advantages, biomarkers generally give us a dichotomous answer—a person was either exposed or not exposed. Biomarkers generally do not shed light on several important questions, such as the following:

What was the total exposure dose?
What was the duration of exposure?
How long ago did the exposure occur?

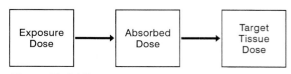

Figure 18–4. What exposures are we trying to measure?

Was the exposure continuous or periodic?

The answers to these questions are crucial in properly interpreting the potential biologic importance of a given exposure.

It should be pointed out that use of biomarkers is not new in epidemiology. In Ecclesiastes it is written: "There is nothing new under the sun."[5] Even before the revolution in molecular biology took place, laboratory techniques were essential in many epidemiologic studies; these included bacterial isolations and cultures, phage typing of organisms, viral isolation, serologic studies, and assays of cholesterol lipoprotein fractions. With the tremendous advances made in molecular biology, a new variety of biomarkers have become available that are relevant to areas such as carcinogenesis. These biomarkers not only identify exposed individuals, but they also cast new light on the pathogenetic process of the disease in question.

META-ANALYSIS

Several scientific questions arise in using epidemiologic data for the formulation of public policy and need to be addressed:

1. Can epidemiologic methods detect small increases in risk?
2. How can we reconcile inconsistencies between animal and human data?
3. How can we use incomplete or equivocal epidemiologic data?
4. How can results be interpreted when epidemiologic studies disagree?

Many of the risks with which we are dealing may be very small, but they may potentially be of great public health importance because of the large numbers of people exposed and a concomitant potential for adverse health effects in many people. However, an observed small increase in relative risk above 1.0 may easily result from bias or other methodologic limitations, and such results must therefore be interpreted with great caution in the absence of replication of the results and other confirmatory evidence.

Given that the results of different epidemiologic studies may not be consistent, and that at times they may be in dramatic conflict, attempts have been made to systematize the process of reviewing the epidemiologic literature on a given topic. This process is called *meta-analysis,* and has been defined as "the statistical analysis of a large collection of analysis results from individual studies for the purpose of integrating the findings."[6] Meta-analysis allows for aggregation of the results of a set of studies with appropriate weighting of each study for the number of subjects sampled and for other characteristics. Meta-analysis can increase the statistical power, particularly for certain outcomes and certain subgroups. It can also help to give an overall perspective on an issue when studies disagree.

However, a number of problems and questions are associated with meta-analysis. First, should only published studies be included in the analysis, or should any available studies be used? Second, how can we handle the problem that the reviewed and aggregated studies may differ considerably in quality? Third, when the relative risks or odds ratios resulting from various studies differ, meta-analysis may mask important differences among individual studies. It is therefore essential that a meta-analysis not replace a rigorous examination of each study included in the analysis, including scrutiny of the results and the methodologic limitations of each study. Fourth, the results of meta-analyses themselves are not always reproducible by other analysts. Finally, meta-analysis is subject to the problem of publication bias, discussed in the next section of this chapter. Figure 18–5 shows the type of diagrammatic presentation that is frequently used to show the results of individual studies as well as the results of the meta-analysis.

Meta-analysis has been most frequently applied to randomized trials, but is being used increasingly to aggregate non-randomized observational studies, including case-control and cohort studies. In the latter instances, the studies do not necessarily share

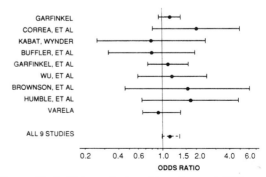

Figure 18–5. Meta-analysis: odds ratios and 95% confidence intervals for nine U.S. epidemiologic studies of the hypothesized association between exposure to environmental tobacco smoke and lung cancer. (From Fleiss JL, Gross AJ: Meta-analysis in epidemiology, with special reference to studies of the association between exposure to environmental tobacco smoke and lung cancer: A critique. J Clin Epidemiol 44:127–139, 1991.)

a common research design. Hence, the question arises as to the necessary degree of similarity between studies to legitimately include them in a meta-analysis. In addition, appropriate control of biases (such as selection bias and misclassification bias) is essential, but often proves a formidable challenge in meta-analyses. In view of the considerations just discussed, meta-analysis remains a subject of considerable controversy.

A final problem with meta-analysis is that in the face of all the difficulties discussed, putting a quantitative imprint on the estimation of a single relative risk or odds ratio from all the studies may lead to a false sense of certainty regarding the magnitude of the risk. People often tend to have an inordinate belief in the validity of findings when a number is attached to them and many of the difficulties which arise in meta-analysis may be ignored as a result.

PUBLICATION BIAS

An earlier chapter discussed the use of twin studies as a means of distinguishing the contributions of environmental and genetic factors to the cause of disease. In that discussion it was mentioned that the degree of concordance and discordance in twins is an important observation for drawing conclusions about the role of genetic factors, but that estimates of concordance reported in the literature may be inflated by publication bias, which is the tendency for articles to be published that report concordance for rare diseases in twin pairs.

Publication bias is not limited to studies of twins; it can occur in any area. It is a particularly important phenomenon in publication of articles regarding environmental risks and in publication of the results of clinical trials. Publication bias may occur because investigators do not submit the results of their studies when the findings do not support "positive" associations and increased risks. In addition, journals may select for publication studies that they believe to be of greatest reader interest, and they may not find studies that report no association to fall in this category. As a result, a literature review that is limited to published articles may preferentially identify studies that report increased risk. Clearly, such a review is highly selective in nature and omits many studies that have obtained what have been called "negative" results (i.e., results showing no effect), which may not have reached publication.

Publication bias therefore has a clear effect on meta-analysis. One approach to this problem is to try to identify unpublished studies and to include them in the analysis. However, the difficulty here is that such studies have not passed journal peer review, and their suitability for inclusion in a meta-analysis is therefore questionable. Regardless of whether we are discussing a traditional type of literature review or a structured meta-analysis, the problem of potential publication bias must be kept in mind.

EPIDEMIOLOGY IN THE COURTS

As mentioned earlier, litigation has become a major path for policy making in the United States. Epidemiology is assuming an ever increasing importance in the legal arena. Particularly in the area of toxic torts, it provides one of the major types of scientific evidence that is relevant to the questions involved. Issues such as effects of dioxin, silicone breast implants, and electromagnetic fields are but a few recent examples.

However, the use of data from epidemiologic studies is not without its problems. Epidemiology answers questions about *groups*, whereas the court often requires information about *individuals*. Furthermore, considerable attention has been directed to the court's interpretation of evidence of causality. Whereas the legal criterion is often "more likely than not"—that is, that the substance or exposure in question is "more likely than not" to have caused a person's disease, epidemiology relies to a great extent on the U.S. Surgeon General's guidelines for causal inferences.[7] It has been suggested that an attributable risk of greater than 50% might constitute evidence of "more likely than not."[8]

Until recently, evidence from epidemiology was only reluctantly accepted in the courts, but this has changed to a point where epidemiologic data are often cited as the only source of relevant evidence in toxic tort cases. For many years, the guiding principle for using scientific evidence in the courts was the Frye test, which stated that for a study to be admissible "it must be sufficiently established to have gained general acceptance in the field in which it belongs."[9] Although terms such as "general acceptance" and "field in which it belongs" were left undefined, it did lead to an assessment of whether the scientific opinion expressed by an expert witness was generally accepted by other professionals in the discipline.

In 1993, in Daubert vs. Merrell Dow Pharmaceuticals,[10] a case in which the plaintiff alleged that a limb deformity at birth was due to ingestion of the drug Bendectin during pregnancy, the U.S. Supreme Court articulated a major change in rules of evidence. The court ruled that "general acceptance" is not a necessary condition for the admissibility of scientific evidence in court. Rather, the trial judge is now assigned the task of ensuring that an expert's testimony rests on a reliable foundation and is relevant to the "task at hand." Thus the judge "must make a preliminary assessment of whether the testimony's underlying reasoning or methodology is scientifically valid and properly can be applied to the facts at issue." Among the considerations cited by the court are whether the theory or technique in question can be and has been tested and whether the methodology has been subjected to peer review and publication.

Given their new responsibilities, judges presiding at trials in which epidemiology is a major source of evidence will need to have a basic knowledge of epidemiologic concepts, including, for example, study design, biases and confounding, and causal inferences, if they are to be able to rule in a sound fashion on whether the approach used by the experts follows accepted "scientific method." Recognizing this need, the Federal Judicial Center has published a Manual on Scientific Evidence for judges that includes a section on Epidemiology.[11] Although it is too early to know what the ultimate effect of the Daubert ruling will be, given the tremendous increase in the use of epidemiology in the courts, the ruling will clearly require enhanced knowledge of epidemiology by many parties involved in legal proceedings that use evidence derived from epidemiologic studies.

POLICY ISSUES REGARDING RISK: WHAT SHOULD THE OBJECTIVES BE?

Public policy is often recognized to be largely made through the processes of legislation and regulation. As discussed earlier, in the United States, litigation has also become an important instrument for developing and implementing public policy. Ideally, each of these processes should reflect societal values and aspirations.

Certain major societal issues must be dealt with in making decisions about risk. Among the questions that must be confronted are the following:

1. What percentage of the population should be protected by the policy?
2. What level of risk is society willing to tolerate?
3. What level of control of risk is society willing to pay for?
4. Who should make decisions about risk?

Although at first glance it might seem appealing to protect the entire population from any amount of risk, in realistic terms this is difficult—if not impossible—to accomplish. Regardless of what we learn from risk data about populations, there are clearly rare individuals who are extraordinarily sensitive to minute concentrations of certain chemicals. If the permissible amount of a chemical is to be set at a level that protects *every* worker, it is possible that entire manufacturing processes may be halted. Similarly, if we demand zero risk for workers or for others who may be exposed, the economic base of many communities might be destroyed. Policymaking therefore requires a balance between what *can* be done and what *should* be done. The degree of priority attached to elimination of all risk and the decision as to what percent of risk should be eliminated clearly are not scientific decisions, but rather depend on societal values. It is hoped that such societal decisions will capitalize on available scientific knowledge in the context of political, economic, ethical, and other considerations.

CONCLUSION

The objectives of epidemiology are to enhance our understanding of the biology and pathogenesis of disease to improve human health and to prevent and treat disease. A thorough understanding of the methodologic issues that arise is essential for the proper interpretation of epidemiologic results as a basis for policy formulation in both the clinical and the public health arenas. The appropriate and judicious use of the results of epidemiologic studies is fundamental to an assessment of risk to human health and to the control of these risks and, concomitantly, to both primary and secondary prevention. Policymakers are often obliged to develop policy in the presence of incomplete or equivocal scientific data. In clinical medicine, both in the diagnostic and the therapeutic processes, decisions are often made with incomplete or equivocal data; this has perhaps been more of an overt impediment in public health and community medicine. No simple set of rules can eliminate this difficulty. As H.L. Mencken wrote: ''There is always an easy solution to every human problem—neat, plausible, and wrong.''[12] A major challenge remains to develop the best process for formulating rational policies under such circumstances, both in clinical medicine and public health.

References

1. Rose G: Sick individuals and sick populations. Int J Epidemiol 14:22–38, 1985.
2. Whelton PK: Epidemiology of hypertension. Lancet 344:101–106, 1994.
3. Committee on the Institutional Means for Assessment of Risks to Public Health: Risk Assessment in the Federal Government: Managing the Process. Washington, DC, National Academy Press, 1983, p 21.
4. Wertheimer N, Leeper E: Electrical wiring configurations and childhood cancer. Am J Epidemiol 109:273–284, 1979.
5. Ecclesiastes 1:9.
6. Glass GV: Primary, secondary and meta-analysis of research. Educ Res 5:3–8, 1976.
7. United States Department of Health, Education and Welfare, Smoking and Health: Report of the Advisory Committee to the Surgeon General. Washington, DC, Public Health Service, 1964.
8. Black B, Lilienfeld DE: Epidemiology proof in toxic tort litigation. Fordham Law Rev 52:732–785, 1984.
9. Frye v. United States, 293F. 1013 (D.C. Cir. 1923).
10. Daubert v. Merrell Dow Pharmaceuticals, Inc., 113 S. Ct. 2786 (1993).,
11. Bailey L, Gordis L, Green M: Reference Guide on Epidemiology, in Reference Manual on Scientific Evidence. Washington, DC, Federal Judicial Center, 1994.
12. Mencken HL: The divine afflatus. The New York Evening Mail, Nov 16, 1917. (Essay reprinted in Mencken HL: Prejudices, series 2. New York, Alfred A. Knopf, 1920.)

CHAPTER 19

Ethical and Professional Issues in Epidemiology

The changing social and scientific context in which epidemiologic research is being conducted has led to new challenges for those working in epidemiology, for those who utilize the results of epidemiologic studies, and for the general public. This chapter reviews some of the ethical and professional issues that are critical both for epidemiologic research and for the application of its results for the improvement of human health.

Clearly, in any scientific discipline, fraud, deceit, or misrepresentation elicit universal disapproval and condemnation from other members of the discipline, from other professionals, and from the lay public. Such issues are not discussed in this chapter. The most difficult ethical dilemmas relating to epidemiology that arise today are likely to be more subtle, involving elements of judgment, philosophy, attitude, and opinion, for which consensus may be more difficult to obtain.

Does epidemiology differ from other scientific disciplines in regard to ethical issues? Although epidemiology shares many problems with other scientific disciplines, it has certain unusual if not unique characteristics. It is a discipline that largely grew out of medicine and public health, and even in its earliest years its findings had immediate policy implications for clinical care or public health action. John Snow's studies of cholera in London and his removal of the handle of the Broad Street pump, whether actually done before or after the crest of the outbreak, reflected the clear policy implications of his work.

The ultimate objective of epidemiology is to improve human health; epidemiology is the basic science of disease prevention. Hence, the relationship of epidemiology to development of public policy is integral to the discipline. As a result, the ethical and professional issues go beyond those that might apply to a scientific discipline such as biophysics or physiology and must be viewed in a broader context. First, epidemiologic findings have direct and often immediate societal relevance. Second, epidemiologic studies are generally funded from public resources. Third, epidemiologic research involves human subjects in one way or another and subjects who participate in epidemiologic studies generally derive no benefit personally from the results of the studies.

This chapter discusses two types of issues: those that relate to the actual conduct of epidemiologic studies and those that relate to broader societal issues, which go beyond the actual epidemiologic research itself.

OBLIGATIONS TO STUDY SUBJECTS

What are the investigator's obligations to the subjects in the non-randomized observational studies with which most epidemiologists generally deal? First, to the greatest extent possible, a truly informed consent, which is consistent with the principle of individual autonomy, should be obtained from every subject. But can a truly informed consent be obtained from a subject in an epidemiologic study? If we believe that a full disclosure of the study's objectives to the subjects will introduce a response bias or another type of bias, clearly the consent will not be a fully "informed" one. Another issue in consent relates to privacy and confidentiality. For many years, in good conscience, epidemiologists assured subjects that their data would be kept confidential, and that this commitment was unqualified. However, research data have become subject to subpoena in recent years, with only a few exceptions. Therefore, the assurance of confidentiality given in informed consent statements must now include qualifications to allow for breaches in confidentiality that could be legally mandated and that would therefore be beyond the control of the investigator. We return to the subject of privacy and confidentiality later in the chapter.

Another issue pertains to balancing the rights of the individual and the welfare of society. In a study of men at high risk for HIV infection, participants were assured of confidentiality. In the interview that was subsequently administered, subjects were asked whether they had donated blood during the previous 2 years. Several subjects who were found to be HIV positive reported having given blood within the 2 years prior to the HIV testing. The concern that emerged was that the donated blood might have been used in a transfusion. Although the blood may have been discarded by the blood bank, there was no way to check on this without breaching confidentiality and violating the original commitment to the subjects. Perhaps the investigators should have anticipated such a problem at the time the interview was developed, prior to obtaining the subjects' informed consent. But even with foresight, such problems arise. In this case, how do we balance the original commitment to the subjects with a need to determine whether anyone had received blood from these donors, so that further transmission of HIV might be prevented?

A third obligation to the subjects relates to communicating the study findings to them. Our approach to this issue may differ depending on whether the subject has been found to have developed a health problem linked to an exposure being studied or whether the subject has only been found to be at increased risk for future development of disease as a result of the exposure. In either case, communicating the results regarding risk to the subjects can be viewed as a possible expression of the ethical principle of beneficence—the obligation of the investigator to help the subjects further their important legitimate interests, such as disease prevention and control, for themselves and their families. However, according to this principle, we must not only provide the benefits such as prevention of disease, but must balance the benefits and costs or harm (principle of utility). For example, if a subject has been exposed to a factor that is shown in a study to be a strong risk factor for cancer of the pancreas, should he be given this information? Given that no effective treatment for pancreatic cancer is available, and that there is no strong evidence that early detection of the disease is beneficial, might we be increasing a person's anxieties by transmitting this information without providing any benefit to the subject?

One can also argue that a participant in any study is entitled to receive the findings of the study even if the findings have no direct bearing on the person's health or even if they may lead to heightened anxiety. Indeed, many epidemiologists now offer all participating subjects the option of requesting a report of the study findings when the study has been completed.

PRIVACY AND CONFIDENTIALITY

Concerns about privacy and confidentiality in our society have increased with the increasing erosion of individual privacy through computerized records. Protection of privacy and confidentiality within the framework of medical investigation, including epidemiologic research, has become an important issue. The origins of such concerns are quite old. Hippocrates wrote in the now commonly used Oath of Physicians: ''that whatsoever I shall see or hear . . . of the lives of men and women . . . which is not fitting to be spoken . . . I will keep inviolably secret. . . .'' As Hippocrates qualified ''whatsoever I shall see or hear'' with the phrase ''which is not fitting to be spoken,'' he apparently considered certain types of information to be of a nature that *is* ''fitting to be spoken.'' Presumably then, under certain circumstances, Hippocrates would have advocated the carefully monitored sharing of personal information in the interest of societal benefit. For example, if a case of smallpox were reported in an American city, Hippocrates would probably support the reporting of this case to health authorities. Thus, individual autonomy regarding privacy and confidentiality is an important principle, but it is not unlimited.

In regard to privacy and confidentiality in epidemiologic studies, attention has focused on use of medical records. Let us ask, first, why medical records are needed in epidemiologic studies. These records are needed for two main purposes:

1. To generate aggregate data and/or to validate information obtained by other means, without contacting patients.
2. To identify individual patients for subsequent follow-up using means such as interviews or blood tests.

Because epidemiology's objectives of improving human health are clearly laudable, one might be tempted at first glance to dismiss any concerns about misuse of medical record data and about intrusions into individual privacy by epidemiologists. However, the words of Supreme Court Justice Louis D. Brandeis ring as true today as when they were first written in 1928:

> *Experience should teach us to be most on guard to protect liberty when the Government's purposes are beneficent. Men born to freedom are naturally alert to repel invasion of their liberty by evil-minded rulers. The greatest dangers to liberty lurk in insidious encroachment by men of zeal, well-meaning but without understanding.*[1]

The ethical principle of autonomy argues strongly for a meaningful informed consent in many areas related to research, including privacy and confidentiality. Therefore, concerns about protection of confidentiality in the research arena are valid. They have led to two major legislative proposals; these might look reasonable at first, but in actuality would seriously damage epidemiologic research and impede progress in both public health and clinical practice. The two proposals are as follows:

1. Patient consent should be required before investigators are allowed access to medical records.
2. Data from medical records should be made available to investigators without any information that would identify an individual.

Both proposals are consistent with the ethical principle of *non-maleficence*—doing no harm—to the subjects participating in a research study. However, if society has a vested interest in the findings from epidemiologic and other biomedical studies, it is necessary to strike a balance between the interests of the individual and those of the community.

Let us consider these two proposals separately. Why would the first proposal, which requires patient consent before investigators gain access to medical records, make many studies impossible?

1. As a first step in a study, records must be reviewed to identify which patients meet the study criteria (for example, which patients have the disease in question and are therefore eligible for inclusion in a case-control study).
2. Many studies are conceived of only many years after a patient was hospitalized, so informed consent could not have been obtained from the patient at that time. By the time the study is later developed, many patients may have died or are not traceable.
3. Certain patients refuse to be interviewed in

epidemiologic studies, but the non-participants can be characterized using data in their medical records so that any biases resulting from their non-participation can be assessed. If records were not available because of patient refusals, a potential selection bias would be introduced, the magnitude and direction of which could not be assessed.

Turning to the second proposal, why is information from medical records that identifies individuals essential for most epidemiologic studies?

1. Review of medical records is often the first step in identifying a group of persons with a disease who will receive subsequent follow-up.
2. Identifying information is essential for linking the records of specific individuals from different sources (such as hospital records, physicians' records, employment records, and death certificates in studies of occupational cancer).

As seen in Figure 19–1, linkage of records is critical for generating unbiased and complete information about each subject, not only in occupational studies (as shown here) but in many types of epidemiologic investigations.

Thus, we see that medical records are essential for epidemiologic studies. Indeed, many significant advances in protecting human health that resulted from epidemiologic research could not have been made if access to medical records had been restricted.[2] At the same time, however, we must be concerned about protecting individual privacy and confidentiality, but without the introduction of new restrictive regulations that would seriously impede epidemiologic research. Effective procedures designed to protect the confidentiality of subjects are currently in force in epidemiologic studies. They include the following:

1. Informed consent is required for all phases of research except review of medical records.
2. All data obtained are stored under lock and key.
3. Only study numbers are used on data forms. The key for linking these numbers to individual names is kept separately under lock and key.
4. Individual identifying information is destroyed at the end of the study unless there is a specific justification for retention. Such retention must be approved by the institutional review board (IRB) or committee on human research.

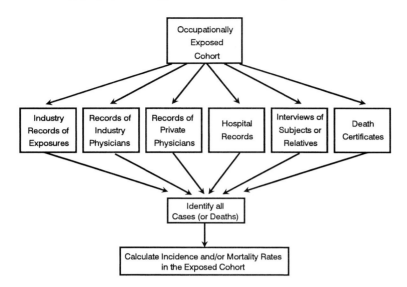

Figure 19–1. Use of record linkage in occupational studies.

5. All results are published only in aggregate or group form—individuals are never identified.

6. Unless essential for the study, individual identifying information is not put on computer tape and individual identifiers are not included in routine tabulations generated from computerized data.

7. The importance of maintaining privacy and confidentiality is regularly emphasized to the research staff.

When people consent to participate in epidemiologic studies, they have voluntarily agreed to some invasion of their privacy for the common good of society, hoping for advances in health promotion and disease prevention as a result of the studies they are making possible. Therefore, investigators have an ethical obligation to protect the privacy and confidentiality of the subjects in these studies to the greatest extent possible. The policies described earlier that are currently in force have been highly successful in achieving this goal. Recognizing the importance of medical records in epidemiologic research and the effectiveness of the measures currently in place, the Privacy Protection Study Commission recommended that patient consent not be required for use of medical records in epidemiologic research.[3]

ACCESS TO DATA

When a study has been completed, who "owns" the data? Who should have access to the data—either "raw" or partially "cooked"—and

under what conditions? We live in an era in which we can be confident that virtually any research data generated that deal with a controversial issue will be reanalyzed by real or alleged experts who support different positions. Some of the relevant questions regarding sharing of data include the following:

1. At what point has a study truly been completed?

2. Should the policy on sharing research data be dependent on who has paid for the study?

3. Should the policy depend on who is requesting the data and on that person's possible motivations in making the request?

4. Under what conditions should identifiers be included with the data?

5. How can the investigator's interests be protected?

6. Who will pay for the expenses involved?

The challenge is to strike a proper balance between the interests of the investigator on the one hand, and those of society on the other hand, for they do not inevitably coincide.

CONFLICT OF INTEREST

Both actual and perceived biases may result from conflict of interest. Such conflict can arise at each stage of a study, from an initial decision as to whether a specific study should be undertaken in the first place through analysis and interpretation of the data and dissemination of the results. Most epidemiologic work in the United States today is performed by epidemiologists who work in academia, industry, or government. These three environments differ in several ways. Funding for epidemiologic research in government and industry is generally internal, whereas academic epidemiologists must seek outside financial support. As a result, research performed by academic epidemiologists is generally subjected to more rigorous peer review as part of the grant application process. Even more important, however, is that the employer of the academic epidemiologist generally has no vested interest in what the results of the study may be. This contrasts with other settings in which the employer may be significantly affected—politically, economically, or legally—by the nature of the findings. Consequently, overt or subtle pressure by an employer not to initiate a study or to prolong the process leading to reporting of the results can introduce a serious bias into reviews of the literature concerning issues such as occupational hazards. Moreover, these biases may be impossible to assess. Although academic settings are not immune to their own problems and pressures, problems relating to epidemiologic research that arise in an academic setting are less likely to be linked to the potential impact of the study's specific findings. Nevertheless, the possibility of conflict of interest relating to any epidemiologic study must be considered, regardless of the specific setting in which the research was conducted. Indeed, such conflict may be related more to sources of funding than to the research setting itself.

It is difficult if not impossible to confront the problem that certain epidemiologic studies may not be initiated because of vested interests and concerns about the potential results of the study. However, efforts should be expended to ensure that the results of the study—whatever they may turn out to be—are published in a peer-reviewed journal in a timely fashion. Sponsorship of the study should be clearly acknowledged in the article that reports the results of the study, as should any financial interests of the investigators or their families that may be affected by the study results.

INTERPRETING FINDINGS

Many of most critical issues regarding how epidemiologic studies are conducted arise in connection with the appropriateness of the study design and the interpretation and reporting of findings. Epidemiologists have often been accused of endlessly reporting new risks, many of which are not confirmed in subsequent studies. The result is that the public finds reported risks all around them, which leads them to become skeptical of newly reported risks and unwilling to take responsibility for their own health care.[4] The question again arises, How do we assess the importance of a single study that shows an increased risk? How many confirmatory studies are needed?

An additional problem is that in earlier years, initial solitary epidemiologic findings or scientific controversies were generally addressed and often resolved within the scientific community before findings were disseminated to the public. Today, both initial unconfirmed reports and scientific controversies are often aired in the press or on television, even before the studies have appeared in peer-reviewed journals. The dilemma is that although enhanced public education and increased public awareness of scientific issues are laudable, anxiety levels are often unjustifiably raised by single studies that are widely reported and that may later be refuted. The problem is exacerbated by a reported bias in newspapers against reporting the results of studies that show no effect.[5]

Furthermore, at what point does a reported trivial increase in risk ratio, even if it is statistically significant, become a biologically significant risk that merits public concern? This relates to the overall issue of public perception of risk. These perceptions are reflected in the data shown in Tables 19–1 and 19–2. For many of the risks listed, the degree of

Table 19–1. Involuntary Risks

Involuntary Risk	Risk of Death per Person per Year
Struck by automobile (United States)	1 in 20,000
Struck by automobile (United Kingdom)	1 in 16,600
Floods (United States)	1 in 455,000
Earthquake (California)	1 in 588,000
Tornados (Midwest)	1 in 455,000
Lightning (United Kingdom)	1 in 10 million
Falling aircraft (United States)	1 in 10 million
Falling aircraft (United Kingdom)	1 in 50 million
Release from an atomic power station	
At site boundary (United States)	1 in 10 million
At 1 km (United Kingdom)	1 in 10 million
Flooding of a dike (The Netherlands)	1 in 10 million
Bites of venomous creatures (United Kingdom)	1 in 5 million
Leukemia	1 in 12,500
Influenza	1 in 5,000
Meteorite	1 in 100 billion

From Dinman BD: The reality and acceptance of risk. JAMA 244:1226, 1980.

Table 19–2. Voluntary Risks

Voluntary Risk	Risk of Death per Person per Year
Smoking: 20 cigarettes/day	1 in 200
Drinking: 1 bottle of wine per day	1 in 13,300
Soccer, football	1 in 25,500
Automobile racing	1 in 1,000
Automobile driving (United Kingdom)	1 in 5,900
Motorcycling	1 in 50
Rock climbing	1 in 7,150
Taking contraceptive pills	1 in 5,000
Power boating	1 in 5,900
Canoeing	1 in 100,000
Horse racing	1 in 740
Amateur boxing	1 in 2 million
Professional boxing	1 in 14,300
Skiing	1 in 430,000
Pregnancy (United Kingdom)	1 in 4,350
Abortion: Legal <12 wk	1 in 50,000
Abortion: Legal >14 wk	1 in 5,900

From Dinman BD: The reality and acceptance of risk. JAMA 244:1226, 1980.

public concern and change in behavior does not seem commensurate with the magnitude of the risk.

If the absolute risk is low, even if the relative risk in exposed individuals is significantly increased, the actual risk to exposed individuals will still be very low. It is interesting that the public often prefers to address "hot" issues (such as a reported risk from alar in apples) for which the evidence may be tenuous while ignoring well-established risk factors such as smoking, alcohol consumption, and sun exposure, for which lifestyle changes that are dependent on individual initiative have been clearly warranted by the available evidence.

Epidemiologists have a major function in communicating health risks and in interpreting epidemiologic data for non-epidemiologists; if epidemiologists do not participate in this activity, it will be left to others with far less training and expertise. This is an essential part of the policy-making process. Studies of human populations often disagree, and epidemiologists often hesitate to draw conclusions on the basis of existing data. In academic settings, epidemiologists can criticize studies and recommend additional research to resolve an issue. However, policy-makers working at the front lines do not have this luxury of delay; they must make immediate decisions (e.g., to regulate or not to regulate). Such decisions should ideally capitalize on epidemiologic information. However, policy-makers cannot act in a rational fashion by merely waiting for findings from future studies to direct their actions regarding current pressing health issues. Epidemiologists must therefore draw the best conclusions possible on the basis of currently available data, fully realizing that a better study, or even a perfect study, may appear tomorrow to contradict today's conclusions.

Epidemiologists have several roles in the process of policy-making, including generating and interpreting the data, presenting specific policy options, projecting the impact of each option, developing specific policy proposals, and evaluating the effects of policies after they have been implemented. Should an epidemiologist be both a researcher and an advocate for a specific policy? Does advocacy for a position imply a loss of objectivity and of scientific credibility? These are difficult questions, but many clear issues, such as the health hazards resulting from cigarette smoking, urgently need the participation of epidemiologists in the struggle to eliminate the source of the danger to the public's health. The question then is not only whether it is ethical for an epidemiologist to be an advocate, but whether it is ethical for an epidemiologist to *not* be an advocate when the evidence of risk is so convincing. Thus, the epidemiologist must serve as an educator as well as a researcher. The epidemiologist's educational efforts are directed at many target populations, including other scientists, other health professionals, legislators, policy-makers, lawyers, judges, and the public. Each group must be dealt with differently, depending on its specific needs and on the objectives toward which the educational effort is directed.

CONCLUSION

The issues facing epidemiology primarily reflect epidemiologists' obligations to subjects and the challenges resulting from the major position that the discipline occupies at the interface of science and public policy. The issues are complex, often subtle, and without simple answers. Given the pivotal position of epidemiology in the development of both clinical and public health policy and its implications for environmental regulation, individual lifestyle changes, and modifications in clinical practice, the findings from epidemiologic studies attract widespread attention and high public visibility. As new questions are addressed by epidemiology in the future, the ethical and professional dilemmas facing the discipline will also continue to evolve. Therefore, a critical need exists for a continuing dialogue between epidemiologists and those who use the results of epidemiologic studies, to ensure that emerging problems will be addressed appropriately and effectively.

References

1. Brandeis L: Dissenting opinion in Olmstead v. United States, 277 U.S. 438 (1928).
2. Gordis L, Gold E: Privacy, confidentiality, and the use of medical records in research. Science 207:153–156, 1980.
3. The Report of The Privacy Protection Study Commission: Personal Privacy in an Information Society. Washington, DC, US Government Printing Office, 1977.
4. Taubes G: Epidemiology faces its limits. Science 269:164–169, 1995.
5. Koren G, Klein N: Bias against negative studies in newspaper reports of medical research. JAMA 13:1824–1826, 1991.

Answers to Review Questions

CHAPTER 2

1. b
2. a
3. b
4. d
5. c

CHAPTER 3

1. 5/1,000
2. 30%
3. c
4. c
5. e
6. e
7. b
8. b
9. d
10. d
11. 9.6/1,000
12. e

CHAPTER 4

1. 72%
2. 84%
3. 69.2%
4. d
5. d
6. b
7. 3.3%
8. b
9. 70%
10. 57%
11. 40%
12. b (intermediate to good)

CHAPTER 5

1. c
2. 54.75%
3. c
4. b
5. c

CHAPTER 7

1. e
2. e
3. c
4. b
5. e
6. b
7. a
8. 57
9. c

CHAPTER 8

1. d
2. a
3. c
4. a
5. c

CHAPTER 9

1. c
2. a
3. c
4. b
5. c
6. d
7. e

CHAPTER 10

1. 15.25
2. e
3. d
4. e
5. e
6. e
7. 4.5
8. 6.33
9. 1:7 (.143)

CHAPTER 11

1. b
2. 27.5/1,000
3. 85%
4. 3.6/1,000
5. 78.3%

CHAPTER 13

1. c
2. a
3. e
4. c
5. b
6. d

CHAPTER 14

1. e
2. c
3. 12
4. 18.7
5. 9
6. 6.2
7. d

CHAPTER 15

1. c
2. b
3. b
4. c
5. c

CHAPTER 16

1. b
2. d
3. b
4. a
5. d

CHAPTER 17

1. a
2. a
3. b
4. c
5. b
6. c
7. c
8. b

Index

Note: Page numbers in *italics* refer to illustrations; page numbers followed by t refer to tables.